T0226637

Updates in Pediatric Otolaryngology

Editors

ROMAINE F. JOHNSON
ELTON M. LAMBERT

OTOLARYNGOLOGIC CLINICS OF NORTH AMERICA

www.oto.theclinics.com

Consulting Editor
SUJANA S. CHANDRASEKHAR

December 2022 • Volume 55 • Number 6

ELSEVIER

1600 John F. Kennedy Boulevard • Suite 1800 • Philadelphia, Pennsylvania, 19103-2899

http://www.oto.theclinics.com

OTOLARYNGOLOGIC CLINICS OF NORTH AMERICA Volume 55, Number 6
December 2022 ISSN 0030-6665, ISBN-13: 978-0-323-94001-6

Editor: Stacy Eastman
Developmental Editor: Diana Grace Ang

© **2022 Elsevier Inc. All rights reserved.**

This periodical and the individual contributions contained in it are protected under copyright by Elsevier, and the following terms and conditions apply to their use:

Photocopying
Single photocopies of single articles may be made for personal use as allowed by national copyright laws. Permission of the Publisher and payment of a fee is required for all other photocopying, including multiple or systematic copying, copying for advertising or promotional purposes, resale, and all forms of document delivery. Special rates are available for educational institutions that wish to make photocopies for non-profit educational classroom use. For information on how to seek permission visit www.elsevier.com/permissions or call: (+44) 1865 843830 (UK)/(+1) 215 239 3804 (USA).

Derivative Works
Subscribers may reproduce tables of contents or prepare lists of articles including abstracts for internal circulation within their institutions. Permission of the Publisher is required for resale or distribution outside the institution. Permission of the Publisher is required for all other derivative works, including compilations and translations (please consult www.elsevier.com/permissions).

Electronic Storage or Usage
Permission of the Publisher is required to store or use electronically any material contained in this periodical, including any article or part of an article (please consult www.elsevier.com/permissions). Except as outlined above, no part of this publication may be reproduced, stored in a retrieval system or transmitted in any form or by any means, electronic, mechanical, photocopying, recording or otherwise, without prior written permission of the Publisher.

Notice
No responsibility is assumed by the Publisher for any injury and/or damage to persons or property as a matter of products liability, negligence or otherwise, or from any use or operation of any methods, products, instructions or ideas contained in the material herein. Because of rapid advances in the medical sciences, in particular, independent verification of diagnoses and drug dosages should be made.

Although all advertising material is expected to conform to ethical (medical) standards, inclusion in this publication does not constitute a guarantee or endorsement of the quality or value of such product or of the claims made of it by its manufacturer.

Otolaryngologic Clinics of North America (ISSN 0030-6665) is published bimonthly by Elsevier, Inc., 360 Park Avenue South, New York, NY 10010-1710. Months of issue are February, April, June, August, October, and December. Business and Editorial Offices: 1600 John F. Kennedy Blvd., Suite 1800, Philadelphia, PA 19103-2899. Customer Service Office: 6277 Sea Harbor Drive, Orlando, FL 32887-4800. Periodicals postage paid at New York, NY and additional mailing offices. Subscription prices are $450.00 per year (US individuals), $1336.00 per year (US institutions), $100.00 per year (US & Canadian student/resident), $576.00 per year (Canadian individuals), $1396.00 per year (Canadian institutions), $628.00 per year (international individuals), $1396.00 per year (international institutions), $270.00 per year (international student/resident). Foreign air speed delivery is included in all *Clinics'* subscription prices. All prices are subject to change without notice. **POSTMASTER:** Send address changes to *Otolaryngologic Clinics of North America*, Elsevier Health Sciences Division, Subscription Customer Service, 3251 Riverport Lane, Maryland Heights, MO 63043. **Telephone: 1-800-654-2452 (U.S. and Canada); 314-447-8871 (outside U.S. and Canada). Fax: 314-447-8029. E-mail: journalscustomerservice-usa@elsevier.com (for print support); journalsonlinesupport-usa@elsevier.com (for online support).**

Reprints. For copies of 100 or more of articles in this publication, please contact the Commercial Reprints Department, Elsevier Inc., 360 Park Avenue South, New York, NY 10010-1710. Tel.: 212-633-3874; Fax: 212-633-3820; E-mail: reprints@elsevier.com.

Otolaryngologic Clinics of North America is also published in Spanish by McGraw-Hill Interamericana Editores S.A., P.O. Box 5-237, 06500 Mexico D.F., Mexico.

Otolaryngologic Clinics of North America is covered in *MEDLINE/PubMed (Index Medicus), Current Contents/Clinical Medicine, Excerpta Medica, BIOSIS, Science Citation Index,* and *ISI/BIOMED.*

Contributors

CONSULTING EDITOR

SUJANA S. CHANDRASEKHAR, MD, FACS, FAAOHNS
Past President, American Academy of Otolaryngology–Head and Neck Surgery, Secretary-Treasurer, American Otological Society, Partner, ENT & Allergy Associates, LLP, Clinical Professor, Department of Otolaryngology–Head and Neck Surgery, Donald and Barbara Zucker School of Medicine at Hofstra/Northwell, Hempstead, New York, USA; Clinical Associate Professor, Department of Otolaryngology–Head and Neck Surgery, Icahn School of Medicine at Mount Sinai, New York, New York, USA

EDITORS

ROMAINE F. JOHNSON, MD, MPH
Professor, Department of Otolaryngology–Head and Neck Surgery, UT Southwestern Medical Center, Dallas, Texas, USA

ELTON M. LAMBERT, MD
Assistant Professor, Division of Otolaryngology, Department of Surgery, Texas Children's Hospital; Bobby R. Alford Department of Otorhinolaryngology and Communicative Sciences, Baylor College of Medicine, Houston, Texas, USA

AUTHORS

IRAM AHMAD, MD, MME
Assistant Professor, Department of Otolaryngology–Head and Neck Surgery, Stanford University, Palo Alto, California, USA

MICHAEL BARTELLAS, MSc (Med), MD
Department of Otolaryngology–Head and Neck Surgery, University of Ottawa, Ottawa, Ontario, Canada

DANIEL C. CHELIUS, MD
Doctor, Associate Professor, Texas Children's Hospital–Pediatric Otolaryngology, Baylor College of Medicine–Otolaryngology, Head and Neck Surgery, Houston, Texas, USA

STEPHEN R. CHORNEY, MD, MPH
Assistant Professor, Department of Otolaryngology, University of Texas Southwestern Medical Center, Division of Pediatric Otolaryngology, Children's Medical Center Dallas, Children's Health Airway Management Program, Department of Pediatric Otolaryngology, Children's Medical Center Dallas, Dallas, Texas, USA

AMY L. DIMACHKIEH, MD
Doctor, Assistant Professor, Texas Children's Hospital–Pediatric Otolaryngology, Baylor College of Medicine–Otolaryngology, Head and Neck Surgery, Houston, Texas, USA

ERIC A. GANTWERKER, MD, MMSc, FACS
Department of Otolaryngology, Pediatric Otolaryngologist, Cohen Children's Medical Center/Long Island Jewish Medical Center at Northwell Health, New Hyde Park, New York, USA; Associate Professor, Department of Otolaryngology, Zucker School of Medicine at Northwell/Hofstra, Hempstead, New York, USA

CHELSEA GATCLIFFE, MD
Division of Pulmonary Medicine, Department of Pediatrics, University of Texas Health Science Center at Houston, Houston, Texas, USA

MARK E. GERBER, MD
Division of Pediatric Otolaryngology–Head and Neck Surgery, Phoenix Children's Hospital, Phoenix, Arizona, USA

CATHERINE K. HART, MD, MS
Division of Pediatric Otolaryngology–Head and Neck Surgery, Cincinnati Children's Hospital Medical Center, Department of Otolaryngology–Head and Neck Surgery, University of Cincinnati College of Medicine, Cincinnati, Ohio, USA

ZHEN HUANG, MD
Department of Otorhinolaryngology–Head and Neck Surgery, University of Texas Health Science Center at Houston, Houston, Texas, USA

JACOB B. HUNTER, MD
Associate Professor, Department of Otolaryngology-Head and Neck Surgery, University of Texas Southwestern Medical Center, Dallas, Texas, USA

AMY HUGHES, MD
Department of Otolaryngology, Connecticut Children's; Division of Otolaryngology, Department of Surgery, UCONN School of Medicine, Hartford, Connecticut, USA

JONATHAN B. IDA, MD, MBA, FAAP, FACS
Associate Professor, Department of Otolaryngology–Head and Neck Surgery, Northwestern University Feinberg School of Medicine, Ann & Robert H. Lurie Children's Hospital of Chicago, Department of Otolaryngology–Head and Neck Surgery, Chicago, Illinois, USA

KRIS R. JATANA, MD, FAAP, FACS
Professor, Department of Otolaryngology–Head and Neck Surgery, Nationwide Children's Hospital and Wexner Medical Center at Ohio State University, Columbus, Ohio, USA

THOMAS JAVENS, BS
Center for Clinical Excellence, Nationwide Children's Hospital, Columbus, Ohio, USA

ZI YANG JIANG, MD
Department of Otorhinolaryngology–Head and Neck Surgery, University of Texas Health Science Center at Houston, Houston, Texas, USA

KAALAN E. JOHNSON, MD
Division of Pediatric Otolaryngology–Head and Neck Surgery, Seattle Children's Hospital, Department of Otolaryngology–Head and Neck Surgery, University of Washington, Seattle, Washington, USA

ROMAINE F. JOHNSON, MD, MPH
Professor, Department of Otolaryngology, University of Texas Southwestern Medical Center, Division of Pediatric Otolaryngology, Children's Medical Center Dallas, Children's Health Airway Management Program, Department of Pediatric Otolaryngology, Children's Medical Center Dallas, Dallas, Texas, USA

ERIN M. KIRKHAM, MD, MPH
Department of Otolaryngology–Head & Neck Surgery, The University of Michigan, Ann Arbor, Michigan, USA

SHELBY KITCHIN, BS
University of Cincinnati College of Medicine, Cincinnati, Ohio, USA

YANN-FUU KOU, MD
Assistant Professor, Department of Otolaryngology, University of Texas Southwestern Medical Center, Division of Pediatric Otolaryngology, Children's Medical Center Dallas, Children's Health Airway Management Program, Department of Pediatric Otolaryngology, Children's Medical Center Dallas, Dallas, Texas, USA

ELTON M. LAMBERT, MD
Assistant Professor, Division of Otolaryngology, Department of Surgery, Texas Children's Hospital; Bobby R. Alford Department of Otorhinolaryngology and Communicative Sciences, Baylor College of Medicine, Houston, Texas, USA

GI SOO LEE, MD, EdM
Department of Otolaryngology and Communication Enhancement, Boston Children's Hospital, Assistant Professor, Department of Otolaryngology–Head and Neck Surgery, Harvard Medical School, Boston, Massachusetts, USA

KENNETH H. LEE, MD
Professor, Department of Otolaryngology–Head and Neck Surgery, University of Texas Southwestern Medical Center, Plano, Texas, USA

JENNIFER M. LAVIN MD, MS, FAAP, FACS
Associate Professor Department of Otolaryngology - Head and Neck Surgery, Northwestern University Feinberg School of Medicine, Ann & Robert H. Lurie Children's Hospital of Chicago, Northwestern University Feinberg School of Medicine, Department of Otolaryngology-Head and Neck Surgery, Chicago, Illinois, USA

SAINITEESH MADDINENI, BS
Medical Student, Department of Otolaryngology–Head and Neck Surgery, Stanford University, Palo Alto, California, USA

TU MAI, MD
Division of Gastroenterology, Department of Pediatrics, University of Texas Health Science Center at Houston, Houston, Texas, USA

JAMES D. PHILLIPS, MD
Monroe Carell Jr Children's Hospital at Vanderbilt, Nashville, Tennessee, USA

PRASANTH PATTISAPU, MD, MPH
Department of Otolaryngology – Head & Neck Surgery, Nationwide Children's Hospital, Department of Otolaryngology e Head & Neck Surgery, The Ohio State University, Center for Surgical Outcomes Research, Nationwide Children's Hospital, Columbus, Ohio, USA

REZA RAHBAR, DMD, MD
Associate Otolaryngologist-in-Chief, Director, Center for Airway Disorders, Co-Director, Head, Neck and Skull Base Surgery Program, Professor of Otolaryngology, Harvard Medical School, Boston, Massachusetts, USA

VIDYA T. RAMAN, MD, MBA
Professor, Department of Anesthesia, Wexner Medical Center at Ohio State University, Columbus, Ohio, USA

NIKHILA P. RAOL, MD, MPH
Department of Otolaryngology–Head and Neck Surgery, Department of Pediatrics, Emory University School of Medicine, Division of Pediatric Otolaryngology, Children's Healthcare of Atlanta, Atlanta, Georgia, USA

CLARE M. RICHARDSON, MD
Division of Pediatric Otolaryngology–Head and Neck Surgery, Seattle Children's Hospital, Department of Otolaryngology–Head and Neck Surgery, University of Washington, Seattle, Washington, USA

SCOTT RICKERT, MD, FACS
Chief, Division of Pediatric Otolaryngology, Associate Professor, Department of Otolaryngology, Pediatrics, and Plastic Surgery, Hassenfeld Children's Hospital at NYU Langone, NYU Langone Health, New York, New York, USA

TARA L. ROSENBERG, MD
Texas Children's Hospital/Baylor College of Medicine, Houston, Texas, USA

KRISTEN L. YANCEY, MD
Neurotology Fellow, Department of Otolaryngology–Head and Neck Surgery, University of Texas Southwestern Medical Center, Dallas, Texas, USA

PENG YOU, MD, FRCSC
Department of Otolaryngology–Head and Neck Surgery, Western University, London, Ontario, Canada

Contents

The purpose of this article is to outline the current state of evaluating children with unilateral hearing loss, with significant focus on cochlear implantation, in terms of reviewing the key points of the history, including the duration of deafness, outlining the recommended audiometric testing battery, and discussing issues related to imaging of the auditory system and related anatomy. In addition, a comprehensive and up-to-date summary of outcomes in terms of speech perception, sound localization, and quality of life for both the child with unilateral hearing loss as well as their parent(s) is reported.

Eustachian tube dysfunction (ETD) is a common middle ear disorder in children that can have a significant impact on the quality of life. This review aims to provide an updated understanding of ETD and its clinical management. We will discuss the pathophysiology and diagnosis of ETD, as well as the medical and surgical treatment of ETD. We will also review studies of both adults and children with ETD, although special attention will be paid to children with ETD.

Drug-induced sleep endoscopy (DISE) is a fiber-optic assessment of the upper airway under sedation can identify dynamic obstruction not seen on awake examination. Frequently used in cases of persistent, postadenotonsillectomy obstructive sleep apnea, the clinical indications for pediatric DISE are expanding to include surgically naïve children. However, there is substantial variation in practice with regard to sedation protocol, scoring, and the interpretation and application of DISE findings. Research in DISE would be strengthened by consensus on anesthetic and scoring protocol, which would facilitate rigorous testing of the predictive value of presurgical DISE findings on postsurgical outcomes.

Drooling and aspiration of saliva can affect the quality of life and morbidity of patients with neuromuscular diseases. Practitioners must differentiate between drooling with and without aspiration of saliva, as the presence of aspiration affects respiratory health. There are several validated drooling scales, but validated assessments for aspiration of saliva are lacking. Once diagnosed, drooling can be treated with rehabilitative therapy, anticholinergics, botulinum toxin to the salivary glands, and surgery. Drooling with aspiration of saliva often requires multidisciplinary engagement to decrease the risk of respiratory complications.

Advances in neonatal and pediatric critical care have resulted in a growing population of medically complex children with a tracheostomy. These children are vulnerable to adverse events from underlying comorbidities, risks of tracheostomy, equipment malfunction, and caregiver inexperience. Multidisciplinary tracheostomy teams have emerged as effective initiatives to address these patient safety concerns. Improvements in quality metrics and clinical outcomes can occur after implementation of a multidisciplinary tracheostomy team. This review provides updates on the evidence for multidisciplinary pediatric tracheostomy teams and offers perspectives on the future direction of these programs.

Pediatric head and neck tumors are uncommon but the consequences of radical resection are extensive. These tumors, benign and malignant, are uniquely challenging because of their proximity to critical functional and neurovascular structures and intimately affect speech, swallowing, voice, breathing, hearing, and vision. In addition, the psychosocial and emotional trauma from the cosmetic and functional consequences can be enduring. Their relative rarity limits surgeon experience and requires a focused effort to develop individual and programmatic expertise. A practiced multidisciplinary team can facilitate smooth preoperative evaluations, efficient coordinated operative procedures, comprehensive rehabilitation, and recovery, as well as optimal oncologic outcomes.

Vascular anomalies of the head and neck is an evolving field, with more recent focus on identifying and understanding the underlying genetic and molecular causes for these lesions. Medical therapies for some of these vascular anomalies have been developed. Many complex vascular anomalies require multimodality therapy, and other lesions could be treated with any of a variety of the available therapies. High-quality outcomes research and establishing clinical practice guidelines to help guide management are essential.

Chronic cough is defined as cough lasting more than 4 weeks in children aged 14 years or older. Normal children, without pathophysiology, can cough up to more than 30 times a day. When cough occurs pathologically, it is often more often and can be divided into specific and nonspecific cough types. Inputs from otolaryngology, pulmonary medicine, and gastroenterology, along with other specialties in an aerodigestive team setting, allow a team approach to consider a wide variety of causes of cough and coordinate diagnostic procedures with treatment.

Three-dimensional printing (3Dp) is a technology with widespread commercial and medical applications. Adoption of 3Dp has occurred in trainee education, along with specific preoperative and perioperative use. This article explores the application of 3Dp within Otolaryngology, with the pediatric population at the forefront. This article will also discuss specific clinical applications, limitations, and potential future applications of this technology.

Congenital tracheal stenosis is a rare but potentially life-threatening condition that is most commonly caused by complete tracheal rings. Slide tracheoplasty was initially introduced as a surgical treatment for congenital tracheal stenosis in 1989 and has significantly improved outcomes and overall survival rates for these patients. It has subsequently been adapted to treat other conditions such as laryngotracheal stenosis, tracheoesophageal fistula, and bronchial stenosis. This article reviews the history, the variety of applications, perioperative management, surgical techniques, potential complications, and new frontiers in slide tracheoplasty surgery.

Enhanced recovery after surgery (ERAS) protocols exist to optimize perioperative care for patients of all ages. The efficacy of ERAS protocols has been studied in various surgical specialties, including pediatric surgery and otolaryngology, but its role in pediatric otolaryngology has not been widely demonstrated in the literature. This review article attempts to assess the current state of ERAS within otolaryngology, pediatric surgery, and more specifically, pediatric otolaryngology to identify opportunities for future development and utilization.

In almost all areas that have been studied, racial, ethnic, socioeconomic, and other disparities have been identified throughout pediatric otolaryngology. This article focuses on some of the most studied areas, including the use of tonsillectomy, ear tubes, cochlear implants, and tracheos-tomies. Disparities are best reduced through multilevel interventions that address policy and upstream determinants of health. However, in some cases, standardization of care through clinical practice guidelines or can reduce disparities in care delivery. Future research in pediatric otolaryn-gology should specifically study disparities, their causes, and how to reduce them.

Patient Safety and Quality Improvement as a formal discipline has become widely established, with hospitals and health systems dedicating signifi-cant resources to improvement science. Physicians have leadership po-tential in quality and safety due to their clinical expertise and influence with both patients and hospital leadership. Success in such a leadership role, however, requires knowledge of the fundamentals of how to navigate an improvement endeavor from inception through implementation, anal-ysis, and sustainment. Herein, the authors introduce the formal process of improvement science, discuss basic principles of change management, and provide a summary of the elements of scholarly writing to facilitate dissemination of knowledge across institutions.

Understanding the principles and theories that are well recognized in adult learning can have a major impact on learning and teaching today. In an era with much less time with trainees and ever-dwindling experiential learning opportunities, the focus should be on maximizing the efficiency and effi-cacy of our everyday teaching. By conceptually understanding the myriad of relevant cognitive theories of adult learning, faculty can transform their teaching and the trainees' learning experiences while modeling and teach-ing the next generation how to invoke these strategies, forever propa-gating better teaching practices.

While the majority of the initial attention to symptomatic COVID-19 focused on adult patients as well as adult critical care and first responders, the pandemic drastically altered care throughout the entire health care in-dustry. COVID-19 has had a profound effect on the treatment and care of pediatric patients within pediatric otolaryngology. The objective of this article is to highlight the unique ramifications of COVID-19 in general and its effect within pediatric otolaryngology, with a focus on the immediate and potential long-term shifts in practice. This article addresses several aspects of care within pediatric otolaryngology including safety, diagnosis, and treatment of COVID-19 detailing the unique effects of the pandemic on the pediatric otolaryngology specialty and opportunities.

OTOLARYNGOLOGIC CLINICS
OF NORTH AMERICA

SERIES OF RELATED INTEREST

Facial Plastic Surgery Clinics
Available at: https://www.facialplastic.theclinics.com/

THE CLINICS ARE AVAILABLE ONLINE!
Access your subscription at:
www.theclinics.com

Foreword

Staying Up-to-Date on Pediatric Otolaryngologic Care

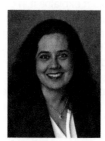

Sujana S. Chandrasekhar, MD, FACS, FAAOHNS
Consulting Editor

Children are not just little adults. We all learned this at the very least on our Pediatrics rotations in medical school, when everyone relied on a well-worn handbook called *The Harriet Lane Handbook*, which is now in its 22nd edition, to ensure child-specific care. I had always imagined that the book was named for a pioneering female pediatrician, but it is, in fact, named for someone who was not a doctor. Harriet Lane was the niece of the 15th (and only bachelor) President of the United States, James Buchanan, and served as his hostess and the First Lady of the United States from 1857 to 1861, when she was in her 20s. She married a bit later in life at age 36, and unfortunately, lost her two young sons within a year of each other to rheumatic fever. At her death in 1903, she left money to endow The Harriet Lane Home for Invalid Children, which opened in 1912. This institution was the first pediatric hospital affiliated with an academic research institution, Johns Hopkins University, and heralded the development of Pediatrics and Pediatric Specialties in the service of the health care of children and their families. *The Handbook* comes from there, now called the Harriet Lane Clinic of the Johns Hopkins Children's Center. Of interest, "Hal," as President Buchanan called her, who had been orphaned at age 11, was also a fierce advocate for Native American living conditions.

Just as we somehow expect all of Pediatrics' knowledge to fit into a lab coat pocket-sized handbook, we also look to a single issue such as this current issue of *Otolaryngologic Clinics of North America* to give us a comprehensive update on all of Pediatric Otolaryngology. And, just like *The Harriet Lane Handbook*, it shouldn't be able to do that, but it does. Guest editors Drs Romaine Johnson and Elton Lambert have ensured that this issue, which happens to also fit into a lab coat pocket, covers the salient details of all that we currently need to know to be up to moment in this field.

Many of the subjects covered in each of the articles merit (or have been covered in) full issues of *Otolaryngologic Clinics of North America* to themselves. The authors of each of

Otolaryngol Clin N Am 55 (2022) xiii–xiv
https://doi.org/10.1016/j.otc.2022.08.001
0030-6665/22/© 2022 Published by Elsevier Inc.

these articles have synthesized the current information and presented it in an easily accessible format. You will see that the clinical subjects range from single-sided hearing loss to Eustachian tube dysfunction to sleep apnea, drooling, and cough. They go on to cover pediatric tracheostomy, including how to ensure maximal safety for the child while minimizing trips back to the health care system. Complex head and neck reconstruction, treatment of vascular anomalies, and tracheoplasty are also addressed. Unfortunately, nearly 3 years into the worldwide pandemic, we know that COVID-19 affects children differently than it does adults, and the article on that subject explains it in detail.

And then there are some not exactly clinical but equally valuable articles. The article on 3D printing takes this option out of fantasy and places it squarely into reality, including outside of academic medical centers. Quality improvement is covered as a stand-alone subject and as part of ERAS (enhanced recovery after surgery). Lack of equity in health care encompasses different components for pediatric specialties compared with their adult counterparts, and appreciation of this as covered in that article is the only way to change it for the better. There is even an article on principles of adult learning from which we can all benefit.

It is a challenge to cover such a diverse topic as Pediatric Otolaryngology updates in a single issue. Drs Johnson and Lambert and all of the authors in this issue have met that challenge beautifully. I hope you enjoy reading this issue as much as I have, and please don't forget to listen to our podcasts—there is one per issue—at www.oto.theclinics.com or wherever you get your podcasts.

Sujana S. Chandrasekhar, MD, FACS, FAAOHNS
Consulting Editor
Otolaryngologic Clinics of North America
Past President
American Academy of Otolaryngology–
Head and Neck Surgery
Secretary-Treasurer
American Otological Society
Partner, ENT & Allergy Associates LLP
18 East 48th Street, 2nd Floor
New York, NY 10017, USA

Clinical Professor, Department of Otolaryngology–
Head and Neck Surgery
Zucker School of Medicine at Hofstra–Northwell
Hempstead, NY, USA

Clinical Associate Professor
Department of Otolaryngology–
Head and Neck Surgery
Icahn School of Medicine at Mount Sinai
New York, NY, USA

Co-Executive Producer and Co-Host, She's On Call

E-mail address:
ssc@nyotology.com

Website:
http://www.ears.nyc

Preface

Updates in Pediatric Otolaryngology

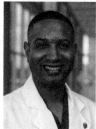 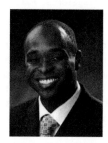

Romaine F. Johnson, MD, MPH   Elton M. Lambert, MD
Editors

It is with great pleasure that we present this issue of *Otolaryngology Clinics of North America* on Updates in Pediatric Otolaryngology. The field of Pediatric Otolaryngology has continued to develop as a specialty shaped by our current health care climate. This issue of *Otolaryngology Clinics of North America* reflects those developments, and the areas that continue to influence the specialty.

We discuss updates on new ways to approach old problems. There is an increasing awareness of the impact of **Single-Sided Deafness** on patients, and the technologies available to treat the condition continue to grow. Children with **Eustachian Tube Dysfunction** now have more options beyond repetitive ventilation tube placement, and the increasing standardization of **Drug-Induced Sleep Endoscopy** protocols and reporting is sure to improve outcomes for children with difficult-to-treat obstructive sleep apnea. **Drooling and Aspiration** afflicts patients with complex dysphagia, and more robust treatment recommendations are now present.

Pediatric Otolaryngology is a team sport, and we highlight our efforts in multidisciplinary care for complex patients. The formation of **Pediatric Tracheostomy Teams** gives these patients a medical home for their tracheostomy tube needs. There is an increased recognition that intensive planning strategies, surgical expertise, and rehabilitative efforts are required for patients who require **Complex Head and Neck Resection and Reconstruction**. We now have more tools in the armamentarium to treat **Vascular Anomalies**, and the coordination of these modalities is needed for optimal patient outcomes. Patients with **Chronic Cough** have many diagnostic and therapeutic dilemmas, and the **Aerodigestive Approach** to these patients can be invaluable.

There are so many areas of innovation within Pediatric Otolaryngology that it is difficult to highlight only a few, such as **3D Printing in Otolaryngology**, which has so many

Otolaryngol Clin N Am 55 (2022) xv–xvi
https://doi.org/10.1016/j.otc.2022.07.017
0030-6665/22/© 2022 Published by Elsevier Inc.

applications across subspecialties. Refinement techniques for **Slide Tracheoplasty** have improved the outcomes in patients with tracheal abnormalities, and protocols for **Enhanced Recovery after Surgery** have transformed perioperative care.

It is vitally important that we examine the areas within Pediatric Otolaryngology that go beyond each clinical and surgical encounter. We cannot achieve **Health Care Equity** without knowing the factors that have contributed to health care inequality and how to combat it. **Quality Improvement** methods seek to optimize patient outcomes within complex health care systems. **Adult Learning** theories allow us to gain better understanding on how to train the next generation of Otolaryngologists and health care professionals.

We have organized a body of work to illustrate the new ways in which our field confronts old problems, how we form multidisciplinary teams to tackle complex problems, to innovate to solve evolving problems, and to continuously learn to solve future problems. We also could a not omit a discussion of the most significant health event in a generation: **COVID-19**, and how it has affected the field of Pediatric Otolaryngology. We would like to sincerely thank our contributing authors for their expertise. We have assembled a team of authors that reflects diversity of Pediatric Otolaryngology that has evolved over time. We would like to thank the readers, whose continuous knowledge-seeking only betters our patients. We hope that you enjoy the articles in the issue and hope that it contributes to the care of your future patients.

Romaine F. Johnson, MD, MPH
Department of Otolaryngology–
Head and Neck Surgery
UT Southwestern Medical Center
2350 North Stemmons Freeway, F6207
Dallas, TX 75019, USA

Elton M. Lambert, MD
Division of Otolaryngology
Department of Surgery
Texas Children's Hospital
Bobby R. Alford Department of Otorhinolaryngology
and Communicative Sciences
Baylor College of Medicine
6701 Fannin Street, D.640
Houston, TX 77030, USA

E-mail addresses:
Romaine.Johnson@UTsouthwestern.edu (R.F. Johnson)
emashela@texaschildrens.org (E.M. Lambert)

Pediatric Single-Sided Deafness

Jacob B. Hunter, MD[a],*, Kristen L. Yancey, MD[a], Kenneth H. Lee, MD[b]

KEYWORDS

- Cochlear implantation • Hearing loss • Unilateral • Child • Speech perception
- Quality of life • Sound localization • Speech

KEY POINTS

- Two manufacturers, Cochlear Corporation (Sydney, Australia) and MED-EL (Innsbruck, Austria), are FDA approved for cochlear implantation in single-sided deafness in children, approved for children aged 5 years or older and with a duration of deafness less than 10 years.
- There is substantial data supporting cochlear implantation in children with unilateral hearing loss younger than 5 years of age.
- Cochlear implantation in pediatric unilateral hearing loss patients can improve speech understanding from the front, as well as when directed to the hearing-impaired ear.
- Assessing quality of life, speech hearing, quality hearing, and spatial hearing have shown significant improvements in children with unilateral hearing loss with a cochlear implant.

INTRODUCTION

Although bilateral hearing loss in children has long been recognized as a cause for speech language delays and impaired academic performance, unilateral hearing loss (UHL) was previously considered to be of little clinical importance. UHL refers to hearing loss on one side with normal hearing in the contralateral ear. In 1984, a seminal article by Bess and Tharpe demonstrated that UHL hinders speech and language development.[1] UHL has deleterious effects on receptive and expressive language skills even when identified early, within the first few months of life.[2] Other functional consequences of UHL include impaired speech understanding in noise and sound localization.[3,4]

Although not as common as bilateral hearing loss in children, UHL has an incidence of 0.6 to 0.7 per 1000 live births according to the Center for Disease Control Early

[a] Department of Otolaryngology-Head and Neck Surgery, University of Texas Southwestern Medical Center, 2001 Inwood Road, Dallas, TX 75390, USA; [b] Department of Otolaryngology-Head and Neck Surgery, University of Texas Southwestern Medical Center, 7609 Preston Road, 3rd Floor, Suite P3500, Plano, TX 75204, USA
* Corresponding author.
E-mail address: jacob.hunter@utsouthwestern.edu

Otolaryngol Clin N Am 55 (2022) 1139–1149
https://doi.org/10.1016/j.otc.2022.07.003
0030-6665/22/© 2022 Elsevier Inc. All rights reserved.

Table 1
Criteria for cochlear implant candidacy for children aged 5 years or older with 10 years or less of single-sided deafness

Manufacturer	PTA[a] (dB HL)	Age	Duration of Deafness
Cochlear Americas	≥90	≥5 y	≥10 y
MED-EL	>80		

FDA, federal drug administration; PTA, pure tone average.

[a] PTA calculated as the average of air conduction thresholds at 500 Hz, 1000 Hz, 2000 Hz, and 4000 Hz.

Hearing Detection and Intervention Database. However, the prevalence of UHL increases to 2.5% to 6% by the time children are in elementary school.[5–7] Thus, routine hearing screening in school-aged children is indicated to capture individuals at-risk of falling short of their academic potential.

The degree of hearing loss in the compromised ear critically affects the options for treatment. Although there are inherent challenges with young children being fitted with and wearing hearing aids, amplification can address mild-to-moderate UHL. However, children with severe to profound UHL, or single-sided deafness (SSD), often cannot benefit from traditional hearing aids, due to functional limitations of the devices.[8] Various audiometric definition of SSD have been reported, both in characterizing the loss in the affected ear and for the contralateral hearing level. Commonly used definitions include pure tone air conduction averages (PTA) greater than 70 dB in the affected ear and PTA less than 20 to 35 dB in the contralateral ear.[9–11] Others have required that thresholds for the contralateral ear be less than 25 dB for all tested frequencies.[12]

For SSD, initial treatment options are limited to a specific type of hearing aid, called a contralateral routing of signal (CROS) aid, and bone conduction systems. Both reroute sound from the side of deafness to the normal hearing ear. Drawbacks include the lack of auditory input to the hearing-impaired ear, preventing restoration of binaural hearing advantages. Moreover, deprivation to the neural pathways can impair normal development of the auditory cortex, leading to irreversible deficits.[13,14]

Nevertheless, hearing aids often are not practical options in young children because they have extremely low compliance for consistent use.[15] Although bone conduction devices are predominantly surgical, there are additional options that hold the bone conducting component against the head but the Food and Drug Administration (FDA) has approved surgically implantable devices that obviate a head band or wearing parts of the device in the ear canal in children aged 5 years or older.[16]

In 2019, the FDA approved cochlear implants (CI) from the MedEl Corporation (MED-EL GmbH, Innsbruck, Austria) to treat children with SSD, followed by the Cochlear Corporation (Cochlear Americas Corporation, Sydney, Australia) in 2022. Candidacy criteria are summarized in **Table 1**. Initial CI outcomes in pediatric SSD have been very favorable.

The purpose of this document is to outline the current state of evaluating children with SSD in terms of reviewing the key points of their history including the duration of their deafness, outlining the recommended audiometric testing, and discussing issues related to imaging of the auditory system and related anatomy. In addition, a comprehensive and up-to-date summary of outcomes in terms of speech perception, sound localization, and quality of life for both the child with SSD as well as their care-giver(s) will be reported.

Evaluation

Clinical presentation

Although up to 35% of pediatric UHL may ultimately be deemed idiopathic, a thorough clinical history should elicit risk factors and possible causes to account for the hearing loss (**Table 2**).[17] Caregivers should be interviewed regarding the following:

- Family history of early onset hearing loss
- Pregnancy complications—maternal infections (eg, cytomegalovirus diagnosed up to 48% of SSD cases),[11,17,18] preterm delivery
- Neonatal history—birth weight, jaundice, hypoxia, intensive care unit stays, intra-venous antibiotics/chemotherapy/other ototoxin exposure, newborn hearing screening, meningitis, syndromic features
- Childhood—developmental milestones including speech and language, routine hearing screenings, vaccination status, ear infections, prior ear surgeries, head injuries, overall coordination, vision concerns, systemic illnesses, and conditions

Table 2
Reported percentages of etiologies of pediatric single-sided deafness (SSD)

Etiology or Risk Factor	
Idiopathic	13%–35%[a,b,c,e,f]
SSNHL	3.3[c]
Prematurity	4%[b]–10%[f]
Family history of early SNHL	6[d]
Congenital	42%[d]
CMV	6%–48%[a,b,c,e,f]
Inner ear malformation	4[b] –36%[a,c,d,e]
Infectious (non-congenital)	
Meningitis	1%–6%[a,b,c,e]
Mumps	6%[b]
Trauma	1%–11%[a,b,c,f]
Ototoxicity	3%[f]
CNS tumor	9%[a]
Auditory neuropathy	2%[b]

CMV, cytomegalovirus; CNS, central nervous system.
Single-sided deafness defined by the following.
[a] ≥70 dB hearing loss in the affected ear and ≤20 dB HL contralaterally. N = 88.
[b] PTA > 70 dB in the affected ear and PTA < 30 dB contralaterally. N = 210.
[c] Majority (>97%) of included patients had ipsilateral PTA ≥ 70 dB and contralateral PTA ≤ 30 dB HL. N = 118.
[d] Hearing levels beyond the testable thresholds in the affected ear and <25 dB at all tested frequencies in the contralateral ear. N = 50 (N = 31 with available imaging for review).
[e] Data reported is from a subset of their unilateral hearing loss sample with at least "severe" sensorineural hearing loss in the affected ear. N = 113.
[f] Click-evoked auditory brainstem responses ≤35 dB normalized hearing level and ≥80 dB contralaterally. Audiometric tests were later performed that confirmed thresholds. N = 31.

Chronic or acute ear disease can place hardware at risk for infection and potentially meningitis following CI.[19] In the setting of recurrent episodes of acute otitis media or eustachian tube dysfunction, some have advocated for ear tubes with low rates of complications either preimplantation or postimplantation.[20,21] In patients with comorbid chronic ear disease, ear canal overclosure with or without mastoid obliteration has been performed to combat recidivism postimplantation.[22]

Imaging

Obtaining computed tomography (CT) temporal bones and/or MRI in the evaluation of pediatric UHL can provide insight into the cause and rule out structural abnormalities that can influence surgical planning and outcomes (**Table 3**). Approximately one-third of 106 pediatric SSD patients were found to have aberrant anatomy on imaging in one recent retrospective review.[9]

Several authors have reported cochlear nerve deficiency (CND), including nerve hypoplasia and aplasia, is the most common radiologic abnormality, occurring in 25% to 48% of the pediatric SSD population.[9–11,23] CND is typically diagnosed on oblique sagittal, T2-weighted MR sequences obtained perpendicular to the meatal plane in the lateral aspect of the internal auditory canal when the cochlear nerve is smaller in caliber relative to the facial nerve.[24] Aplasia is designated when no cochlear nerve is identifiable. CND is also often correlated with cochlear aperture stenosis, encountered with a pooled frequency of 44% on CT in 2019 systematic review of pediatric unilateral sensorineural hearing loss (SNHL).[25] CND has been reported more often in UHL compared with bilateral congenital SNHL (50% of 56 vs 5.3% of 114 cases)[26] and portends poorer implant performance.[27]

Notably, ophthalmologic pathologic condition has been reported in 67% of children with unilateral CND but concomitant syndromes are uncommon.[23] Nonetheless, routine ophthalmologic evaluation has been recommended for all pediatric patients presenting with SSD.[28] Given vestibular end organ dysfunction has been reported in 17% to 48% of pediatric SSD patients, vestibular evaluations should also be considered, especially in patients with potential comorbid visual impairments.[29,30]

Postmeningitis profound hearing loss and labyrinthitis ossificans can occasionally occur unilaterally.[9,31] Some degree of cochlear ossification has been reported in approximately 34% of high-resolution CTs (HRCT) for pediatric hearing loss following meningitis.[32] If considering CI, T2-weighted-MRI can be useful in detecting the presence of fluid signal within the cochlea to suggest patency.[33] There is a critical time period for implantation following meningitis to increase the likelihood that an implant can be successfully inserted within the scala tympani. Mild degrees of cochlear ossification have been detected on HRCT within a week of meningitis diagnosis.[34] However, surgeons should anticipate the potential need for drilling out the basal turn, or incomplete or scala vestibuli insertions.[35]

Although a 2019 systematic review (N = 1,504) on the clinical utility of imaging in pediatric UHL did not find evidence to support a strong clinical recommendation for obtaining imaging, the authors reported imaging suggested underlying causes in a pooled frequency of approximately 35% and 37% of CTs and MRIs, respectively.[25] Diagnostic yield from imaging has also been found to be higher for congenital UHL than bilateral cases.[36] As in adults, tumors and other isolated lesions of the central nervous system can also be identified on imaging.

Audiometric testing

As in bilateral pediatric hearing loss, early identification is crucial. Fortunately, the implementation of universal newborn hearing screening has also led to increased

Table 3
Reported frequencies of imaging abnormalities related to hearing loss in pediatric patients with unilateral sensorineural hearing loss[c], and single-sided deafness,[9,11,12] N (%)

Study	Common Cavity			Cochlear Dysplasia			Cochlear Hypoplasia			Incomplete Partition — IP-I			Incomplete Partition — IP-II			Incomplete Partition — IP-I or IP-II			EVA			CND[a]			Cochlear Aperture Stenosis			IAC Stenosis or Absence		
	CT	MRI	NS	CT	MRI	NS	CT	MRI	NS	CT	MRI	NS	CT	MRI	NS	CT	MRI	NS	CT	MRI	NS	CT	MRI	NS	CT	MRI	NS	CT	MRI	NS
Dewyer et al,[9] 2022				1 (1)								1 (1)											8 (9)	22 (25)	14 (16)[b]					
Lin et al,[12] 2021															1 (3)									9 (29)						
Cushing et al,[11] 2019						3 (4)	3 (4)		8 (10)			2 (2)			2 (2)									32 (39)						
Ropers et al,[23] 2019	2 (1–3)	0 (0–2)		12 (8–17)	1 (0–3)		3 (0–7)	4 (1–13)		3 (1–4)	0 (0–7)		6 (2–10)	2 (0–6)		10 (7–13)	2 (0–6)		7[d] (4–11)	12[d] (3–22)		-	16 (3–29)		44[e] (36–53)		-	9[f] (5–14)	-	

CI, cochlear implant; CND, cochlear nerve deficiency; CT, computed tomography; EVA, enlarged vestibular aqueduct; IAC, internal auditory canal; IP, incomplete partition; MRI, magnetic resonance imaging; NS, not specified; SCC, semicircular canal.

a CND includes cochlear nerve aplasia or hypoplasia.
b Cochlear aperture stenosis defined as <1.7 mm.
c Percentages represent pooled frequencies (95% confidence interval) as reported in this systematic review.
d Various definitions of EVA were used including: >0.9 mm, >1.5 mm, and >2.0 mm.
e Various definitions of stenosis were used including: <1.4 mm, <1.5 mm (most common), and <1.7 mm.
f Various definitions of stenosis were used including: <2.0 mm, <3.0 mm (most common), and <3.8 mm.

detection rates of UHL.[37] A multidisciplinary approach can provide resources to assist with speech and language development (eg, enrollment in dedicated speech language therapy, individualized education plans at school) beyond aural rehabilitation alone.

Assessing for UHL in the pediatric population is challenging. If unable to participate in behavioral audiometry, corrected thresholds based on evoked auditory brainstem responses are often obtained and may require general anesthesia. In older children, reliance on and compensation with the normal hearing ear may lead to delayed detection. Dewyer and colleagues[9] reviewed 181 children diagnosed with SSD and reported the median age of the first audiogram was 7 years (interquartile range [IQR] = 5–10y). In contrast, the proportion of pediatric SSD attributable to congenital cases has been estimated as high as 42%.[12]

Currently, there are no known genetic mutations specific to UHL, and hereditary etiologies are estimated to be 2.5 times as common in bilateral compared with UHL.[38] The most common abnormality on genetic testing is heterozygous mutations of connexin 26. Monoallelic GJB2 mutations have been detected in 12% to 29% of pediatric UHL cases.[12,39] In bilateral SNHL, genetic testing can account for the cause of up to 30%, with bi-allelic connexin 26 mutations being more common.[40,41]

Criteria for candidacy. At the time of this writing, 2 manufacturers, Cochlear Corporation and MED-EL, are FDA approved for CI in SSD in children aged 5 years or older and with a duration of deafness 10 years or less (**Table 1**). Although it is speculated that the lower age limit is the result of theoretical safety concerns, there is an imminent need to revise the stringent criteria for CI for pediatric SSD, earlier implantation positively affects outcomes, coinciding with auditory pathway maturation with binaural processing.[42]

Duration of absent aural stimulation. The FDA's inclusion of "duration of deafness" within candidacy criteria is inherently problematic because it is reliant on imperfect methods of detection. All efforts should be made to minimize the duration of absent aural stimulation, highlighting the need for revision of current SSD CI criteria.

Outcomes

There is no direct data comparing objective or subjective outcomes with CROS hearing aids, bone conduction systems, and CI in children with UHL. However, Zhan and colleagues[43] performed a retrospective review of 108 pediatric SSD subjects, 3 of which underwent CI, and the remaining subjects either observed the hearing loss, or pursued hearing aids, a CROS device, or a bone-conduction system. Although all 3 CI recipients used the device at least 6 hours daily, 84.7% of the remaining subjects with devices reported 6 hours or less of daily use.[43]

With little objective data for pediatric UHL patients with a traditional CROS or bone-conduction device, the focus of this section will be devoted to CI outcomes. Direct comparison among studies is limited by varying definitions of congenital deafness, as well as a variety of speech perception tests, quality-of-life instruments, and speaker arrangements.

Speech perception

Most studies assess speech perception testing from a 3-speaker set up, with speakers positioned in front of the subject, and then at 90° on either side. In this arrangement, speech and noise are both presented from the front speaker, in addition to speech to the normal hearing ear and implanted ear. This also enables assessment of spatial release from masking. In the most recent systematic review and meta-analysis regarding CI outcomes in pediatric SSD, Benechetrit and colleagues[44] summarized 8 studies (N = 49 children) with speech perception in noise. Following CI, 79.6% of children experienced improved speech perception in noise.[44] Deep and colleagues[45] assessed 8 SSD children (≤12 years old) with a mean follow-up of 3.4 years and found a 49% improvement in mean WRS in the CI-only condition.

Many studies use the 3-speaker arrangement, including one study demonstrating that all subjects showed significant improvement in the speech reception threshold when speech was presented from the front, with no significant difference between groups.[46] In another study including 9 children who demonstrated hearing loss after 4 years of age, there were significant improvements when speech was presented to the CI side. In contrast, Thomas and colleagues[47] observed speech comprehension in noise was significantly improved with the CI in all 3 testing conditions. In summary, CI in pediatric SSD patients can improve speech understanding from the front, as well as when directed to the hearing-impaired ear.

Duration of auditory deprivation. Many studies do not specify the duration of deafness, perhaps better termed the duration of auditory deprivation, which is arguably the most important outcome variable. Zeitler and colleagues[48] assessed 9 SSD CI users with a median follow-up 12.3 months and a median duration of deafness of 2.9 years (range, 0.8–9.5 years). In the CI-only condition, AzBio scores ranged from 69% to 99%, with a median score of 82% (N = 3).[48] However, one child implanted at 9.5 years of age did not have any speech perception improvement.[48]

In arguably the most comprehensive study to date, Brown and colleagues'[49] Childhood Unilateral Hearing Loss (CUHL) trial provides strong support for implantation younger than 5 years of age. Twenty children (ages 3.5–6.5 years) were implanted, with speech perception less than 30% in the ear to be implanted.[49] At 12 months, consonant-nucleus-consonant (CNC) scores significantly improved from 1% to 50%.[49] They found significant improvement regarding head shadow and summation benefits at 6 months, with squelch effect seen at 12 months.[49] Although current FDA approval limits CI to children *older* than 5 years, these studies underscore the additional benefit children receive with earlier implantation.

Localization

With binaural hearing providing localization abilities, several studies have explored localization abilities of SSD pediatric CI recipients. Most studies calculate the root mean square difference in degrees between correct speaker identification with and without the CI. In the CUHL trial, Brown and colleagues[49] reported an average improvement of 17° at 3 months, increasing to an average improvement of 26° at 9 months after activation. Rahne and Plontke observed that localization improved in all subjects, reaching 32° at 12 months, although no further improvement was noted.[46] Although these studies all show improvements in localization for pediatric SSD patients with CI, potential differences in auditory deprivation and age at implantation could account for differences between studies.

Quality of life

Although quality-of-life outcomes are becoming more pervasive in clinical practice, reports are still limited. Given most quality-of-life instruments are designed for adults, pediatric studies have either modified adult instruments and/or assessed parental interpretation of their child's experience and quality of life. Arndt and colleagues[50] observed that parental evaluations of children with hearing loss beyond 4 years of age were higher than the pediatric patients' self-evaluations, whereas parents and children had similar evaluations in kids who lost their hearing at a younger age. Assessing parents, Thomas and colleagues[47] reported a significant improvement in all Speech, Spatial, and Qualities of Hearing Scale (SSQ) subscales following CI, although SSQ scores were not correlated with localization and speech perception results.

In the CUHL trial, Brown and colleagues[49] used the Bern Benefit in Single-Sided Deafness Questionnaire, with 19 of the 20 subjects reporting that hearing was "much easier with their cochlear implant than without." They additionally used the Speech, Spatial, and Qualities of Hearing Scale for Children with Impaired Hearing, designed specifically for children based on the adult version.[49] Assessing all sub-scales, speech hearing, quality hearing, and spatial hearing all showed significant improvements, with spatial hearing demonstrating the largest gain.[49] On further analysis, the authors noted that the greatest gains were in distance and movement of sound, localization, speech in noise, speech in speech, listening effort, and processing multiple speech streams.[49]

Additional outcomes

Similar to adult CI literature, trends in data logging have been evaluated, with greater use believed to translate to greater benefit. Deep and colleagues[45] reported that 9 of 13 CI recipients wore their device more than 7 h/d, with one user using it less than 1 h/d but without associations to speech perception outcomes. Polonenko and colleagues[51] found a 10% increase in CI "experience was associated with an additional 0.02 hours of CI use," and "as CI experience increased, the frequency of coil-offs decreased."

With respect to speech and language, pediatric CI recipients demonstrate normal development with good auditory memory in a study by Ehrmann-Mueller and colleagues.[52] In another study, Sangen and colleagues[3] explored longitudinal linguistic outcomes in 18 SSD children, including 6 CI recipients, in comparison with a normal hearing cohort. Patients implanted with CI were comparable to the normal hearing cohort, with diverse outcomes in those who did not obtain a CI.[3]

In the Cochlear Implant for Children and One Deaf Ear Study, 34 children were identified to be CI candidates. Fifteen children were subsequently implanted and compared with the 16 children that deferred implantation, in addition to a normal hearing cohort.[18] Compared with the normal hearing cohort, children with SSD and a CI had similar grammar scores, whereas children with SSD and without a CI had significantly worse grammar scores, compared with both the normal hearing controls and unilateral CI recipients.[18]

Although tinnitus outcomes are commonly reported in the adult SSD literature, little data exist within the pediatric literature. Although Ehrmann-Mueller and colleagues had no reports of tinnitus before or after CI, Zeitler and colleagues noted complete resolution in 50%, with partial suppression in the remaining patients when using a CI.[48,52]

DISCLOSURE

The authors have noting to disclose.

REFERENCES

1. Bess FH, Tharpe AM. Unilateral hearing impairment in children. Pediatrics 1984; 74(2):206–16.

2. Fitzpatrick EM, Gaboury I, Durieux-Smith A, et al. Auditory and language outcomes in children with unilateral hearing loss. Hear Res 2019;372:42–51.

3. Sangen A, Royackers L, Desloovere C, et al. Single-sided deafness affects language and auditory development - a case-control study. Clin Otolaryngol 2017; 42(5):979–87.

4. Bess FH, Tharpe AM, Gibler AM. Auditory performance of children with unilateral sensorineural hearing loss. Ear Hear 1986;7(1):20–6.

5. Bess FH, Dodd-Murphy J, Parker RA. Children with minimal sensorineural hearing loss: prevalence, educational performance, and functional status. Ear Hear 1998; 19(5):339–54.

6. Shargorodsky J, Curhan SG, Curhan GC, et al. Change in prevalence of hearing loss in US adolescents. JAMA 2010;304(7):772–8.

7. Ross DS, Visser SN, Holstrum WJ, et al. Highly variable population-based prevalence rates of unilateral hearing loss after the application of common case definitions. Ear Hear 2010;31(1):126–33.

8. Bagatto M, DesGeorges J, King A, et al. Consensus practice parameter: audiological assessment and management of unilateral hearing loss in children. Int J Audiol 2019;58(12):805–15.

9. Dewyer NA, Smith S, Herrmann B, et al. Pediatric Single-sided deafness: a review of prevalence, radiologic findings, and cochlear implant candidacy. Ann Otol Rhinol Laryngol 2022;131(3):233–8.

10. Usami SI, Kitoh R, Moteki H, et al. Etiology of single-sided deafness and asymmetrical hearing loss. Acta Otolaryngol 2017;137(sup565):S2–7.

11. Cushing SL, Gordon KA, Sokolov M, et al. Etiology and therapy indication for cochlear implantation in children with single-sided deafness : retrospective analysis. HNO 2019;67(10):750–9.

12. Lin PH, Hsu CJ, Lin YH, et al. Etiologic and audiologic characteristics of patients with pediatric-onset unilateral and asymmetric sensorineural hearing loss. JAMA Otolaryngol Head Neck Surg 2017;143(9):912–9.

13. Kral A, Heid S, Hubka P, et al. Unilateral hearing during development: hemispheric specificity in plastic reorganizations. Front Syst Neurosci 2013;7:93.

14. Gordon K, Henkin Y, Kral A. Asymmetric hearing during development: the aural preference syndrome and treatment options. Pediatrics 2015;136(1):141–53.

15. Fitzpatrick EM, Gaboury I, Durieux-Smith A, et al. Parent report of amplification use in children with mild bilateral or unilateral hearing loss. J Am Acad Audiol 2019;30(2):93–102.

16. Branemark Bone Anchored Hearing Aid (BAHA) System. K984162. In: US Food and Drug Administration's letter providing permission to Nobel Biocare USA to market their bone anchored hearing aid. The paperwork noting the 5 years and older limit is authored by Nobel Biocare USA, Inc. Rockville, MD: U.S. Food and Drug Administration; 1999 (FDA) 510(k).

17. van Wieringen A, Boudewyns A, Sangen A, et al. Unilateral congenital hearing loss in children: challenges and potentials. Hear Res 2019;372:29–41.

18. Arras T, Boudewyns A, Dhooge I, et al. Assessment of receptive and expressive language skills among young children with prelingual single-sided deafness managed with early cochlear implantation. JAMA Netw Open 2021;4(8): e2122591.

19. Hellingman CA, Dunnebier EA. Cochlear implantation in patients with acute or chronic middle ear infectious disease: a review of the literature. Eur Arch Otorhinolaryngol 2009;266(2):171–6.

20. Kennedy RJ, Shelton C. Ventilation tubes and cochlear implants: what do we do? Otology & Neurotology 2005;26(3):438–41.

21. Baranano CF, Sweitzer RS, Mahalak ML, et al. The management of myringotomy tubes in pediatric cochlear implant recipients. Arch Otolaryngol Head Neck Surg 2010;136(6):557–60.

22. Bernardeschi D, Nguyen Y, Smail M, et al. Middle ear and mastoid obliteration for cochlear implant in adults: indications and anatomical results. Otology & neurotology 2015;36(4):604–9.

23. Clemmens CS, Guidi J, Caroff A, et al. Unilateral cochlear nerve deficiency in children. Otolaryngol Head Neck Surg 2013;149(2):318–25.

24. Miyasaka M, Nosaka S, Morimoto N, et al. CT and MR imaging for pediatric cochlear implantation: emphasis on the relationship between the cochlear nerve canal and the cochlear nerve. Pediatr Radiol 2010;40(9):1509–16.

25. Ropers FG, Pham ENB, Kant SG, et al. Assessment of the Clinical Benefit of Imaging in Children With Unilateral Sensorineural Hearing Loss: A Systematic Review and Meta-analysis. JAMA Otolaryngol Head Neck Surg 2019;145(5):431–43.

26. Nakano A, Arimoto Y, Matsunaga T. Cochlear nerve deficiency and associated clinical features in patients with bilateral and unilateral hearing loss. Otology & neurotology 2013;34(3):554–8.

27. Chung J, Jang JH, Chang SO, et al. Does the width of the bony cochlear nerve canal predict the outcomes of cochlear implantation? Biomed Res Int 2018;2018: 5675848.

28. Haffey T, Fowler N, Anne S. Evaluation of unilateral sensorineural hearing loss in the pediatric patient. Int J Pediatr Otorhinolaryngol 2013;77(6):955–8.

29. Sokolov M, Gordon KA, Polonenko M, et al. Vestibular and balance function is often impaired in children with profound unilateral sensorineural hearing loss. Hear Res 2019;372:52–61.

30. Wolter NE, Cushing SL, Vilchez-Madrigal LD, et al. Unilateral hearing loss is associated with impaired balance in children: a pilot study. Otology & Neurotology. 2016;37(10):1589–95.

31. Buch K, Baylosis B, Fujita A, et al. Etiology-specific mineralization patterns in patients with labyrinthitis ossificans. AJNR Am J Neuroradiol 2019;40(3):551–7.

32. Durisin M, Bartling S, Arnoldner C, et al. Cochlear osteoneogenesis after meningitis in cochlear implant patients: a retrospective analysis. Otology & Neurotology 2010;31(7):1072–8.

33. Booth TN, Roland P, Kutz JW Jr, et al. High-resolution 3-D T2-weighted imaging in the diagnosis of labyrinthitis ossificans: emphasis on subtle cochlear involvement. Pediatr Radiol 2013;43(12):1584–90.

34. Durisin M, Buchner A, Lesinski-Schiedat A, et al. Cochlear implantation in children with bacterial meningitic deafness: The influence of the degree of ossification and obliteration on impedance and charge of the implant. Cochlear Implants Int 2015;16(3):147–58.

35. Singhal K, Singhal J, Muzaffar J, et al. Outcomes of cochlear implantation in patients with post-meningitis deafness: a systematic review and narrative synthesis. J Int Adv Otol 2020;16(3):395–410.

36. Preciado DA, Lim LH, Cohen AP, et al. A diagnostic paradigm for childhood idiopathic sensorineural hearing loss. Otolaryngol Head Neck Surg 2004;131(6): 804–9.

37. Ghogomu N, Umansky A, Lieu JE. Epidemiology of unilateral sensorineural hearing loss with universal newborn hearing screening. Laryngoscope 2014;124(1): 295–300.

38. van Beeck Calkoen EA, Engel MSD, van de Kamp JM, et al. The etiological evaluation of sensorineural hearing loss in children. Eur J Pediatr 2019;178(8): 1195–205.

39. Gruber M, Brown C, Mahadevan M, et al. The yield of multigene testing in the management of pediatric unilateral sensorineural hearing loss. Otology & Neurotology 2016;37(8):1066–70.

40. Wiley S, Arjmand E, Jareenmeinzen D, et al. Findings from multidisciplinary evaluation of children with permanent hearing loss. Int J Pediatr Otorhinolaryngol 2011;75(8):1040–4.

41. Lin JW, Chowdhury N, Mody A, et al. Comprehensive diagnostic battery for evaluating sensorineural hearing loss in children. Otol Neurotol 2011;32(2):259–64.

42. Park LR, Gagnon EB, Brown KD. The limitations of FDA criteria: inconsistencies with clinical practice, findings, and adult criteria as a barrier to pediatric implantation. Semin Hear 2021;42(4):373–80.

43. Zhan KY, Findlen UM, Allen DZ, et al. Therapeutic challenges and clinical characteristics of single-sided deafness in children. Int J Pediatr Otorhinolaryngol 2020; 135:110116.

44. Benchetrit L, Ronner EA, Anne S, et al. Cochlear implantation in children with single-sided deafness: a systematic review and meta-analysis. JAMA Otolaryngol Head Neck Surg 2021;147(1):58–69.

45. Deep NL, Gordon SA, Shapiro WH, et al. Cochlear implantation in children with single-sided deafness. Laryngoscope 2021;131(1):E271–7.

46. Rahne T, Plontke SK. Functional result after cochlear implantation in children and adults with single-sided deafness. Otology & Neurotology. 2016;37(9):e332–40.

47. Thomas JP, Neumann K, Dazert S, et al. Cochlear implantation in children with congenital single-sided deafness. Otology & Neurotology 2017;38(4):496–503.

48. Zeitler DM, Sladen DP, DeJong MD, et al. Cochlear implantation for single-sided deafness in children and adolescents. Int J Pediatr Otorhinolaryngol 2019;118: 128–33.

49. Brown KD, Dillon MT, Park LR. Benefits of Cochlear Implantation in Childhood Unilateral Hearing Loss (CUHL Trial). Laryngoscope 2022;132(Suppl 6):S1–18.

50. Arndt S, Prosse S, Laszig R, et al. Cochlear implantation in children with single-sided deafness: does aetiology and duration of deafness matter? Audiol Neurootol 2015;20(Suppl 1):21–30.

51. Polonenko MJ, Papsin BC, Gordon KA. Children with single-sided deafness use their cochlear implant. Ear Hear 2017;38(6):681–9.

52. Ehrmann-Mueller D, Kurz A, Kuehn H, et al. Usefulness of cochlear implantation in children with single sided deafness. Int J Pediatr Otorhinolaryngol 2020;130: 109808.

Updates in Eustachian Tube Dysfunction

Sainiteesh Maddineni, BS, Iram Ahmad, MD, MME*

KEYWORDS

- Eustachian tube dysfunction • Middle ear disorder • Otitis media
- Conductive hearing loss • Cholesteatoma • Pediatric

KEY POINTS

- Eustachian tube dysfunction (ETD) is a common middle ear pathology often affecting children.
- Data on medical management of ETD does not have a clear consensus, but current data suggests that current medical treatments for ETD may not be robust in all children. Consideration of these data should be taken before prescribing pharmacologic therapy.
- ETD is associated with sequelae like otitis media, tympanic membrane retraction, cholesteatoma, and conductive hearing loss.
- The medical management of ETD is not always effective, and surgical options are available based on patient presentation.
- Greater resesarch on etiologies, diagnostics, and treatment of children with ETD is necessary.

ANATOMY AND PHYSIOLOGY OF THE EUSTACHIAN TUBE

The Eustachian tube (ET) is found below the skull base and consists of an osseous posterolateral segment and a cartilaginous anteromedial segment. The cartilaginous component is suspended from the skull base and comprises approximately 2/3 of the length of the ET while 1/3 is osseous. The longitudinal axis of the ET is shallower in children and may contribute to the common sequelae of ETD in children via impaired drainage of middle ear fluid. The ET is also shorter in children compared to adults.[1,2] The main function of the ET is to equalize pressure between the middle ear and the atmosphere.[1,3] The ET is capable of dilation, and this action is controlled primarily by the tensor veli palatini (TVP) with assistance from the levator veli palatini (LVP). The ET is collapsed at rest and opens involuntarily during swallowing but can also voluntarily open through swallowing or yawning, activating the TVP.[1,2,4] The ET has

Department of Otolaryngology–Head & Neck Surgery, Stanford University, Stanford, CA 94305, USA
* Corresponding author.
E-mail address: iramnahmad@stanford.edu

Otolaryngol Clin N Am 55 (2022) 1151–1164
https://doi.org/10.1016/j.otc.2022.07.010
0030-6665/22/© 2022 Elsevier Inc. All rights reserved.

oto.theclinics.com

ciliated epithelium that enables mucociliary clearance of middle ear fluid while providing a barrier to the entry of pathogens from the nasopharynx.[1,3]

EPIDEMIOLOGY

Eustachian tube dysfunction (ETD) is a common pathology, especially in pediatric populations. The prevalence of ETD in children is estimated to be around 4–20%.[5–7] ETD is more prevalent in children than adults, and there are an average of 0.77 adult visits for ETD for every pediatric visit.[8] Otitis media with effusion (OME) and tympanic membrane retraction are possible sequelae of ETD, and there were on average 2.6 million visits per year related to ETD, OME, and tympanic membrane retraction in patients under the age of 20, based on analysis of United States population data between 2005 and 2012. In the pediatric population, more males are affected with ETD (55.72%).[9] Given the large prevalence of ETD and its sequelae in pediatric patients, a deep understanding of its pathophysiology and management is essential for otolaryngologists.

ETIOLOGY AND PATHOPHYSIOLOGY

Most cases of ETD may not have a definitive etiology identified other than the aforementioned anatomic challenges that children face. Commonly the ETD resolves before a cause is identified.[10] The 3 subtypes of ETD that have been described are: obstructive (dilatory), patulous, and baro-challenge-induced.[8,10,11]

Obstructive or Dilatory

Obstructive (also referred to as dilatory) ETD refers to an ET that is occluded and unable to effectively dilate.[8,10] The most common reason for the impairment of ET dilation is the inflammation of the mucosa of the cartilaginous ET.[12] In young children, this can be caused by frequent infections and exposure in daycare, adenoid hypertrophy with obstruction, and bottle feeding. The horizontal anatomy of the ET in children can propagate the effects of these etiologies. Gastroesophageal and laryngoesophageal reflux are also linked to an increased risk of ETD. Gastroesophageal reflux is common in infants and toddlers, and may contribute to the increased prevalence of ETD in children.[13,14] Further research investigating this mechanism of reflux triggering ETD is needed.[14]

Infection and allergy have also been supported as etiologies of acute, obstructive ETD. Similar to reflux, infection can trigger inflammation within the ET lumen that leads to impaired dilation and obstruction.[11] Allergic rhinitis has also been reported as an etiology for ETD, although this association has been controversial. Treatment of ETD with intranasal corticosteroids to alleviate allergic rhinitis has not been efficacious in improving symptoms of ETD.[7] Unfortunately, little data are available on patients with concurrent allergic rhinitis and ETD to differentiate the effect of corticosteroid treatment between rhinitis and ETD. There is also a need for further research on the mechanistic link between allergies and ETD.[7]

Patulous

In contrast to the failure of the ET to dilate in obstructive ETD, patulous ETD is characterized by an excessively patent ET that does not sufficiently constrict and is relatively less common than obstructive ETD.[8,10] The majority of cases of patulous ETD do not have a clear etiology.[11] One retrospective study reported a variety of comorbidities found in patients with patulous ETD. Allergy, stress, and anxiety were specifically noted to be risk factors for sustained contraction of the TVP, which leaves the ET dilated for a prolonged time and contributes to the development of patulous ETD.[15] Additionally, recent weight loss has been identified as an additional risk factor. However, regaining the weight is not a reliable method of resolving patulous ETD.[11,15]

Baro-Challenge-Induced

Baro-challenge-induced ETD is a situational presentation of ETD in which sudden changes in atmospheric pressure can affect ET function. Specifically, deep-sea diving or descent from high altitudes are common examples of situations that can induce baro-challenge-induced ETD.[8] Children with this subtype of ETD usually present without symptoms and a normal otoscopic and tympanometry examination at normal atmospheric pressure.[16] However, a major baro-challenge episode can trigger middle ear effusion and hemotympanum.[11] Baro-challenge-induced ETD is thought to arise from localized inflammation of ET mucosa due to stress induced by repeated pressure changes.[8]

Risk Factors

Congenital malformations can be major predisposing factors for ETD in the pediatric population. Children with cleft palate are more likely to have abnormal dilatory function of the ET that can result in functionally obstructive ETD.[17,18] Specifically, children with cleft palate have reduced dilatory function of the TVP, contributing to ETD.[19] Furthermore, ET function may improve after palatoplasty if the integrity of the TVP is maintained, but this is not a consistent result.[19,20] Patients with Down Syndrome have a high rate of ETD. In children with Down syndrome, the TVP may be normal, but the ET itself may be narrower due to their craniofacial anatomy.[21–23] The cartilaginous portion of the ET can also be weaker and more collapsible, contributing to this structural abnormality and resulting ETD.[24]

Several additional risk factors are thought to contribute to the pathogenesis of ETD. Children with obstructive sleep apnea have been found to have greater prevalence of ETD, due to the involvement of the adenoids and tonsils, which can influence the onset and duration of ETD in children.[6,25] Because ETD is associated with enlarged adenoids in children, adenoidectomy can help treat ETD.[26,27] Chronic sinusitis is also associated with an increased rate of ETD in children, but this association weakens with age, suggesting that growth leads to anatomical changes that mitigate the risk of ETD.[28] Environmentally, children who were exposed to tobacco smoke had higher odds of ETD.[29] Finally, a diagnosis of granulomatous disease, cystic fibrosis, Samter's triad, primary ciliary dyskinesia, or Kartagener's syndrome has also been reported as risk factors for ETD in children.[12]

EUSTACHIAN TUBE DYSFUNCTION SEQUELAE

While ETD itself can be a symptomatic pathology, it is also associated as an etiology or comorbidity for other common childhood ear pathologies.

Otitis Media

One of the most common sequelae of ETD is otitis media (OM), a collection of middle ear inflammatory diseases common in children. Acute OM is a complication of ETD that may develop following the inflammation associated with a viral upper respiratory tract infection or an episode of allergic rhinitis.[30,31] Normally, the ET can effectively protect the middle ear from infection through a combination of mucociliary clearance and antimicrobial proteins. However, children are at higher risk of middle ear infection given their environment, and the shorter, more horizontal structure of the ET that permits more facile pathogen entry. Viral infection of the ET mucosa also triggers the release of inflammatory mediators that can increase bacterial colonization of the ET and middle ear, contributing to ETD and acute OM. Furthermore, viruses can impede effective mucociliary clearance, further contributing to ETD.[32] These inflammatory processes can correspond to obstructive ETD, as previously discussed.

Tympanic Membrane Retraction and Cholesteatoma

ETD is associated with tympanic membrane retraction and development of an associated squamous epithelial cyst known as a cholesteatoma that can damage the middle or inner ear.[8,10] In ETD, increased middle ear negative pressure can result in the retraction of the tympanic membrane.[33,34] This retracted membrane can then be trapped in a retraction pocket and form a cholesteatoma sac, where trapped skin cells and debris can accumulate as the pocket deepens and grows an epithelial cyst known as a cholesteatoma. Cholesteatoma can also form in children without tympanic membrane retraction but instead are born with skin cells trapped behind the tympanic membrane.[35] Cholesteatoma can be infected or expand into the middle ear and other spaces, causing serious symptoms such as hearing loss.[33] Importantly, tympanic membrane retraction does not confirm a diagnosis of ETD, even though ETD can cause tympanic membrane retraction.[26] Episodes of otitis media, independent of ETD, can also contribute to tympanic membrane retraction.[36–38] Cholesteatoma is significantly associated with a stenotic ET seen in obstructive ETD. Yet, patulous ETD in combination with habitual sniffing is also associated with cholesteatoma.[12,39]

Conductive Hearing Loss

Conductive hearing loss (CHL) can be a direct result of ETD or its associated sequelae, including otitis media and cholesteatoma.[8,40,41] CHL caused by acute OM and OME is often transient and recovers with the treatment of the underlying OM. Often, the CHL in patients with ETD is of mild to moderate severity.[11] Children with unilateral cleft palate are twice as likely to have CHL in the ear ipsilateral to the cleft lip and palate compared to their contralateral ear.[42] This is because ETD is more common and prominent in children with cleft palate.[43] CHL can prove to be a major quality of life issue for children afflicted by ETD and its sequelae, making it an important to diagnose in a timely manner.

DIAGNOSIS OF EUSTACHIAN TUBE DYSFUNCTION
Clinical Presentation

Each subset of ETD has its own characteristic clinical presentations. Symptoms that suggest ETD, in general, include: pressure in the ear, aural fullness; popping, pain, or discomfort in the ear; muffled hearing; and autophony.[11] Obstructive ETD can present with aural fullness, pain, altered or muffled hearing, and tinnitus.[11,44] Patients may also attempt a Valsalva maneuver or jaw-thrust in an attempt to equalize middle ear and atmospheric pressures.[11] In baro-challenge-induced ETD, patients may only experience the aural symptoms described previously during situations of rapid pressure changes, especially with exposure to high pressures. However, the pain associated with baro-challenge-induced ETD could be related to factors beyond ETD alone, and the clinical presentation of patients with this subset of ETD can be complex.[45] Patulous ETD can present with similar symptoms, and patients can present with positional autophony, audible breathing, pulsatile tinnitus that synchronizes with breathing, a sense of pressure in the ear, and hearing loss.[12,42] Overall, different subtypes of ETD present with similar symptoms but can subtly vary, providing clinicians with important diagnostic clues. Additionally, ETD presentation is not limited to the aforementioned symptoms, and pediatric clinicians should be careful and thorough about diagnosing ETD since it can present with other, less common symptoms.[26]

Diagnostics

A child's clinical presentation in combination with additional tests can help make a diagnosis of ETD. For suspected obstructive ETD, the clinician should evaluate the patient's symptoms and confirm negative pressure in the middle ear. The latter can be achieved via otoscopy or tympanogram measurement.[11] As a caveat, one study of 250 patients did report that those with symptoms consistent with ETD sometimes had tympanometric peak pressures that were considered normal. Furthermore, when compared to a patient survey of symptoms, TPP had a specificity of 53.2% and a negative predictive value of only 40.9%, suggesting that it is not a robust diagnostic tool.[46] However, tympanometry is routinely used as part of ETD diagnosis in children, including those with congenital risk factors, like cleft palate and Down syndrome.[25,47] The diagnosis of baro-challenge-induced ETD especially relies on patient history as patients may present with a normal tympanic membrane and feel asymptomatic during a clinic visit. However, middle ear effusion or hemotympanum may be present in these patients as further support for the diagnosis of baro-challenge-induced ETD. In patulous ETD, tympanic membrane excursion can be noticed during otoscopy or tympanometry while the patient breaths. For suspected ETD in general, audiometry can be helpful in some instances in which patients are experiencing conductive hearing loss, and nasopharyngoscopy can be utilized to possibly identify an etiology for the patient's ETD and may help confirm the diagnosis.[11]

Functional Tests or Scores

Several functional tests and composite scoring systems have been developed to aid in the diagnosis of ETD, and a few have been consistently used in otology research or clinical practice. The ETDQ-7 questionnaire was originally developed to quantify the severity of common symptoms associated with ETD.[48] The ETS-7 test was introduced as a successor to the ETDQ-7 and relies on more objective measurements to diagnose ETD. Specifically, it incorporates clinical symptoms and examination, multiple tympanogram measurements at various pressures, and tympanometry analysis. The ETS-7 achieved a reported sensitivity ranging from 73% to 96% and specificity of 60% to 96%, but further validation in children alone is needed.[49] ETS-7 has since been extended to other studies, including one study that used ETS-7 to identify a positive association between obstructive sleep apnea and ETD in adults.[50] ETS-7 benefits from its quantitative metrics, as patient-reported outcome measures have been shown to have little diagnostic value. Rather, tests of ET opening, like tympanometry, in combination with clinical assessment provide the most accurate diagnoses, as there is still no universal consensus on a gold standard diagnostic test.[51,52]

Imaging

Radiologic imaging has also been explored as a diagnostic tool for ETD. Traditionally, CT and MRI have been useful to analyze the anatomy of the ET in detail.[53] Imaging of ET patency is possible via cine x-ray or scintigraphy, but a contrast agent is necessary for such studies.

Obstructive ETD can be imaged with CT scans. Key features of obstructive ETD on CT imaging include a narrowing of the ET osseous portion and the tube having a shallower angle. Patulous ETD has also been identified on CT imaging, which can show abnormal ET patency via reconstruction perpendicular to the ET long axis. However, patulous ETD can improve in the supine position often assumed during CT scans, and CT imaging of patients in the seated position while performing a Valsalva maneuver can improve imaging and diagnosis of patulous ETD.[53–55] However, data on the efficacy of Valsalva CT are conflicting, with studies showing its ability to identify obstructed parts of the ET lumen but the results of the imaging not correlating well with functional tests like the ETS-7.[56,57] Valsalva MRI could confirm the opening of the ET, but data on its usage in patients with ETD specifically are necessary.[53] More information on Valsalva CT or MRI is necessary to understand its role in the diagnostic workup of ETD. Ultimately, a combination of clinical examination, diagnostic tests, and imaging may prove most useful in establishing a clear diagnosis of ETD in children.

SURGICAL MANAGEMENT OF EUSTACHIAN TUBE DYSFUNCTION
Nondefinitive Surgical Approaches

Surgical treatment of ETD can involve alleviating symptoms associated with increased negative pressure in the middle ear. Myringotomy with tympanostomy tube placement can alleviate symptoms of obstructive ETD by permitting ventilation through the tympanic membrane but does not address the underlying ETD itself.[44] Tympanostomy tube placement is instead a common surgery in children to alleviate associated OME.[58] Similarly, myringotomy and grommet placement can alleviate symptoms of patulous ETD but is not curative.[12] Additionally, adenoidectomy in children with adenoid hypertrophy could significantly improve ETS-7 score and treat ETD.[27]

Patulous Eustachian Tube Dysfunction Surgical Approaches

Patulous ETD involves several unique surgical approaches to treatment, including reconstructive procedures and implants to restore physiologic ET function. Reconstruction can involve instilling a submucosal graft to modify the abnormal concavity of the ET anterolateral wall that occurs in patulous ETD.[59] Specifically, a submucosal flap is raised and autologous cartilage, collagen, or a different implant can be placed, such as a Vox implant, which consists of polydimethylsiloxane dissolved in polyvinyl-pyrrolidone hydrogel.[60–62] In addition to the reconstruction of the ET, implants can be inserted into the ET lumen. The Kobayashi plug is inserted through the tympanic membrane into the ET and has shown 83% efficacy in patients with chronic, patulous ETD.[54,63] Moreover, shim insertion with IV catheters into the ET lumen can also help treat patulous ETD.[64]

Additionally, injection of bulking agents can help treat patulous ETD. Injection of a calcium hydroxyapatite filler can be utilized to provide bulk to the ET.[59,64,65] Fat grafting is an option with the cauterization of the ET lumen to promote scarring and closure.[59,66] Complete ET occlusion is only considered in rare cases of persistent autophony.[64] Comparing these different treatment options, complete obliteration of the ET was most effective at symptom alleviation, followed by shim insertion and ET reconstruction. Hydroxyapatite filler injection was worst at symptom alleviation.[67]

Eustachian Tube Dilation

Tuboplasty is a surgical procedure to dilate an obstructed ET via balloon dilation. Balloon dilation of the Eustachian tube (BDET) is an effective treatment modality for patients with persistent, obstructive ETD who may also present with barotrauma and serous OM.[68,69] BDET was shown to have better therapeutic efficacy compared to medical intervention in RCTs of adult patients, and also shows better long-term data compared to medical therapy.[69–72] Before recommending BDET as an option, clinicians should perform a clinical examination with nasal endoscopy to ensure that the patient does not have patulous ETD. Additionally, nasal endoscopy allows the clinician to confirm the obstruction of the ET, plan their transnasal approach for tuboplasty, and identify potential etiologies for ETD that can be managed nonsurgically.[44] After undergoing BDET, a patient's ability to perform a modified Valsalva is an indicator of therapeutic benefit from surgery.[44]

In children specifically, BDET shows therapeutic benefit. Children with chronic ETD show the alleviation of symptoms comparable to tympanostomy tubes, and improvement in tympanograms to a normal Type A after BDET.[73-76] These findings are supported by a meta-analysis showing that BDET generally improves symptoms, but is a second-line therapy in most studies. Currently, Eustachian tube dilation is not FDA approved for patients under 18 and is not routinely performed in children. Children have narrower cartilaginous portions of the ET that lead to shorter distances between the cartilaginous ET and carotid canal.[77] As a result, care and consideration for the proximity of the carotid canal must be taken for children undergoing off-label treatment. Additional, higher quality data are needed before BDET can be established as the first-line standard of care.[74]

Instead of BDET, lasers can also be utilized to perform tuboplasty by ablating the epipharyngeal opening of the ET.[78] Laser tuboplasty has been shown to help with chronic, obstructive ETD.[12] However, in a meta-analysis of BDET and laser tuboplasty, BDET showed greater improvement of ETS score and tympanometry measurements compared to laser tuboplasty. Yet, the lack of abundant data precludes any definitive conclusion on whether BDET is consistently superior to laser tuboplasty.[78]

NONSURGICAL MANAGEMENT OF EUSTACHIAN TUBE DYSFUNCTION

The nonsurgical management of ETD includes a variety of pharmacologic approaches with few nonmedication approaches. Clinicians should differentiate between obstructive and patulous ETD before initiating medical therapy. Medications for ETD include nasal steroids, antihistamines, and systemic decongestants.[12] Regarding corticosteroids, a study of dexamethasone in children found improvement in ETD symptoms such as negative ear pressure, but dexamethasone should only be used for a limited period of time given that it can increase cortisol levels.[79] However, a randomized, controlled trial (RCT) of intranasal steroid sprays in adults and children found no benefit in the treatment of ETD.[80] Moreover, a trial of topical decongestants found that patients only with very high middle ear pressures had any benefit.[81] This finding is backed up by a systematic review that found only mild, short-term improvements in the middle ear for patients receiving topical decongestants. However, intranasal fluticasone was associated with a reduced need for tympanostomy tubes in children, although children with cleft lip, cleft palate, or Down syndrome may not benefit from this steroid due to their underlying anatomical malformations driving ETD.[82]

In patulous ETD specifically, estrogen nasal drops or potassium iodide administered orally can trigger inflammation and swelling of the ET opening. Other medications include hydrochloric acid, chlorobutanol, and benzyl alcohol, but these treatments may not be effective in all patients with patulous ETD.[12] In sequelae such as OME in children, a primary goal is to limit chronic inflammation of the middle ear until a child's growth could correct any relevant anatomic issues that cause ETD. This can be achieved using many of the pharmaceuticals discussed, as well as antibiotics and mucolytics. Yet, these options may also not have long-term efficacy in treating OME.[83]

Overall, the data on the efficacy of medications for ETD can be scattered without consensus. A recent meta-analysis of medical treatment of ETD found that only 50.3% of patients had improvement in ETD symptoms, and scores on the ETDQ-7

Table 1
Summary of clinical management of ETD

Type of ETD	Description	Clinical Presentation	Surgical Treatment	Medical Treatment
Obstructive/Dilatory	Occluded ET or poor dilation	Aural fullness, tinnitus, pain in ears, altered hearing; patients attempt Valsalva for comfort	Tympanostomy tube placement, balloon dilation	Nasal steroids, antihistamines, decongestants, Politzer, Otovent
Patulous	ET too dilated or poor constriction	Autophony, audible breathing, tinnitus with breathing, hearing loss, pressure in ears	Tympanostomy tube placement, filler or fat injections, implants (Vox), reconstruction	Inflammatory agents such as estrogen or potassium iodide
Baro-Challenge-Induced	ET dysfunction due to changes in pressure	Symptoms mainly experienced during pressure changes (flights, diving, etc...)	Tympanostomy tube placement	Nasal steroids, antihistamines, decongestants, Politzer, Otovent

functional survey did not improve.[84] Moreover, the finding that intranasal corticosteroids are not effective is consistent across multiple studies.[84–86] Nonmedication approaches such as Politzer devices and Valsalva therapy have also not shown significant efficacy.[84] For children with barotrauma who need to equalize pressure, the Otoventautoinflation system can be used under parental supervision, but is mainly for short-term alleviation.[12] Ultimately, nonsurgical interventions for ETD do not appear to be effective currently, and additional work is needed in developing this treatment area.[12,87]

DISCUSSION

In this review, we have considered the various subsets of ETD, including obstructive, patulous, and baro-challenge-induced. We have discussed the clinical presentation, possible etiologies, and the pathophysiology of ETD, including its associated complications, especially with respect to children. Finally, we reviewed the diagnosis and management of ETD. **Table 1** summarizes key points about ETD discussed in this review.

There is still a need for higher-quality studies on ETD. Hypothesized etiologies of ETD should be investigated further, as there are many associations but limited mechanistic studies that confirm risk factors as etiologies. Moreover, additional data and RCTs on medical interventions and surgical interventions are necessary to provide children and their families with additional, effective treatment options for ETD. Greater research on diagnostics can also help identify a gold standard test that can be reliably used in all clinic settings, not solely in specialized ENT clinics or research labs. Importantly, more studies in children specifically can guide pediatric clinicians on the best, evidence-based approaches to the treatment of ETD.

DISCLOSURE

The Authors have nothing to disclose.

CLINICS CARE POINTS

- Clinical presentation of different types of ETD may have overlapping symptoms. Otoscopy and tympanometry can be useful initial diagnostic tools for suspected ETD. No gold standard functional score exists, but ETS-7 may emerge as a useful scoring metric as further validation studies are done.

- Data on medical management of ETD does not have a clear consensus, but current data suggests that current medical treatments for ETD may not be robust in all children. Consideration of these data should be taken before prescribing pharmacologic therapy.

- Initial surgical management of ETD generally involves tympanostomy tube placement. Given the different surgical treatments for obstructive and patulous ETD, identification of the type of ETD a patient presents with is important.

REFERENCES

1. Tysome JR, Sudhoff H. the role of the eustachian tube in middle ear disease. Adv Otorhinolaryngol 2018;81:146–52.
2. Leuwer R. Anatomy of the eustachian tube. Otolaryngol Clin North Am 2016; 49(5):1097–106.

3. Casale J, Hatcher JD. Physiology, Eustachian Tube Function. In: StatPearls. StatPearls Publishing; 2022. Available at: http://www.ncbi.nlm.nih.gov/books/NBK532284/. Accessed January 30, 2022.

4. Georgakopoulos B, Borger J. Anatomy, head and neck, tensor veli palatini muscle. In: StatPearls. StatPearls Publishing; 2022. Available at: http://www.ncbi.nlm.nih.gov/books/NBK544302/. Accessed January 30, 2022.

5. Kim AS, Betz JF, Goman AM, et al. Prevalence and population estimates of obstructive eustachian tube dysfunction in US adolescents. JAMA Otolaryngology–Head Neck Surg 2020;146(8):763–5.

6. Robison JG, Wilson C, Otteson TD, et al. Increased eustachian tube dysfunction in infants with obstructive sleep apnea. Laryngoscope 2012;122(5):1170–7.

7. Juszczak HM, Loftus PA. Role of allergy in eustachian tube dysfunction. Curr Allergy Asthma Rep 2020;20(10):54.

8. Hamrang-Yousefi S, Ng J, Andaloro C. Eustachian tube dysfunction. In: StatPearls. StatPearls Publishing; 2022. Available at: http://www.ncbi.nlm.nih.gov/books/NBK555908/. Accessed February 1, 2022.

9. Vila PM, Thomas T, Liu C, et al. The burden and epidemiology of eustachian tube dysfunction in adults. Otolaryngol Head Neck Surg 2017;156(2):278–84.

10. Poe D. Eustachian tube dysfunction. UpToDate. Available at: https://www.uptodate.com/contents/eustachian-tube-dysfunction. Accessed February 1, 2022.

11. Schilder A, Bhutta M, Butler C, et al. Eustachian tube dysfunction: consensus statement on definition, types, clinical presentation and diagnosis. Clin Otolaryngol 2015;40(5):407–11.

12. Sudhoff HH, Mueller S. Treatment of pharyngotympanic tube dysfunction. Auris Nasus Larynx 2018;45(2):207–14.

13. Grimmer JF, Poe DS. Update on eustachian tube dysfunction and the patulous eustachian tube. Curr Opin Otolaryngol Head Neck Surg 2005;13(5):277–82.

14. Karkos PD, Assimakopoulos D, Issing WJ. Pediatric middle ear infections and gastroesophageal reflux. Int J Pediatr Otorhinolaryngol 2004;68(12):1489–92.

15. Ward BK, Ashry Y, Poe DS. patulous eustachian tube dysfunction: patient demographics and comorbidities. Otol Neurotol 2017;38(9):1362–9.

16. Utz ER, LaBanc AJ, Nelson MJ, et al. Balloon dilation of the eustachian tube for baro-challenge-induced otologic symptoms in military divers and aviators: a retrospective analysis. Ear Nose Throat J 2020. https://doi.org/10.1177/0145561320938156. 0145561320938156.

17. Doyle WJ, Cantekin EI, Bluestone CD. Eustachian tube function in cleft palate children. Ann Otol Rhinol Laryngol 1980;89(3_suppl):34–40.

18. Kraus F., Hagen R., Shehata-Dieler W., Middle-ear effusion in children with cleft palate: congenital or acquired?, J Laryngol Otol, 136 (2), 2022, 137–140.

19. Heidsieck DSP, Smarius BJA, Oomen KPQ, et al. The role of the tensor veli palatini muscle in the development of cleft palate-associated middle ear problems. Clin Oral Investig 2016;20:1389–401.

20. Smith TL, Diruggiero DC, Jones KR. Third place — resident clinical science award 1994: recovery of eustachian tube function and hearing outcome in patients with cleft palate. Otolaryngol Head Neck Surg 1994;111(4):423–9.

21. Ramia M, Musharrafieh U, Khaddage W, et al. Revisiting down syndrome from the ENT perspective: review of literature and recommendations. Eur Arch Otorhinolaryngol 2014;271(5):863–9.

22. Shibahara Y, Sando I. Congenital anomalies of the eustachian tube in Down syndrome. Histopathologic case report. Ann Otol Rhinol Laryngol 1989;98(7 Pt 1): 543–7.
23. Brown PM, Lewis GT, Parker AJ, et al. The skull base and nasopharynx in Down's syndrome in relation to hearing impairment. Clin Otolaryngol Allied Sci 1989; 14(3):241–6.
24. Ghadersohi S, Ida JB, Bhushan B, et al. Outcomes of tympanoplasty in children with down syndrome. Int J Pediatr Otorhinolaryngol 2017;103:36–40.
25. Funamura JL, Said M, Lin SJ, et al. Eustachian tube dysfunction in children with cleft palate: a tympanometric time-to-event analysis. Laryngoscope 2020;130(4): 1044–50.
26. Alper CM, Teixeira MS, Richert BC, et al. Presentation and eustachian tube function test results in children evaluated at a specialty clinic. Laryngoscope 2019; 129(5):1218–28.
27. Manno A, Iannella G, Savastano V, et al. Eustachian tube dysfunction in children with adenoid hypertrophy: the role of adenoidectomy for improving ear ventilation. Ear Nose Throat J 2021. https://doi.org/10.1177/0145561321989455. 145561321989455.
28. Leo G, Piacentini E, Incorvaia C, et al. Sinusitis and Eustachian tube dysfunction in children. Pediatr Allergy Immunol 2007;18(s18):35–9.
29. Patel MA, Mener DJ, Garcia-Esquinas E, et al. Tobacco smoke exposure and eustachian tube disorders in us children and adolescents. PLoS One 2016;11(10): e0163926.
30. Harmes K, Blackwood RA, Burrows H, et al. Otitis media: diagnosis and treatment. AFP 2013;88(7):435–40.
31. Fireman P. Otitis media and eustachian tube dysfunction: Connection to allergic rhinitis. J Allergy Clin Immunol 1997;99(2):s787–97.
32. Schilder AGM, Chonmaitree T, Cripps AW, et al. Otitis media. Nat Rev Dis Primers 2016;2(1):16063.
33. Holt JJ. Cholesteatoma and Otosclerosis: Two slowly progressive causes of hearing loss treatable through corrective surgery. Clin Med Res 2003;1(2):151–4.
34. Kuo CL. Etiopathogenesis of acquired cholesteatoma: prominent theories and recent advances in biomolecular research. Laryngoscope 2015;125(1):234–40.
35. Cholesteatoma. Otolaryngology — Head & Neck Surgery. Available at: https:// med.stanford.edu/ohns/OHNS-healthcare/earinstitute/conditions-and-services/ conditions/cholesteatoma.html. Accessed March 19, 2022.
36. Bayoumy AB, Veugen CCAFM, Rijssen LB, et al. The natural course of tympanic membrane retractions in the posterosuperior quadrant of pars tensa: a watchful waiting policy. Otology & Neurotology. 2021;42(1):e50.
37. Ruah CB, Schachern PA, Paparella MM, et al. Mechanisms of Retraction Pocket Formation in the Pediatric Tympanic Membrane. Arch Otolaryngology–Head Neck Surg 1992;118(12):1298–305. https://doi.org/10.1001/archotol.1992. 01880120024005.
38. Redaelli de Zinis LO, Nassif N, Zanetti D. Long-term results and prognostic factors of underlay myringoplasty in pars tensa atelectasis in children. JAMA Otolaryngology–Head Neck Surg 2015;141(1):34–9.
39. Ohta S, Sakagami M, Suzuki M, et al. Eustachian tube function and habitual sniffing in middle ear cholesteatoma. Otology & Neurotology. 2009;30(1):48–53.
40. Sooriyamoorthy T, De Jesus O. Conductive Hearing Loss. In: StatPearls. StatPearls Publishing; 2022. Available at: http://www.ncbi.nlm.nih.gov/books/ NBK563267/. Accessed February 6, 2022.

41. Nieto H, Dearden J, Dale S, et al. Paediatric hearing loss. BMJ 2017;356:j803.
42. Hu A, Shaffer AD, Jabbour N. eustachian tube dysfunction in children with unilateral cleft lip and palate: differences between ipsilateral and contralateral ears. Cleft Palate Craniofac J 2020;57(6):723–8.
43. Goldman JL, Martinez SA, Ganzel TM. Eustachian tube dysfunction and its sequelae in patients with cleft palate. South Med J 1993;86(11):1236–7.
44. Tucci DL, McCoul ED, Rosenfeld RM, et al. Clinical consensus statement: balloon dilation of the eustachian tube. Otolaryngol Head Neck Surg 2019;161(1):6–17.
45. Smith ME, Bance M, Tysome JR. Eustachian tube function in patients with symptoms on baro-challenge. Audiol Neurootol 2020;25(5):249–57.
46. Parsel SM, Unis GD, Souza SS, et al. Interpretation of normal and abnormal tympanogram findings in eustachian tube dysfunction. Otolaryngol Head Neck Surg 2021;164(6):1272–9.
47. Mitchell S, Mitchell S. Middle ear pressure changes over time in children with down syndrome. doi:10.23937/2572-4193.1510043
48. Teixeira MS, Swarts JD, Alper CM. Accuracy of the ETDQ-7 Questionnaire for Identifying Persons with Eustachian Tube Dysfunction. Otolaryngol Head Neck Surg 2018;158(1):83–9.
49. Schröder S, Lehmann M, Sauzet O, et al. A novel diagnostic tool for chronic obstructive eustachian tube dysfunction—the eustachian tube score. Laryngoscope 2015;125(3):703–8.
50. Magliulo G, de Vincentiis M, Iannella G, et al. Eustachian tube evaluation in patients with obstructive sleep apnea syndrome. Acta Oto-Laryngologica. 2018; 138(2):159–64.
51. Smith ME, Takwoingi Y, Deeks J, et al. Eustachian tube dysfunction: a diagnostic accuracy study and proposed diagnostic pathway. PLoS One 2018;13(11): e0206946.
52. Smith Me, Tysome Jr. Tests of Eustachian tube function: a review. Clin Otolaryngol 2015;40(4):300–11.
53. Smith ME, Scoffings DJ, Tysome JR. Imaging of the Eustachian tube and its function: a systematic review. Neuroradiology 2016;58(6):543–56.
54. Kikuchi T, Oshima T, Ogura M, et al. Three-dimensional computed tomography imaging in the sitting position for the diagnosis of patulous eustachian tube. Otol Neurotol 2007;28(2):199–203.
55. Tarabichi M, Najmi M. Visualization of the eustachian tube lumen with Valsalva computed tomography. Laryngoscope 2015;125(3):724–9.
56. Angeletti D, Pace A, Iannella G, et al. Chronic obstructive Eustachian tube dysfunction: CT assessment with Valsalva maneuver and ETS-7 score. PLoS One 2021;16(3):e0247708.
57. Lee S, Oh SJ, Choi SW, et al. The usefulness of Valsalva computed tomography as an assessment tool for the Eustachian tube. Am J Otolaryngol 2020;41(4): 102499.
58. Spaw M, Camacho M. Tympanostomy Tube. In: StatPearls. StatPearls Publishing; 2022. Available at: http://www.ncbi.nlm.nih.gov/books/NBK565858/. Accessed March 20, 2022.
59. Poe DS. Diagnosis and management of the patulous eustachian tube. Otology & Neurotology 2007;28(5):668–77.
60. Yañez C, Pirrón JA, Mora N. Curvature inversion technique: a novel tuboplastic technique for patulous eustachian tube—a preliminary report. Otolaryngol Head Neck Surg 2011;145(3):446–51.

61. Teschner M. Evidence and evidence gaps in the treatment of Eustachian tube dysfunction and otitis media. GMS Curr Top Otorhinolaryngol Head Neck Surg 2016;15:Doc05.
62. Koltsidopoulos P, Skoulakis C. Current treatment options for patulous eustachian tube: a review of the literature. Ear Nose Throat J 2020. https://doi.org/10.1177/0145561320932807. 0145561320932807.
63. Sato T, Kawase T, Yano H, et al. Trans-tympanic silicone plug insertion for chronic patulous Eustachian tube. Acta Oto-Laryngologica. 2005;125(11):1158–63.
64. Adil E, Poe D. What is the full range of medical and surgical treatments available for patients with Eustachian tube dysfunction? Curr Opin Otolaryngol Head Neck Surg 2014;22(1):8–15.
65. Vaezeafshar R, Turner JH, Li G, et al. Endoscopic hydroxyapatite augmentation for patulous Eustachian tube. Laryngoscope 2014;124(1):62–6.
66. Doherty JK, Slattery WH. Autologous fat grafting for the refractory patulous eustachian tube. Otolaryngol Head Neck Surg 2003;128(1):88–91.
67. Ward BK, Chao WC, Abiola G, et al. Twelve-month outcomes of Eustachian tube procedures for management of patulous Eustachian tube dysfunction. Laryngoscope 2019;129(1):222–8.
68. Huisman JML, Verdam FJ, Stegeman I, et al. Treatment of Eustachian tube dysfunction with balloon dilation: A systematic review. Laryngoscope 2018; 128(1):237–47.
69. Plaza G, Navarro JJ, Alfaro J, et al. Consensus on treatment of obstructive Eustachian tube dysfunction with balloon Eustachian tuboplasty. Acta Otorrinolaringol Esp (Engl Ed 2020;71(3):181–9.
70. Meyer TA, O'Malley EM, Schlosser RJ, et al. A randomized controlled trial of balloon dilation as a treatment for persistent eustachian tube dysfunction with 1-year follow-up. Otol Neurotol 2018;39(7):894–902.
71. Poe D, Anand V, Dean M, et al. Balloon dilation of the eustachian tube for dilatory dysfunction: a randomized controlled trial. Laryngoscope 2018;128(5):1200–6.
72. Anand V, Poe D, Dean M, et al. Balloon dilation of the eustachian Tube: 12-month follow-up of the randomized controlled trial treatment group. Otolaryngol Head Neck Surg 2019;160(4):687–94.
73. Toivonen J, Kawai K, Gurberg J, et al. Balloon dilation for obstructive eustachian tube dysfunction in children. Otol Neurotol 2021;42(4):566–72.
74. Saniasiaya J, Kulasegarah J, Narayanan P. Outcome of eustachian tube balloon dilation in children: a systematic review. Ann Otol Rhinol Laryngol 2021. https://doi.org/10.1177/00034894211041340. 00034894211041340.
75. Aboueisha MA, Attia AS, McCoul ED, et al. Efficacy and safety of balloon dilation of eustachian tube in children: Systematic review and meta-analysis. Int J Pediatr Otorhinolaryngol 2022;154:111048.
76. Leichtle A, Hollfelder D, Wollenberg B, et al. Balloon Eustachian Tuboplasty in children. Eur Arch Otorhinolaryngol 2017;274(6):2411–9.
77. Noonan KY, Linthicum FH, Lopez IA, et al. a histopathologic comparison of eustachian tube anatomy in pediatric and adult temporal bones. Otol Neurotol 2019; 40(3):e233–9.
78. Wang TC, Lin CD, Shih TC, et al. Comparison of balloon dilation and laser eustachian tuboplasty in patients with eustachian tube dysfunction: a meta-analysis. Otolaryngol Head Neck Surg 2018;158(4):617–26.
79. Shapiro GG, Bierman CW, Furukawa CT, et al. Treatment of persistent eustachian tube dysfunction in children with aerosolized nasal dexamethasone phosphate versus placebo. Ann Allergy 1982;49(2):81–5.

80. Gluth MB, McDonald DR, Weaver AL, et al. Management of eustachian tube dysfunction with nasal steroid spray: a prospective, randomized, placebo-controlled trial. Arch Otolaryngology–Head Neck Surg 2011;137(5):449–55.

81. Jensen JH, Leth N, Bonding P. Topical application of decongestant in dysfunction of the Eustachian tube: a randomized, double-blind, placebo-controlled trial. Clin Otolaryngol Allied Sci 1990;15(3):197–201.

82. Crowson MG, Ryan MA, Ramprasad VH, et al. Intranasal fluticasone associated with delayed tympanostomy tube placement in children with eustachian tube dysfunction. Int J Pediatr Otorhinolaryngol 2017;94:121–6.

83. Simon F, Haggard M, Rosenfeld RM, et al. International consensus (ICON) on management of otitis media with effusion in children. Eur Ann Otorhinolaryngol Head Neck Dis 2018;135(1, Supplement):S33–9.

84. Mehta NK, Ma C, Nguyen SA, et al. medical management for eustachian tube dysfunction in adults: a systematic review and meta-analysis. Laryngoscope 2021. https://doi.org/10.1002/lary.29878.

85. Norman G, Llewellyn A, Harden M, et al. Systematic review of the limited evidence base for treatments of Eustachian tube dysfunction: a health technology assessment. Clin Otolaryngol 2014;39(1):6–21.

86. Llewellyn A, Norman G, Harden M, et al. Interventions for adult Eustachian tube dysfunction: a systematic review. Health Technol Assess 2014;18(46):1–180, v-vi.

87. Robes C, Tillett JS. Pharmacologic Therapy for Eustachian Tube Dysfunction. AFP 2013;87(12):883–8.

Pediatric Drug-Induced Sleep Endoscopy

Erin M. Kirkham, MD, MPH

KEYWORDS

- Sleep endoscopy • Obstructive sleep apnea • Tonsillectomy • DISE • Pediatric

KEY POINTS

- Experts agree that drug-induced sleep endoscopy (DISE) is indicated for cases of persistent obstructive sleep apnea after adenotonsillectomy (AT).
- DISE has the potential to benefit surgically naive patients who have risk factors for AT failure by facilitating a patient-centered treatment plan.
- Research on the predictive value of DISE for surgical outcomes in children would be facilitated by consensus on scoring system and anesthetic protocol.

INTRODUCTION

Obstructive sleep apnea (OSA) is characterized by repetitive upper airway collapse that restricts airflow and leads to sleep disruption, gas exchange abnormalities, and derangements in multiple organ systems. Children with OSA frequently exhibit snoring, agitated sleep, nighttime wakefulness, excessive daytime sleepiness, hyperactivity, and inattention. OSA occurs in 1% to 4% of children and if left untreated can negatively affect behavior, cognition, health, and quality of life.[1–11] The sequelae of untreated pediatric OSA results in a 226% increase in health-care utilization.[12,13] Of particular public health concern, OSA disproportionately affects already vulnerable health populations, including obese children and those of Black race and disadvantaged communities.[14–16]

Overnight monitored polysomnography is the gold standard diagnostic test for OSA but does not yield specific information about the underlying cause of upper airway obstruction. The most common cause of OSA in children is adenotonsillar hypertrophy and current guidelines recommend AT as first-line treatment in children.[17,18] Because awareness of pediatric OSA has increased, the frequency of AT has increased, and it is now the second-most common procedure performed in US children.[17,19–21] Although AT is curative in many cases, pooled data from a meta-analysis demonstrated that 34% of healthy, normal-weight children have moderate-to-severe persistent OSA after

Department of Otolaryngology - Head & Neck Surgery, The University of Michigan, 1540 East Hospital Dr CW 5-702, SPC 4241, Ann Arbor, MI 48109, USA
E-mail address: ekirkham@umich.edu

Otolaryngol Clin N Am 55 (2022) 1165–1180
https://doi.org/10.1016/j.otc.2022.07.004
0030-6665/22/© 2022 Elsevier Inc. All rights reserved.

oto.theclinics.com

AT.[22] In children with specific comorbidities, that number increases to 62%.[22] Comorbidities such as obesity, muscle tone abnormalities, and craniofacial anomalies can play a significant role in OSA in some children.[23] Other risk factors for persistent post-AT OSA include older age,[24,25] Black race,[26,27] obesity,[24,26,28–32] severe baseline OSA,[24,32,33] and major medical comorbidities (eg, Down syndrome, craniofacial disorders, and neuromuscular conditions).[34–37] Guidelines recommend treating persistent OSA with continuous positive airway pressure (CPAP) but CPAP adherence rates in children can be as low as 33%, leading to referral back to the otolaryngologist for additional surgical options.[38–40]

Persistent post-AT OSA is frequently due to residual, untreated upper airway obstruction that can be identified by drug-induced sleep endoscopy (DISE).[41–43] DISE is a fiber-optic assessment of the upper airway under sedation that identifies dynamic obstruction not seen on awake endoscopy or clinical examination.[44] First described by Croft and Pringle in 1991, DISE has been used in adults with OSA to guide surgical treatment for more than 2 decades.[44–46] Clinically significant obstruction can occur in children at sites of the airway aside from the tonsils and adenoids.[41–43] As such, DISE has become a useful tool to identify patterns and sites of obstruction that contribute to OSA in children in order to develop a patient-specific treatment plan.

Overall, DISE is a safe procedure, with no reports of severe morbidity or mortality to date. Complications of DISE can include epistaxis and rarely laryngospasm and desaturation.[47,48] Even children with medical comorbidities can safely be discharged after DISE when performed without additional procedures. Other modalities for assessment of sites of upper airway obstructive have been described, which include pharyngeal pressure catheters,[49] sleep fluoroscopy,[50–52] cine computed tomography,[53] plain film X-rays,[54] and both standard and cine MRI.[55–58] No method has been as widely adopted in practice as DISE, likely due to the ease of use, safety profile, and the direct visual information provided. DISE offers an advantage over other modalities in that it uses simple equipment readily available and familiar to the otolaryngologist. In addition, surgical intervention can be performed under the same anesthetic based on the information gathered. This approach serves to minimize anesthetic exposure and is often preferred by families for ease of scheduling. DISE has grown in popularity among providers and has become common practice among pediatric otolaryngologists within the past 5 years. However, there is substantial variation in practice with regard to indications, sedation protocol, scoring, and the utility of DISE in the improvement of postsurgical outcomes.[59,60]

DISCUSSION
Indications

Experts agree that DISE is indicated for cases of persistent OSA after adenotonsillectomy (AT).[60] This consensus is supported by multiple retrospective series of DISE-assisted surgery for persistent post-AT OSA, which consistently demonstrate that DISE can diagnose sites of residual obstruction and facilitate surgical treatment that significantly reduces OSA burden.[61–72] Some surgeons suggest that DISE can also be used to spare surgically naïve patients from interventions that may not help them and/or direct surgery only at levels that seem problematic.[68,73] Indeed, DISE has proven to be a useful tool to identify obstruction at sites other than the tonsils and adenoids.[74,75] However, the literature is mixed as to whether this information changes initial management in surgically naïve patients to a significant degree. In otherwise healthy, surgically naïve patients, DISE changes the surgical decision-making in

25% to 35% of cases, so the majority still undergoes tonsillectomy with or without adenoidectomy.[68,76,77] Thus many argue that DISE before AT in children without risk factors for persistence is not efficient or cost effective due to the high frequency of adenotonsillar obstruction in this population.[68,78]

It stands to reason that DISE has a greater potential to benefit surgically naive patients who have risk factors for AT failure. Studies of DISE before AT in children at risk for AT failure have demonstrated: 1) the majority has a significant degree of collapse outside the adenotonsillar region and 2) AT alone results in at best modest improvement in OSA.[64,79,80] In a retrospective analysis of DISE-assisted surgery in 62 surgically naïve children with OSA who had risk factors for OSA persistence, 58% underwent treatment other than AT. OSA improved significantly after DISE-directed surgery from 22 to 7 obstructive events per hour. It is notable that children who underwent AT alone experienced less improvement overall than those who underwent non-AT intervention, likely due to residual obstruction left untreated. This suggests that obstruction at non-AT levels of the airway that is left untreated by AT may predict worse post-AT outcomes. This has been the case in adults with OSA, in which significant tongue base obstruction on preoperative DISE predicts upper pharyngeal surgery failure.[81] However the degree, pattern and sites of obstruction that may predict AT failure in children remains an open question.

In a recent consensus statement on pediatric DISE, experts agreed that DISE is useful in surgically naïve children without tonsillar hypertrophy, although there was no consensus as to what constitutes "small tonsils."[60] In general, tonsil size correlates with the degree of obstruction seen on DISE at the lateral pharyngeal walls.[68,82] Miller and colleagues found that children with OSA who have grade 1+ or 2+ tonsils exhibit greater obstruction at other levels of the airway, particularly the tongue base.[82] Williamson and colleagues found a similar pattern in a series limited to children with 1+ tonsils.[73] In a prospective cohort study of surgically naïve children at risk for persistent post-AT OSA, Lam and colleagues showed that assessment of tonsillar collapse during DISE better predicts the outcome of AT alone than awake clinical examination.[83] In a series of DISE-directed surgery in children with small tonsils, subjects improved on average from severe-to-moderate OSA.[65] In a retrospective study that used DISE to determine need for tonsillectomy in children with small tonsils, Chen and colleagues found that 78% of children with grade 2 tonsils and 19% with grade 1 tonsils had tonsillar obstruction on DISE that was not immediately apparent on awake examination.[84] Children in the DISE-directed surgery group experienced significant improvements in OSA compared with a control group of children with small tonsils whose parents declined DISE and opted for adenoidectomy alone. Considered together, the evidence suggests that for children with OSA without tonsillar hypertrophy, the potential benefits of DISE may outweigh the risks.

Use of DISE in children has expanded to surgically naive patients at high risk for persistent OSA due not only to small tonsils but also to severe baseline disease (apnea-hypopnea index [AHI] >10 events per hour), obesity, Down syndrome, craniofacial anomalies, and/or neuromuscular disorders.[60,61,69,85–87] DISE also has a role for infants with OSA to diagnose sleep-state laryngomalacia and has been used more recently in older children with Down syndrome to determine candidacy for hypoglossal nerve stimulation.[43,61,76,77,88–90] DISE is not recommended for children without PSG-confirmed OSA, an AHI less than 2 events/h, or in surgically naïve children with OSA who do not have risk factors for post-AT persistence.[59,60]

Scoring

Pediatric DISE findings have been reported via 7 separate scoring systems (**Table 1**).[91–93] Of these, 5 were developed in the pediatric population.[68,92,94–96] The

Table 1
Comparison of scoring scales for pediatric drug-induced sleep endoscopy

	Nasal Cavity	Nasopharynx/ Adenoid	Palate/ Velum	Lateral Pharynx/ Oropharynx/ Tonsils	Tongue Base	Hypopharynx	Epiglottis/ Supraglottis/ Larynx
Bachar[91]	1–2	–	1–2	–	1–2	1–2	1–2
Boudewyns[68]	–	0–3	0–1	0–3	0–2	–	0–1
Chan-Parikh[95]	–	0–3	0–3	0–3	0–3	–	0–3
Carr[96]	0–2	0–2	0–2	0–2	0–2[b]	–	0–2[†]
Fishman[92]	0–3	0–3	–	0–3	0–3	–	0–3
SERS[94]	0–2	0–2	0–2	0–2	–	0–2	–
VOTE[a,93]	–	–	0–2	0–2	0–2	–	0–2

VOTE, velum, oropharynx, tongue base, and epiglottis; SERS, sleep endoscopy rating scale.
[a] Includes qualitative description of pattern of collapse at each level.
[b] Tongue base and lingual tonsils are scored independently.
[†] Epiglottis, aryepiglottic folds and arytenoids are each scored independently.

scoring systems differ in the levels of the airway included and the scoring scale applied at each level. In addition, some incorporate qualitative assessment of the pattern of collapse, whereas others rely on a numerical grade alone. Of the 6 scoring systems, the VOTE is the most widely published but it does not include assessment of the nasopharynx (adenoids) or larynx, which are common sites of obstruction in pediatric OSA.[97]

An ideal scoring system would allow the surgeon to systematically document pertinent information on surgically actionable levels of the airway, have high interrater and intrarater reliabilities, good test–retest reliability, and predictive value for postsurgical outcome. No scoring system has been thoroughly validated in the pediatric population to date. Fishman and colleagues reported that sleep endoscopy scores did not reliably predict OSA severity, although it was more reliable than awake endoscopy. They found moderate–good interrater reliability at most levels of the airway assessed.[92] Dahl and colleagues showed that the Chan-Parikh total score had a significant correlation with obstructive AHI and saturation nadir.[98] Lam and colleagues found that their Sleep Endoscopy Rating Scale (SERS) total score correlated significantly with obstructive AHI and that a SERS total score greater than 6 had a sensitivity of 82%, specificity of 88%, and correctly classified 84% of patients. Intrarater and interrater reliabilities were substantial-to-excellent and fair-to-substantial, respectively.[94] Somewhat contrary to these original reports, Tejan and colleagues applied 6 pediatric DISE scoring systems to the same group of patients and did not find significant correlations between any of the total scores and pre-DISE polysomnography parameters.[99] It remains unclear whether a holistic total score is useful to the surgeon, or whether complete obstruction at a given level or levels is most predictive of postsurgical outcome. The evolving field of pediatric sleep surgery would benefit from consensus on a single universally adopted pediatric DISE scoring system, which would facilitate prospective data collection and comparison across studies. Until that time, regardless of the scoring system they choose, surgeons should document the pattern and severity of obstruction of the nasal cavities, nasopharynx, soft palate/velum, pharyngeal airway (including lateral oropharyngeal wall), tongue base, and supraglottic larynx.[60] Subglottic assessment is low yield and unnecessary in patients without risk factors for tracheal pathologic condition.[100]

ANESTHETIC PROTOCOL

DISE requires a balanced state in which patients are sedated to the point that they do not react to the intranasal scope yet are not so deeply anesthetized that they cannot maintain spontaneous breathing for long enough to capture upper airway dynamics. Although no anesthetic can replicate sleep, the ideal drug is safe, efficient, and can be reliably titrated to a state that mimics sleep. Anesthetic drugs have variable impact on airway muscle tone, reflexes, and respiratory drive (**Table 2**). Thus, the anesthetic protocol may affect DISE findings and their predictive value but this has not been rigorously tested. The most common agents used for pediatric DISE are intravenous (IV) propofol and IV dexmedetomidine (DEX), with no consensus on drug choice.[60] Propofol is a gamma-aminobutyric acid ($GABA_A$) receptor complex agonist/N-methyl-D-aspartate receptor (NMDA) receptor antagonist that suppresses sleep-like electroenchelalography (EEG) activity.[101] DEX is a selective alpha-2 adrenergic receptor agonist that produces sedation with some EEG characteristics that overlap those of natural sleep.[101–103] In a recent international Delphi consensus statement on the diagnosis and management of pediatric OSA, 58% of pediatric otolaryngologists reported that they used propofol for DISE while 50% reported they used DEX.[104] The overlapping

Table 2
Anesthetic drugs, upper airway impact, and role in pediatric drug-induced sleep endoscopy

Drug	Role in Pediatric DISE and Rationale	Upper Airway (UA) Impact
Sevoflurane	Inhaled induction → painless IV placement Typically avoided as a sole agent for DISE Con: Unpredictable pharmacokinetics Con: Open airway exposes staff to exhaled gas	↓ UA muscle activity, ↑ UA collapse[121–124] ↓ UA cross-sectional area with ↑ dose[125]
Propofol	Continuous IV anesthetic Pro: Rapid pharmacokinetics[105–107] and titration Con: Suppresses sleep-like EEG activity[101] Con: May exaggerate UA obstruction relative to sleep	↓ UA cross-sectional area with ↑ dose[114–116,126]
Dexmedetomidine	Continuous IV anesthetic Pro: Some EEG features of natural sleep[102,127] and titration Con: Slower pharmacokinetics[113] and titration Con: May improve UA obstruction relative to sleep	Minimal effect on UA cross-sectional area[118,128] Preserved UA reflexes[129]/respiratory drive[112]
Ketamine	IV bolus given in combination with IV infusion Pro: Rapid pharmacokinetics Pro: Deepens anesthesia without obstruction/apnea Con: May improve UA obstruction relative to sleep	Minimal effect on respiratory drive[130] ↑ UA dilator (genioglossus) activity
Opioids	Avoided ↑ risk of obstruction and apnea[127,131]	↓ UA reflexes[132] ↓ respiratory drive[127,131]
Benzodiazepines	Avoided ↑ risk of obstruction[133]	↑ UA resistance[134] ↓ UA diameter[135]
Topical anesthetics	Avoided ↑ risk of obstruction[136]	↑ UA resistance[137,138] ↓ UA dilator activity[136]

percentages indicate that some surgeons use both routinely. Use of both drugs has been reported in pediatric DISE research with similar frequency.[65,66,68,69,71,76–78,82,94] Studies that have compared propofol versus DEX suggest that propofol provides more reliable sedation,[105–107] whereas DEX yields greater respiratory stability (see **Table 2**).[108–116] Both drugs are equally safe for use in the pediatric operating room. Although propofol yields lower blood pressure and DEX a lower heart rate, these hemodynamic differences are of questionable clinical significance.[108,117–120] Although the airway must be carefully managed during the procedure with pauses to maintain patency with an oral airway device, jaw-thrust maneuver, or bag-masking as needed for brief desaturations, no study to date has reported any severe respiratory events with either drug.

Additional considerations unique to pediatric anesthesia merit comment. As standard of care, young children who present for airway evaluation undergo inhaled mask induction with a volatile agent to facilitate painless, atraumatic IV placement. The inhalant is quickly discontinued, and an IV anesthetic is initiated and titrated to maintain anesthesia with spontaneous respiration. A minority of surgeons perform DISE under inhaled anesthetic alone.[104] This is not ideal for multiple reasons. First, inhaled anesthetics have unpredictable pharmacokinetics and are more difficult to titrate to a sleep-like state for DISE than IV agents. This can increase the risk of apnea and airway obstruction.[121–124] Second, operating room staff are exposed to the volatile gas because it is exhaled from the patient's open airway during endoscopy, which is an occupational safety concern. Additional drugs such as benzodiazepines (anxiolytics), opioids (systemic analgesics), and lidocaine (topical analgesic) that are commonly given during pediatric anesthesia are generally avoided during DISE because they are not strictly necessary and may affect the upper airway (see **Table 1**). Ketamine is a dissociative IV anesthetic with minimal effect on respiratory drive that is commonly used for DISE in addition to the IV infusion. Ketamine has a rapid onset and can quickly deepen the plane of anesthesia to avoid reaction to scope insertion without precipitating apnea. Although it may be an efficient way to achieve sedation, ketamine increases the activity of upper airway dilators and may prevent observation of the obstruction that occurs during sleep, although this has not been rigorously tested.[130,139]

Direct comparisons of DEX and propofol for use in adult DISE suggest a higher frequency of respiratory depression, oxygen desaturation, and tongue base obstruction with propofol than DEX.[109–111,140,141] However, these results do not necessarily extrapolate to children due to anatomic and physiologic differences between adult and pediatric airways. A retrospective review in children did not find a statistically significant difference in the odds of 50% or greater obstruction at the tongue base between DEX and propofol with or without adjustment for potential confounders.[142] This study was limited by the lack of standardization of anesthetic protocol, DISE technique, and a heterogenous patient population with respect to age, comorbidities, and previous AT. The high potential for confounding and bias limits the conclusions that can be drawn from this retrospective study and highlights the need for a prospective comparison of DISE anesthetics in children.

SUMMARY

The current standard-of-care AT fails to resolve OSA in 25% to 75% of children and follow-up after AT varies widely.[24,26,28,32] Many children are never assessed for persistent disease and carry the burden of undertreated OSA as they grow, with unknown (but almost certainly negative) consequences to their health, psychosocial development, school performance, and future success. If clinically significant obstruction can be detected and treated either before or after AT, children may have greater rates of resolution of OSA and its symptoms, leading to reduced burden on the healthcare system and society. DISE has emerged as an important tool that can inform an efficient, patient-centered treatment plan. DISE-assisted surgery has become necessary in cases of post-AT OSA and may in fact be a better alternative to standard-of-care AT, especially in high-risk groups. However, many questions regarding timing of DISE, patient selection, ideal scoring method, and threshold for operative intervention remain unanswered because no controlled studies of DISE-assisted surgery in children have been conducted. Fundamental questions cannot be answered without consensus on optimal anesthetic protocol and scoring system. This will facilitate standardization and rigorous assessment of the predictive value of presurgical DISE findings on postsurgical outcomes.

CLINICS CARE POINTS

- Surgeons should consider drug-induced sleep endoscopy (DISE)-directed surgery in children with persistent, postadenotonsillectomy obstructive sleep apnea who refuse or fail positive pressure therapy.

- Surgeons may consider DISE in surgically naïve children with risk factors for postadenotonsillectomy sleep apnea, which include small tonsils, severe baseline disease (apnea-hypopnea index >10 events per hour), obesity, Down syndrome, craniofacial anomalies, and/or neuromuscular disorders.

- Intravenous dexmedetomidine or propofol (both with and without ketamine) are both valid choices for DISE.

- Regardless of the scoring system they choose, surgeons should document the pattern, and severity of obstruction of the nasal cavities, nasopharynx, soft palate/velum, pharyngeal airway (including lateral oropharyngeal wall), tongue base, and supraglottic larynx.

DISCLOSURE

E.M. Kirkham, MD, MPH is an author for UpToDate and is supported by the National Heart Lung and Blood Institute of the National Institutes of Health (K23HL153897).

REFERENCES

1. Chervin RD, Ruzicka DL, Giordani BJ, et al. Sleep-disordered breathing, behavior, and cognition in children before and after adenotonsillectomy. Pediatrics 2006;117(4):e769–78.
2. Mulvaney SA, Goodwin JL, Morgan WJ, et al. Behavior problems associated with sleep disordered breathing in school-aged children–the Tucson children's assessment of sleep apnea study. J Pediatr Psychol 2006;31(3):322–30.
3. Mitchell RB, Kelly J. Quality of life after adenotonsillectomy for SDB in children. Otolaryngol Head Neck Surg 2005;133(4):569–72.
4. Mitchell RB, Kelly J. Behavior, neurocognition and quality-of-life in children with sleep-disordered breathing. Int J Pediatr Otorhinolaryngol 2006;70(3):395–406.
5. Garetz SL, Mitchell RB, Parker PD, et al. Quality of life and obstructive sleep apnea symptoms after pediatric adenotonsillectomy. Pediatrics 2015;135(2):e477–86.

6. Baldassari CM, Mitchell RB, Schubert C, et al. Pediatric obstructive sleep apnea and quality of life: a meta-analysis. Otolaryngol Head Neck Surg 2008;138(3): 265–73.

7. Bixler EO, Vgontzas AN, Lin HM, et al. Blood pressure associated with sleep-disordered breathing in a population sample of children. Hypertension 2008; 52(5):841–6.

8. Galland BC, Tripp EG, Gray A, et al. Apnea-hypopnea indices and snoring in children diagnosed with ADHD: a matched case-control study. Sleep & breathing = Schlaf & Atmung 2011;15(3):455–62.

9. O'Brien LM, Holbrook CR, Mervis CB, et al. Sleep and neurobehavioral characteristics of 5- to 7-year-old children with parentally reported symptoms of attention-deficit/hyperactivity disorder. Pediatrics 2003;111(3):554–63.

10. O'Brien LM, Gozal D. Autonomic dysfunction in children with sleep-disordered breathing. Sleep 2005;28(6):747–52.

11. Teo DT, Mitchell RB. Systematic review of effects of adenotonsillectomy on cardiovascular parameters in children with obstructive sleep apnea. Otolaryngol Head Neck Surg 2013;148(1):21–8.

12. Reuveni H, Simon T, Tal A, et al. Health care services utilization in children with obstructive sleep apnea syndrome. Pediatrics 2002;110(1 Pt 1):68–72.

13. Tarasiuk A, Greenberg-Dotan S, Simon-Tuval T, et al. Elevated morbidity and health care use in children with obstructive sleep apnea syndrome. Am J Respir Crit Care Med 2007;175(1):55–61.

14. Chervin RD, Clarke DF, Huffman JL, et al. School performance, race, and other correlates of sleep-disordered breathing in children. Sleep Med 2003;4(1):21–7.

15. Redline S, Tishler PV, Schluchter M, et al. Risk factors for sleep-disordered breathing in children. Associations with obesity, race, and respiratory problems. Am J Respir Crit Care Med 1999;159(5 Pt 1):1527–32.

16. Wang R, Dong Y, Weng J, et al. Associations among Neighborhood, Race, and Sleep Apnea Severity in Children. A Six-City Analysis. Ann Am Thorac Soc 2017; 14(1):76–84.

17. Baugh RF, Archer SM, Mitchell RB, et al. Clinical practice guideline: tonsillectomy in children. Otolaryngol Head Neck Surg 2011;144(1 Suppl):S1–30.

18. Marcus CL, Brooks LJ, Draper KA, et al. Diagnosis and management of childhood obstructive sleep apnea syndrome. Pediatrics 2012;130(3):576–84.

19. Boss EF, Marsteller JA, Simon AE. Outpatient tonsillectomy in children: demographic and geographic variation in the United States, 2006. J Pediatr 2012; 160(5):814–9.

20. Bhattacharyya N, Lin HW. Changes and consistencies in the epidemiology of pediatric adenotonsillar surgery, 1996-2006. Otolaryngol Head Neck Surg 2010;143(5):680–4.

21. Erickson BK, Larson DR, St Sauver JL, et al. Changes in incidence and indications of tonsillectomy and adenotonsillectomy, 1970-2005. Otolaryngol Head Neck Surg 2009;140(6):894–901.

22. Friedman M, Wilson M, Lin HC, et al. Updated systematic review of tonsillectomy and adenoidectomy for treatment of pediatric obstructive sleep apnea/hypopnea syndrome. Otolaryngol Head Neck Surg 2009;140(6):800–8.

23. Katz E. Pathophysiology of pediatric obstructive sleep apnea: putting it all together. In: Kheirandish-Gozal L, Gozal D, editors. Sleep disordered breathing in children. New York (NY): Springer Science; 2012. p. 153–9.

24. Bhattacharjee R, Kheirandish-Gozal L, Spruyt K, et al. Adenotonsillectomy outcomes in treatment of obstructive sleep apnea in children: a multicenter retrospective study. Am J Respir Crit Care Med 2010;182(5):676–83.

25. Imanguli M, Ulualp SO. Risk factors for residual obstructive sleep apnea after adenotonsillectomy in children. Laryngoscope 2016;126(11):2624–9.

26. Marcus CL, Moore RH, Rosen CL, et al. A randomized trial of adenotonsillectomy for childhood sleep apnea. N Engl J Med 2013;368(25):2366–76.

27. Amin R, Anthony L, Somers V, et al. Growth velocity predicts recurrence of sleep-disordered breathing 1 year after adenotonsillectomy. Am J Respir Crit Care Med 2008;177(6):654–9.

28. Mitchell RB, Kelly J. Outcome of adenotonsillectomy for obstructive sleep apnea in obese and normal-weight children. Otolaryngol Head Neck Surg 2007; 137(1):43–8.

29. Costa DJ, Mitchell R. Adenotonsillectomy for obstructive sleep apnea in obese children: a meta-analysis. Otolaryngol Head Neck Surg 2009;140(4):455–60.

30. O'Brien LM, Sitha S, Baur LA, et al. Obesity increases the risk for persisting obstructive sleep apnea after treatment in children. Int J Pediatr Otorhinolaryngol 2006;70(9):1555–60.

31. Scheffler P, Wolter NE, Narang I, et al. Surgery for obstructive sleep apnea in obese children: literature review and meta-analysis. Otolaryngol Head Neck Surg 2019;160(6). 194599819829415.

32. Tauman R, Gulliver TE, Krishna J, et al. Persistence of obstructive sleep apnea syndrome in children after adenotonsillectomy. J Pediatr 2006;149(6):803–8.

33. Mitchell RB. Adenotonsillectomy for obstructive sleep apnea in children: outcome evaluated by pre- and postoperative polysomnography. Laryngoscope 2007;117(10):1844–54.

34. Thottam PJ, Choi S, Simons JP, et al. Effect of adenotonsillectomy on central and obstructive sleep apnea in children with down syndrome. Otolaryngol Head Neck Surg 2015;153(4):644–8.

35. Sudarsan SS, Paramasivan VK, Arumugam SV, et al. Comparison of treatment modalities in syndromic children with obstructive sleep apnea–a randomized cohort study. Int J Pediatr Otorhinolaryngol 2014;78(9):1526–33.

36. Lam DJ, Jensen CC, Mueller BA, et al. Pediatric sleep apnea and craniofacial anomalies: a population-based case-control study. Laryngoscope 2010; 120(10):2098–105.

37. Marcus CL, Keens TG, Bautista DB, et al. Obstructive sleep apnea in children with Down syndrome. Pediatrics 1991;88(1):132–9.

38. Marcus CL, Rosen G, Ward SL, et al. Adherence to and effectiveness of positive airway pressure therapy in children with obstructive sleep apnea. Pediatrics 2006;117(3):e442–51.

39. Nixon GM, Mihai R, Verginis N, et al. Patterns of continuous positive airway pressure adherence during the first 3 months of treatment in children. J Pediatr 2011; 159(5):802–7.

40. Machaalani R, Evans CA, Waters KA. Objective adherence to positive airway pressure therapy in an Australian paediatric cohort. Sleep Breath 2016;20(4): 1327–36.

41. Lin AC, Koltai PJ. Persistent pediatric obstructive sleep apnea and lingual tonsillectomy. Otolaryngol Head Neck Surg 2009;141(1):81–5.

42. Chan DK, Truong MT, Koltai PJ. Supraglottoplasty for occult laryngomalacia to improve obstructive sleep apnea syndrome. Arch Otolaryngol Head Neck Surg 2012;138(1):50–4.

43. Mase CA, Chen ML, Horn DL, et al. Supraglottoplasty for sleep endoscopy diagnosed sleep dependent laryngomalacia. Int J Pediatr Otorhinolaryngol 2015; 79(4):511–5.

44. Croft CB, Pringle M. Sleep nasendoscopy: a technique of assessment in snoring and obstructive sleep apnoea. Clin Otolaryngol Allied Sci 1991;16(5):504–9.

45. Charakorn N, Kezirian EJ. Drug-induced sleep endoscopy. Otolaryngol Clin North Am 2016;49(6):1359–72.

46. Atkins JH, Mandel JE. Drug-induced sleep endoscopy: from obscure technique to diagnostic tool for assessment of obstructive sleep apnea for surgical interventions. Curr Opin Anaesthesiol 2018;31(1):120–6.

47. Bergeron M, Lee DR, DeMarcantonio MA, et al. Safety and cost of drug-induced sleep endoscopy outside the operating room. Laryngoscope 2020;130(8): 2076–80.

48. Collu MA, Esteller E, Lipari F, et al. A case-control study of Drug-Induced Sleep Endoscopy (DISE) in pediatric population: a proposal for indications. Int J Pediatr Otorhinolaryngol 2018;108:113–9.

49. Dedhia RC, Seay EG, Schwartz AR. Beyond VOTE: The New Frontier of Drug-Induced Sleep Endoscopy. ORL 2022;84(4):296–301.

50. Gibson SE, Myer CM 3rd, Strife JL, et al. Sleep fluoroscopy for localization of upper airway obstruction in children. Ann Otol Rhinol Laryngol 1996;105(9): 678–83.

51. Felman AH, Loughlin GM, Leftridge CA Jr, et al. Upper airway obstruction during sleep in children. AJR Am J Roentgenol 1979;133(2):213–6.

52. Fernbach SK, Brouillette RT, Riggs TW, et al. Radiologic evaluation of adenoids and tonsils in children with obstructive sleep apnea: plain films and fluoroscopy. Pediatr Radiol 1983;13(5):258–65.

53. Haponik EF, Smith PL, Bohlman ME, et al. Computerized tomography in obstructive sleep apnea. correlation of airway size with physiology during sleep and wakefulness. Am Rev Respir Dis 1983;127(2):221–6.

54. Sedaghat AR, Flax-Goldenberg RB, Gayler BW, et al. A case-control comparison of lingual tonsillar size in children with and without Down syndrome. Laryngoscope 2012;122(5):1165–9.

55. Nandalike K, Shifteh K, Sin S, et al. Adenotonsillectomy in obese children with obstructive sleep apnea syndrome: magnetic resonance imaging findings and considerations. Sleep 2013;36(6):841–7.

56. Fricke BL, Donnelly LF, Shott SR, et al. Comparison of lingual tonsil size as depicted on MR imaging between children with obstructive sleep apnea despite previous tonsillectomy and adenoidectomy and normal controls. Pediatr Radiol 2006;36(6):518–23.

57. Donnelly LF, Shott SR, LaRose CR, et al. Causes of persistent obstructive sleep apnea despite previous tonsillectomy and adenoidectomy in children with down syndrome as depicted on static and dynamic cine MRI. AJR Am J Roentgenol 2004;183(1):175–81.

58. Shott SR, Donnelly LF. Cine magnetic resonance imaging: evaluation of persistent airway obstruction after tonsil and adenoidectomy in children with down syndrome. Laryngoscope 2004;114(10):1724–9.

59. Friedman NR, Parikh SR, Ishman SL, et al. The current state of pediatric drug-induced sleep endoscopy. Laryngoscope 2017;127(1):266–72.

60. Baldassari CM, Lam DJ, Ishman SL, et al. Expert consensus statement: pediatric drug-induced sleep endoscopy. Otolaryngol Head Neck Surg 2021;165(4). 5778–591.194599820985000.

61. Park JS, Chan DK, Parikh SR, et al. Surgical outcomes and sleep endoscopy for children with sleep-disordered breathing and hypotonia. Int J Pediatr Otorhinolaryngol 2016;90:99–106.
62. Lin AC, Koltai PJ. Sleep endoscopy in the evaluation of pediatric obstructive sleep apnea. Int J Pediatr 2012;2012:576719.
63. Coutras SW, Limjuco A, Davis KE, et al. Sleep endoscopy findings in children with persistent obstructive sleep apnea after adenotonsillectomy. Int J Pediatr Otorhinolaryngol 2018;107:190–3.
64. Truong MT, Woo VG, Koltai PJ. Sleep endoscopy as a diagnostic tool in pediatric obstructive sleep apnea. Int J Pediatr Otorhinolaryngol 2012;76(5):722–7.
65. Miller C, Kirkham E, Ma CC, et al. Polysomnography outcomes in children with small tonsils undergoing drug-induced sleep endoscopy-directed surgery. Laryngoscope 2018;129(12):2771–4.
66. He S, Peddireddy NS, Smith DF, et al. Outcomes of drug-induced sleep endoscopy-directed surgery for pediatric obstructive sleep apnea. Otolaryngol Head Neck Surg 2018;158(3):559–65.
67. Durr ML, Meyer AK, Kezirian EJ, et al. Drug-induced sleep endoscopy in persistent pediatric sleep-disordered breathing after adenotonsillectomy. Arch Otolaryngol Head Neck Surg 2012;138(7):638–43.
68. Boudewyns A, Verhulst S, Maris M, et al. Drug-induced sedation endoscopy in pediatric obstructive sleep apnea syndrome. Sleep Med 2014;15(12):1526–31.
69. Akkina SR, Ma CC, Kirkham EM, et al. Does drug induced sleep endoscopy-directed surgery improve polysomnography measures in children with Down Syndrome and obstructive sleep apnea? Acta Otolaryngol 2018;138(11):1009–13.
70. Esteller E, Villatoro JC, Aguero A, et al. Outcome of drug-induced sleep endoscopy-directed surgery for persistent obstructive sleep apnea after adenotonsillar surgery. Int J Pediatr Otorhinolaryngol 2019;120:118–22.
71. Wootten CT, Chinnadurai S, Goudy SL. Beyond adenotonsillectomy: outcomes of sleep endoscopy-directed treatments in pediatric obstructive sleep apnea. Int J Pediatr Otorhinolaryngol 2014;78(7):1158–62.
72. Socarras MA, Landau BP, Durr ML. Diagnostic techniques and surgical outcomes for persistent pediatric obstructive sleep apnea after adenotonsillectomy: A systematic review and meta-analysis. Int J Pediatr Otorhinolaryngol 2019;121:179–87.
73. Williamson A, Coutras SW, Carr MM. Sleep Endoscopy Findings in Children With Obstructive Sleep Apnea and Small Tonsils. Ann Otol Rhinol Laryngol 2021;131(8):851–8, 34894211045645.
74. Wilcox LJ, Bergeron M, Reghunathan S, et al. An updated review of pediatric drug-induced sleep endoscopy. Laryngoscope Investig Otolaryngol 2017;2(6):423–31.
75. Manickam PV, Shott SR, Boss EF, et al. Systematic review of site of obstruction identification and non-CPAP treatment options for children with persistent pediatric obstructive sleep apnea. Laryngoscope 2016;126(2):491–500.
76. Boudewyns A, Van de Heyning P, Verhulst S. Drug-induced sedation endoscopy in children <2 years with obstructive sleep apnea syndrome: upper airway findings and treatment outcomes. Eur Arch Otorhinolaryngol 2017;274(5):2319–25.
77. Boudewyns A, Saldien V, Van de Heyning P, et al. Drug-induced sedation endoscopy in surgically naive infants and children with obstructive sleep apnea: impact on treatment decision and outcome. Sleep Breath 2018;22(2):503–10.

78. Gazzaz MJ, Isaac A, Anderson S, et al. Does drug-induced sleep endoscopy change the surgical decision in surgically naive non-syndromic children with snoring/sleep disordered breathing from the standard adenotonsillectomy? A retrospective cohort study. J Otolaryngol Head Neck Surg 2017;46(1):12.

79. Maris M, Verhulst S, Saldien V, et al. Drug-induced sedation endoscopy in surgically naive children with Down syndrome and obstructive sleep apnea. Sleep Med 2016;24:63–70.

80. Raposo D, Menezes M, Rito J, et al. Drug-induced sleep endoscopy in pediatric obstructive sleep apnea. Otolaryngol Head Neck Surg 2021;164(2):414–21.

81. Green KK, Kent DT, D'Agostino MA, et al. Drug-induced sleep endoscopy and surgical outcomes: a multicenter cohort study. Laryngoscope 2019;129(3): 761–70.

82. Miller C, Purcell PL, Dahl JP, et al. Clinically small tonsils are typically not obstructive in children during drug-induced sleep endoscopy. Laryngoscope 2017;127(8):1943–9.

83. Lam DJ, Krane NA, Mitchell RB. Relationship between drug-induced sleep endoscopy findings, tonsil size, and polysomnographic outcomes of adenotonsillectomy in children. Otolaryngol Head Neck Surg 2019;161(3):507–13.

84. Chen J, He S. Drug-induced sleep endoscopy-directed adenotonsillectomy in pediatric obstructive sleep apnea with small tonsils. PLoS One 2019;14(2): e0212317.

85. Hyzer JM, Milczuk HA, Macarthur CJ, et al. Drug-induced sleep endoscopy findings in children with obstructive sleep apnea with vs without obesity or down syndrome. JAMA Otolaryngol Head Neck Surg 2021;147(2):175–81.

86. Lookabaugh S, McKenna M, Karelsky S, et al. Drug-induced sleep endoscopy findings in surgically-naive obese vs non-obese children. Int J Pediatr Otorhinolaryngol 2020;138:110289.

87. Filipek N, Kirkham E, Chen M, et al. Drug-induced sleep endoscopy directed surgery improves polysomnography measures in overweight and obese children with obstructive sleep apnea. Acta Oto-Laryngologica. 2020;1–6.

88. Smith JL 2nd, Sweeney DM, Smallman B, et al. State-dependent laryngomalacia in sleeping children. Ann Otol Rhinol Laryngol 2005;114(2):111–4.

89. Sivan Y, Ben-Ari J, Soferman R, et al. Diagnosis of laryngomalacia by fiberoptic endoscopy: awake compared with anesthesia-aided technique. Chest 2006; 130(5):1412–8.

90. Digoy GP, Shukry M, Stoner JA. Sleep apnea in children with laryngomalacia: diagnosis via sedated endoscopy and objective outcomes after supraglottoplasty. Otolaryngol Head Neck Surg 2012;147(3):544–50.

91. Bachar G, Nageris B, Feinmesser R, et al. Novel grading system for quantifying upper-airway obstruction on sleep endoscopy. Lung 2012;190(3):313–8.

92. Fishman G, Zemel M, DeRowe A, et al. Fiber-optic sleep endoscopy in children with persistent obstructive sleep apnea: inter-observer correlation and comparison with awake endoscopy. Int J Pediatr Otorhinolaryngol 2013;77(5):752–5.

93. Kezirian EJ, Hohenhorst W, de Vries N. Drug-induced sleep endoscopy: the VOTE classification. Eur Arch Otorhinolaryngol 2011;268(8):1233–6.

94. Lam DJ, Weaver EM, Macarthur CJ, et al. Assessment of pediatric obstructive sleep apnea using a drug-induced sleep endoscopy rating scale. Laryngoscope 2016;126(6):1492–8.

95. Chan DK, Liming BJ, Horn DL, et al. A new scoring system for upper airway pediatric sleep endoscopy. JAMA Otolaryngol Head Neck Surg 2014;140(7): 595–602.

96. Williamson At, Ibrahim SR, Coutras SW, et al. Pediatric drug-induced sleep endoscopy: technique and scoring system. Cureus 2020;12(10):e10765.

97. Amos JM, Durr ML, Nardone HC, et al. Systematic review of drug-induced sleep endoscopy scoring systems. Otolaryngol Head Neck Surg 2018;158(2):240–8.

98. Dahl JP, Miller C, Purcell PL, et al. Airway obstruction during drug-induced sleep endoscopy correlates with apnea-hypopnea index and oxygen nadir in children. Otolaryngol Head Neck Surg 2016;155(4):676–80.

99. Tejan J, Medina M, Ulualp SO. Comparative assessment of drug-induced sleep endoscopy scoring systems in pediatric sleep apnea. Laryngoscope 2019; 129(9):2195–8.

100. Bliss M, Yanamadala S, Koltai P. Utility of concurrent direct laryngoscopy and bronchoscopy with drug induced sleep endoscopy in pediatric patients with obstructive sleep apnea. Int J Pediatr Otorhinolaryngol 2018;110:34–6.

101. Purdon PL, Sampson A, Pavone KJ, et al. Clinical Electroencephalography for Anesthesiologists: Part I: Background and Basic Signatures. Anesthesiology 2015;123(4):937–60.

102. Nelson LE, Lu J, Guo T, et al. The alpha2-adrenoceptor agonist dexmedetomidine converges on an endogenous sleep-promoting pathway to exert its sedative effects. Anesthesiology 2003;98(2):428–36.

103. Shteamer JW, Dedhia RC. Sedative choice in drug-induced sleep endoscopy: A neuropharmacology-based review. Laryngoscope 2017;127(1):273–9.

104. Benedek P, Balakrishnan K, Cunningham MJ, et al. International Pediatric Otolaryngology group (IPOG) consensus on the diagnosis and management of pediatric obstructive sleep apnea (OSA). Int J Pediatr Otorhinolaryngol 2020;138:110276.

105. Char D, Drover DR, Motonaga KS, et al. The effects of ketamine on dexmedetomidine-induced electrophysiologic changes in children. Paediatr Anaesth 2013;23(10):898–905.

106. Schuttler J, Ihmsen H. Population pharmacokinetics of propofol: a multicenter study. Anesthesiology 2000;92(3):727–38.

107. Wu J, Mahmoud M, Schmitt M, et al. Comparison of propofol and dexmedetomedine techniques in children undergoing magnetic resonance imaging. Paediatr Anaesth 2014;24(8):813–8.

108. Kandil A, Subramanyam R, Hossain MM, et al. Comparison of the combination of dexmedetomidine and ketamine to propofol or propofol/sevoflurane for drug-induced sleep endoscopy in children. Paediatr Anaesth 2016;26(7):742–51.

109. Cho JS, Soh S, Kim EJ, et al. Comparison of three sedation regimens for drug-induced sleep endoscopy. Sleep Breath 2015;19(2):711–7.

110. Chattopadhyay U, Mallik S, Ghosh S, et al. Comparison between propofol and dexmedetomidine on depth of anesthesia: A prospective randomized trial. J Anaesthesiol Clin Pharmacol 2014;30(4):550–4.

111. Kuyrukluyildiz U, Binici O, Onk D, et al. Comparison of dexmedetomidine and propofol used for drug-induced sleep endoscopy in patients with obstructive sleep apnea syndrome. Int J Clin Exp Med 2015;8(4):5691–8.

112. Ebert TJ, Hall JE, Barney JA, et al. The effects of increasing plasma concentrations of dexmedetomidine in humans. Anesthesiology 2000;93(2):382–94.

113. Petroz GC, Sikich N, James M, et al. A phase I, two-center study of the pharmacokinetics and pharmacodynamics of dexmedetomidine in children. Anesthesiology 2006;105(6):1098–110.

114. Evans RG, Crawford MW, Noseworthy MD, et al. Effect of increasing depth of propofol anesthesia on upper airway configuration in children. Anesthesiology 2003;99(3):596–602.

115. Crawford MW, Rohan D, Macgowan CK, et al. Effect of propofol anesthesia and continuous positive airway pressure on upper airway size and configuration in infants. Anesthesiology 2006;105(1):45–50.

116. Machata AM, Kabon B, Willschke H, et al. Upper airway size and configuration during propofol-based sedation for magnetic resonance imaging: an analysis of 138 infants and children. Paediatr Anaesth 2010;20(11):994–1000.

117. Mahmoud M, Gunter J, Donnelly LF, et al. A comparison of dexmedetomidine with propofol for magnetic resonance imaging sleep studies in children. Anesth Analg 2009;109(3):745–53.

118. Mahmoud M, Jung D, Salisbury S, et al. Effect of increasing depth of dexmedetomidine and propofol anesthesia on upper airway morphology in children and adolescents with obstructive sleep apnea. J Clin Anesth 2013;25(7):529–41.

119. Watt S, Sabouri S, Hegazy R, et al. Does dexmedetomidine cause less airway collapse than propofol when used for deep sedation? J Clin Anesth 2016;35: 259–67.

120. Kamal K, Asthana U, Bansal T, et al. Evaluation of efficacy of dexmedetomidine versus propofol for sedation in children undergoing magnetic resonance imaging. Saudi J Anaesth 2017;11(2):163–8.

121. Bruppacher H, Reber A, Keller JP, et al. The effects of common airway maneuvers on airway pressure and flow in children undergoing adenoidectomies. Anesth Analg 2003;97(1):29–34, table of contents.

122. Eastwood PR, Szollosi I, Platt PR, et al. Collapsibility of the upper airway during anesthesia with isoflurane. Anesthesiology 2002;97(4):786–93.

123. Arai YC, Fukunaga K, Ueda W, et al. The endoscopically measured effects of airway maneuvers and the lateral position on airway patency in anesthetized children with adenotonsillar hypertrophy. Anesth Analg 2005;100(4):949–52.

124. Reber A, Paganoni R, Frei FJ. Dynamic imaging of the pediatric upper airway during general anesthesia. J Clin Monit Comput 1998;14(3):199–202.

125. Crawford MW, Arrica M, Macgowan CK, et al. Extent and localization of changes in upper airway caliber with varying concentrations of sevoflurane in children. Anesthesiology 2006;105(6):1147–52 [discussion: 1145A].

126. Kellner P, Herzog B, Plossl S, et al. Depth-dependent changes of obstruction patterns under increasing sedation during drug-induced sedation endoscopy: results of a German monocentric clinical trial. Sleep Breath 2016;20(3):1035–43.

127. Hsu YW, Cortinez LI, Robertson KM, et al. Dexmedetomidine pharmacodynamics: part I: crossover comparison of the respiratory effects of dexmedetomidine and remifentanil in healthy volunteers. Anesthesiology 2004;101(5): 1066–76.

128. Mahmoud M, Radhakrishman R, Gunter J, et al. Effect of increasing depth of dexmedetomidine anesthesia on upper airway morphology in children. Paediatr Anaesth 2010;20(6):506–15.

129. Mahmoud M, Ishman SL, McConnell K, et al. Upper airway reflexes are preserved during dexmedetomidine sedation in children with down syndrome and obstructive sleep apnea. J Clin Sleep Med 2017;13(5):721–7.

130. Miller AC, Jamin CT, Elamin EM. Continuous intravenous infusion of ketamine for maintenance sedation. Minerva Anestesiol 2011;77(8):812–20.

131. Abrams JT, Horrow JC, Bennett JA, et al. Upper airway closure: a primary source of difficult ventilation with sufentanil induction of anesthesia. Anesth Analg 1996;83(3):629–32.

132. Tagaito Y, Isono S, Nishino T. Upper airway reflexes during a combination of propofol and fentanyl anesthesia. Anesthesiology 1998;88:1459–66.

133. Litman RS, Kottra JA, Berkowitz RJ, et al. Upper airway obstruction during midazolam/nitrous oxide sedation in children with enlarged tonsils. Pediatr Dent 1998;20(5):318–20.

134. Oshima T, Masaki Y, Toyooka H. Flumazenil antagonizes midazolam-induced airway narrowing during nasal breathing in humans. Br J Anaesth 1999;82(5): 698–702.

135. Shorten GD, Opie NJ, Graziotti P, et al. Assessment of upper airway anatomy in awake, sedated and anaesthetised patients using magnetic resonance imaging. Anaesth Intensive Care 1994;22(2):165–9.

136. Berry RB, McNellis MI, Kouchi K, et al. Upper airway anesthesia reduces phasic genioglossus activity during sleep apnea. Am J Respir Crit Care Med 1997; 156(1):127–32.

137. Beydon L, Lorino AM, Verra F, et al. Topical upper airway anaesthesia with lidocaine increases airway resistance by impairing glottic function. Intensive Care Med 1995;21(11):920–6.

138. Berry RB, Kouchi KG, Bower JL, et al. Effect of upper airway anesthesia on obstructive sleep apnea. Am J Respir Crit Care Med 1995;151(6):1857–61.

139. Eikermann M, Grosse-Sundrup M, Zaremba S, et al. Ketamine activates breathing and abolishes the coupling between loss of consciousness and upper airway dilator muscle dysfunction. Anesthesiology 2012;116(1):35–46.

140. Capasso R, Rosa T, Tsou DY, et al. Variable findings for drug-induced sleep endoscopy in obstructive sleep apnea with propofol versus dexmedetomidine. Otolaryngol Head Neck Surg 2016;154(4):765–70.

141. Padiyara TV, Bansal S, Jain D, et al. Dexmedetomidine versus propofol at different sedation depths during drug-induced sleep endoscopy: a randomized trial. Laryngoscope 2020;130(1):257–62.

142. Kirkham EM, Hoi K, Melendez JB, et al. Propofol versus dexmedetomidine during drug-induced sleep endoscopy (DISE) for pediatric obstructive sleep apnea. Sleep Breath 2020;25(2):757–65.

Drooling and Aspiration of Saliva

Amy Hughes, MD[a,b], Elton M. Lambert, MD[c,d],*

KEYWORDS

- Drooling • Sialorrhea • Aspiration of saliva • Submandibular gland excision
- Duct ligation • Botulinum toxin injections to the salivary glands

KEY POINTS

- Drooling is the unintentional loss of saliva from the oral cavity, and can occur with or without associated aspiration.
- Aspiration of saliva can lead to pulmonary complications including chronic cough, aspiration pneumonia and recurrent respiratory hospitalizations.
- Botulinum toxin injection to the salivary glands is an effective treatment for drooling.
- Surgical procedures for drooling include submandibular gland excision, submandibular duct ligation or rerouting and parotid duct ligation and re-routing with various combinations of procedures described in the literature.
- Drooling with associated aspiration requires a multidisciplinary approach to control respiratory complications.

BACKGROUND

Drooling, or sialorrhea, is a common problem among children and young adults with cerebral palsy (CP) and other neuromuscular diseases. It is estimated that 40% of children across the full range of CP severity have difficulty with sialorrhea, with a prevalence of 80% among those children with more severe forms of CP.[1] Drooling is typically not due to excess saliva production but usually occurs in the setting of poor oral motor control, weakness of the bulbar and facial musculature, abnormal swallowing mechanisms combined with a reduced swallowing frequency, and malocclusion.[2] Sialorrhea secondary to hypersecretion may occur in patients with active

Off-label use of formulations of botulinum toxin injections to the salivary glands will be discussed, but all recommendations related to this are evidenced-based.
[a] Department of Otolaryngology, Connecticut Children's, Division of Otolaryngology, UCONN School of Medicine, 282 Washington Street, Hartford, CT 06106, USA; [b] Department of Surgery, UCONN School of Medicine, 282 Washington Street, Hartford, CT 06106, USA; [c] Division of Otolaryngology, Department of Surgery, Texas Children's Hospital; [d] Department of Otolaryngology, Baylor College of Medicine, 6701 Fannin Street D. 640, Houston, TX, 77030, USA
* Corresponding author. Department of Otolaryngology, Baylor College of Medicine, 6701 Fannin Street D. 640, Houston, TX, 77030.
E-mail address: emashela@texaschildrens.org

Otolaryngol Clin N Am 55 (2022) 1181–1194
https://doi.org/10.1016/j.otc.2022.07.007
0030-6665/22/© 2022 Elsevier Inc. All rights reserved.

dental concerns, esophageal reflux disease, patients on antiepileptic and/or antipsychotic medications, or from frequent oral stimulation/mouthing.[1,3] The degree of sialorrhea may vary day to day, depending on patient factors such as their level of fatigue, head positioning, dosing of anticholinergics, and neurologic status.

Sialorrhea is classified as being anterior or posterior. The term "drooling" typically refers to the more clinically apparent anterior sialorrhea, when patients have spillage of saliva from the mouth. Although anterior drooling does not usually have significant medical repercussions, it can have an associated social stigma and significantly affect the child and family psychosocially.[4] In contrast, posterior drooling may be more difficult to diagnose if it is not associated with visible drooling, but it can have more serious physiologic sequelae due to aspiration of saliva and exacerbation of chronic lung disease. Lower respiratory tract infections are the leading cause of death in children with CP. Clinicians need to be aware of the differing manifestations of anterior and posterior drooling as well as the management options, as these can vary as well.

Assessment

Clinical evaluation of children with sialorrhea should be conducted using a multidisciplinary approach with good communication between members of the health care team. As with any patient, a thorough clinical history and physical examination should be completed. Assessment should include an evaluation for exacerbating factors such as poor oral health or malocclusion, oropharyngeal dysphagia, allergies, gastroesophageal reflux disease, nasal or airway obstruction, medication side effects, as well as patient trunk and head positioning to be sure that these factors have been optimized.

Providers should also assess respiratory health to determine the presence of posterior drooling. Questioning regarding frequent gurgling, coughing, choking, as well as a history of recurrent respiratory infections suggest salivary aspiration. However, a multidisciplinary team to rule out airway abnormalities, such as laryngeal clefts or tracheoesophageal fistula, as causes for respiratory infection is paramount. Bedside flexible fiberoptic nasopharyngoscopy and laryngoscopy can play an important role in diagnosing posterior drooling by allowing providers to witness episodes of salivary aspiration. In addition, flexible endoscopic evaluation of swallowing (FEES) in patients able to eat orally and the modified Evan's blue dye test in NPO patients can assess aspiration of food boluses and secretions, respectively.[5]

Radionuclide salivagrams are performed by tracing technetium 99m sulfur colloid from the oral cavity to the esophagus or respiratory tract (**Fig. 1**). Aspiration on salivagram is associated with increased risk of chronic respiratory infections/pneumonia and reactive airway exacerbations.[6] Salivagrams do not distinguish between salivary aspiration due to excessive saliva versus dysphagia only.

Quantitative assessment tools may be used to evaluate the extent, severity, and impact of drooling. **Table 1** outlines commonly used subjective and objective scales for measurement of anterior drooling.[7–9] There are no validated scales for assessment of symptoms from aspiration of saliva; however, Shoval and colleagues described a nonvalidated scale, which is shown in **Table 2**.[10] The Murray Secretion Scale is validated and predicts aspiration risk due to excessive secretions in the hypopharynx (**Table 3**); this has not been studied in children.[11] Implementation of these measures into practice allows providers to establish a baseline for comparison following interventions.

Once a provider has classified the severity and type of sialorrhea that is present, treatment should be initiated.

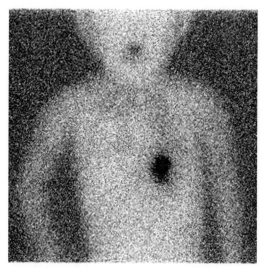

Fig. 1. Nuclear aspiration study of a 5-year-old girl with choking on secretions but no obvious drooling. Sulfur colloid was administered in the mouth with accumulation of radiotracer into the left lower lung field.

Therapeutic Options

Multiple interventions are available for sialorrhea management. In individuals with anterior drooling and mild-to-moderate dysfunction who are able to participate in their care, providers may consider behavioral therapy, oral motor therapy, and oral appliances; although these interventions have low-level evidence supporting their role, they have shown effectiveness.[12,13] For the management of anterior drooling, posterior drooling, or a combination of both, pharmacologic interventions, botulinum toxin injections into the salivary glands, and surgical procedures should be considered.

Pharmacologic Interventions

Anticholinergic medications are the most commonly prescribed medications for drooling management. These medications work by inhibiting the parasympathetic stimulation of the salivary glands, thereby reducing saliva production. Although most of the patients may have trialed medications before an otolaryngologic evaluation, being familiar with the commonly prescribed medications is important.

The most commonly used anticholinergic agents include glycopyrrolate and scopolamine. In 2012, a randomized, placebo-controlled phase III clinical trial examining the efficacy of glycopyrrolate solution showed that patients taking glycopyrrolate had a significantly higher response rate than patients in the placebo group.[14] The most frequently reported side effects included dry mouth, constipation, and vomiting. A prospective study from 2000 showed similar improvement but found a dose-dependent increase in adverse events. Twenty percent of children discontinued the medication due to behavioral problems, constipation, xerostomia, or urinary retention.[15] Compared with glycopyrrolate, hyoscine hydrobromide (scopolamine) has a less favorable side-effect profile. The Drooling Reduction Intervention randomized trial compared the efficacy and acceptability of scopolamine patches and glycopyrrolate liquid on drooling in children with neurodisability.[16] Their results showed a clinically and statistically significant reduction in drooling (measured by the drooling impact

Table 1
Anterior drooling assessment tools[7-9]

Tool	Length	Measure	Set-Up	Scale	Overall Score
Drooling Rating Scale (DRS)	8-item scale	Physical and psychosocial domains	Two parts 1) Description of drooling in prior week in 4 situations; measured 0 (excessive dryness) to 3 (continuous drool) 2) 5 min intervals tid × 7 d, count number of saliva swallows	Likert-type scale Ordinal numbers	1) 0–3 (lower less severe) 2) Counting number of dry swallows
Drooling Severity and Frequency Scale(DSFS)		Physical	Two parts 1) Assess severity from dry (never drools) to profuse (wet) 2) Assess frequency of drooling (never, occasional, frequent, constant)	4- and 5-point Likert-type scale	Ranges 2–9, lower less severity and frequency
Drooling Impact Scale (DIS)	10 items	Physical and psychosocial	Assesses frequency, severity, embarrassment, and family impact of drooling; data referring to past	Likert-type scales (10 points) Ordinal scales	Ranges 0–100, higher score, more severe impact
Teacher Drooling Scale (TDS)		Physical	Assess severity from dry (no drooling) to profuse (constant, always wet)	Likert-type scale	Range 1–5, lower less severe
Drooling Quotient (DQ)		Objective, direct observational method	DQ10 measures observation of drool (new saliva at lip margin or dropping from chin/mouth) at 15-s intervals over 10 min at rest and during activity DQ5 same measure over 5 min rather than 10 min	Ordinal numbers	
Visual Analog Scale (VAS)		Physical	Severity as perceived by parents 0 (no drool) –100 (excessive drool)	Likert-type scale	Range 0–100, lower less severe

Table 2	
Posterior drooling scale[10]	
0	No choking or coughing
1	Choking/ coughing while lying down
2	Choking/coughing while sitting Up
3	One aspiration pneumonia in the last 12 mo
4	Two or more aspiration pneumonias in the last 12 mo

scale) at week 4 for both medications; however, there was a 42% increased chance of continuing treatment at week 12 in the glycopyrrolate group compared with scopolamine. The authors recommended glycopyrrolate as the first-line anticholinergic medication.[16]

Inhaled ipratropium bromide (Atrovent) and sublingual atropine ophthalmic drops are 2 additional medications that may be initiated for drooling management. In general, fewer studies examining their efficacy have been performed, and although some of the results have been promising, these are not as widely used.[17]

Intraglandular Botulinum Toxin Injections

Botulinum toxin injected into the salivary glands results in an inhibition of presynaptic release of acetylcholine in parasympathetic fibers without causing the systemic anticholinergic side effects seen with the prescribed medications. The injections are commonly performed using ultrasound (US) guidance under general or local anesthesia, with injections targeted at the submandibular glands or parotid glands alone or in combination (**Fig. 2**).[18] A systematic review published by Rodwell and colleagues in 2012 found variation in the doses and dilutions of botulinum toxin used. Onabotulinum toxin A Botox brand was the most commonly injected toxin type. The reported median total dose was 70 units (10–100U), and the median total toxin dose per gland was 25 units (5–25U). The median maximal dilution of Botox was 28.1 units/mL (25–100 U/mL). The maximum effect is typically seen between 2 and 8 weeks, with the improvement lasting between 4 and 6 months.[19]

The benefits of botulinum toxin injections have been published in cohort studies, systematic reviews, and randomized controlled trials. Studies examining the efficacy of botulinum toxin injections to the bilateral parotid and submandibular glands demonstrate an improved response with injection of all 4 glands versus parotid or submandibular gland injections alone.[20,21] In 2008, Reid and colleagues compared outcomes

Table 3	
Murray secretion scale[11]	
0	Most normal rating. No visible secretions anywhere in the hypopharynx or some transient bubbles visible in the valleculae and pyriform sinuses
1	Deeply pooled bilateral secretions in the valleculae and pyriform sinuses and ending the observation segment with no visible secretions
2	Any secretions that changed from a "1" rating to a "3" rating during the observation period
3	Most severe rating. Any secretions in laryngeal vestibule. Pulmonary secretions were included if not cleared by swallowing or coughing

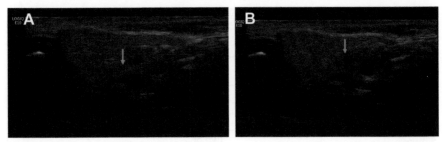

Fig. 2. (*A*) US-guided submandibular gland botulinum toxin injection. (*B*) Botulinum toxin seen diffusing into the submandibular gland.

following bilateral parotid and submandibular gland botulinum toxin injections between a treatment group and control group. Using the drooling impact scale, they found a satisfactory response rate in approximately 68% of patients. Sixteen percent experienced thickened saliva; increased difficulty with swallowing was also mentioned.[22] Jongerius and colleagues compared outcomes between submandibular botulinum toxin injections and scopolamine treatment in a controlled clinical trial.[23] Findings included a significant decrease in drooling measured by the drooling quotient that persisted up to 24 weeks in 50% of patients. Botulinum toxin injections had a more favorable side-effect profile than scopolamine, with 71% of patients taking scopolamine experiencing moderate-to-severe side effects. Only 5 (11%) patients experienced side effects from botulinum toxin. Lastly, Rodwell's systematic review suggested a moderate to strong reduction in drooling following BoNT injections.[19]

Although adverse reactions are uncommon following botulinum toxin injections, US guidance seems to mitigate risk by providing injectors the opportunity to properly position the needle into the salivary gland and diminish the risk of diffusion or injection into adjacent musculature.[24,25] Reported adverse events include xerostomia, thickened saliva, and mild-to-moderate dysphagia, with the most significant risk including severe dysphagia resulting in aspiration pneumonia. Van Hulst and colleagues reported transient oral motor dysfunction in 33% of patients in their cohort study. This dysfunction is most commonly presented within 1 week and resolved by 4 weeks.[26]

Surgical Techniques

Surgical interventions may be considered in patients with profuse, consistent anterior drooling despite conservative treatment; patients who are unable to tolerate side effects of anticholinergic medications; and/or patients with persistent posterior drooling who are at risk for developing or who have chronic lung disease. Goals of surgical management include (1) redirecting salivary flow through rerouting or (2) eliminating salivary flow through ligation of salivary ducts or elimination of salivary glands. The most commonly performed procedures include salivary duct ligation (2, 3, or 4 duct), submandibular duct (SMD) rerouting ± sublingual gland excision, and submandibular gland (SMG) excision ± parotid duct ligation or rerouting (PDL, PDR).

Duct Ligation

Salivary duct ligation is a more minimally invasive surgical approach. This surgical approach is performed intraorally and involves circumferential isolation and either clip or suture ligation of the submandibular and/or parotid ducts. Two, three, or four duct ligations have been described, and the reported surgical efficacy varies greatly, with a range of postoperative improvement from 50% to 81%.[27,28] The largest concern with duct ligation is the risk of duct recannulation and drooling recurrence. Following submandibular duct ligation, Bekkers and colleagues reported a significant decrease in the visual analog scale (VAS) and drooling quotient at 8 weeks, but by 32 weeks there was a significant increase again suggesting recurrence. Martin and colleagues reported a recurrence rate of 68.8% in their group of 16 patients.[29] Khan and colleagues had a more favorable result, with improvement persisting past 1 year in 76% of their patients; however, caregiver satisfaction was only 53% at most recent patient follow-up.[30] Suggested causes for recurrence include the upregulation of the sublingual and minor salivary glands versus the redevelopment of salivary pathways.[27]

Bilateral Submandibular Gland Excision

Bilateral submandibular gland excision (SMGE) with parotid duct rerouting was first presented as a surgical treatment of drooling in 1977.[31] Today bilateral SGME is more commonly performed either in isolation or combined with parotid duct ligation. Success rates for bilateral SMGE with PDL or rerouting have ranged from 75% to 100%.[28,32] Noonan and colleagues tracked lower respiratory tract infections and found significantly fewer infections following surgery.[33] Reviews of SMGE without parotid duct intervention report a 62% to 66% success rate.[28] A review looking at both subjective and objective results after SMGE alone found a significant reduction in drooling in 62% of participants at 32 weeks.[34] There has been a move toward earlier and more definitive surgical intervention with SMGE with or without PDL in patients with posterior drooling who require intensive care unit care, noninvasive ventilation, or tracheotomy.[35]

Submandibular Duct Rerouting with Sublingual Gland Excision for Anterior Drooling

Submandibular duct relocation may be considered in patients with anterior drooling that have an intact swallow. The goal of surgery is to relocate the submandibular duct papillae to the base of tongue to allow saliva to flow posteriorly into the oropharynx and trigger the swallow reflux. If performed in the correct patient population, success rates range from 58% to 100%, with most of the studies concluding that SMDR is safe and effective.[28,36] In a cohort study of 91 patients, at 32 weeks 66% of their patients had a 50% reduction in Drooling Quotient scores and 73.6% had a reduction of 2 SD in VAS score. The authors found that children aged 12 years and older had a more favorable outcome and recommended waiting until this age.[37] Complications include floor of mouth edema, lingual nerve injury, ranula (blocked sublingual gland) formation, and xerostomia. SMDR is commonly combined with sublingual gland excision, which decreases the risk of ranula formation.[38]

DISCUSSION
Controversies in Choosing Drooling Surgery

As previously outlined, surgeons have several options in drooling management, with interventions broadly divided into excision procedures and duct procedures (ligation and rerouting). How does one choose among them?

A balance must be struck between the desired effects of reduction in saliva, improvement in quality of life, and morbidity of aspiration and the potential side effects of xerostomia, perioperative complications, and aesthetic considerations. Although not fully elucidated, surgical interventions may also affect dental health by changing the amount of saliva and its chemical composition.[39,40] Mucous plugging in tracheostomy patients may be another concern.

Despite these potential adverse events, undertreatment of drooling has consequences on quality of life and in those with salivary aspiration-respiratory morbidity. The issue of needing additional procedures and associated anesthesia in this complex patient population should also not be overlooked, with the goal of definitive surgical treatment often the best one.

Reed and colleagues in their systematic review note that drooling procedures have an overall success rate of 81.6%, ranging from 64.1% for 4-duct ligation to 87.8% for bilateral SMGE with bilateral PDR.[28] With the surgeon having to balance outcomes and side effects of treatments, choosing a surgery for drooling can be daunting. Two major questions have arisen in the literature and are addressed here.

What additional benefit do parotid duct drooling procedures confer on submandibular gland/duct procedures?

In answering the first question, it is important to consider the basics. The submandibular gland produces most of the resting saliva; drooling can be considered a resting saliva issue; therefore, many advocate that a submandibular gland procedure alone may be adequate. Thangirala and colleagues showed no additional benefit in parent's perception of success when PDL was added to SMGE for drooling. Patients in the SMGE + PDL group, however, had more surgical site complications, most of which were minor including facial swelling.[41] Schild and colleagues in their systematic review showed no difference in drooling control when comparing SMGE alone, SMGE + PDR, and SMGE + PDL.[42] Complications rates were harder to compare, but SMGE + PDL patients had higher rates of xerostomia and parotitis compared with SMGE + PDR patients.

Submandibular duct ligation (SMDL) versus 4-duct ligation (4DL) has also been compared. Becmeur and colleagues noted similar salivary control rates for SMDL versus 4DL.[43] Advocates for SMDL tout its shorter procedure time and lack of parotitis as advantages. Although SMDL alone has been shown to be effective for control of drooling,[44] surgeons should be aware of the high recurrence rate.[27] A recent publication by Delsing and colleagues concluded that although SMDL reduced signs and symptoms of posterior drooling, the greatest effect was seen after SMGE.[38]

Combined submandibular gland and parotid duct procedures represent a viable option for patients when compared with SMG procedures alone. The success rate of 4DL can be as high as 93% depending on the authors' definition of success.[30,45] SMGE + PDL's success rates are as high as 87%.[46,47] SMG-alone procedures for drooling can have a failure rate as high as 40%.[41,44] The question becomes what percentage of these failures are due to lack of including a PD procedure versus other factors such as patient selection, progression of neuromuscular disease, or recanalization in the case of SMDL. Both authors will add PDL to SMGE in cases of drooling with chronic aspiration of saliva.[48] These patients have a higher morbidity of potential drooling procedure failure, are generally a higher anesthetic risk, and are typical NPO, so the impact on mastication from xerostomia is a nonissue as opposed to those who have oral intake. Those without aspiration of saliva are managed with a stepwise approach with SMGE only and subsequent PDL if needed.[34]

What are the advantages and disadvantages of duct ligation versus duct rerouting procedures?

When considering DL versus duct rerouting/relocation (DR) procedures, it is almost universally accepted that patients with chronic aspiration or who are at risk of aspiration should not undergo DR procedures.[49] Advocates for DR procedures note the lower xerostomia and sialadenitis risk, while offering good saliva control rates.[42] DR procedures are more technically demanding and have been criticized for increased scarring in the floor of mouth in SMGDR and oropharynx in PGDR. Opponents also note that scarring and fibrosis of the duct after DR in essence "ligates" the duct as salivary gland hypofunctioning results as in DL procedures.[50] In patients with an intact swallow and lower level of physical impairment, DR procedures remain a viable option for drooling without aspiration of saliva.

Drooling Procedures and Aspiration of Saliva

Chronic aspiration of saliva negatively affects pulmonary health through mechanisms not completely understood. Amylase, lysozyme, and other salivary enzymes may injure respiratory epithelium, but seeding by oral flora also promotes infection.[50] Although aspiration pneumonia is a sequalae of salivary aspiration; chronic cough, need for inhaled bronchodilators and corticosteroids, chronic respiratory failure, frequent hospitalizations, and increased tracheostomy secretions in tracheostomy patients can be present.[51]

Providers may have a difficult time differentiating between patients with excessive saliva who overcome airway protection mechanisms versus those with a normal amount of saliva with poor airway protection mechanisms. Alternately, there are patients in whom saliva control does not affect respiratory morbidity.[41] A multidisciplinary approach can assist in addressing this issue. Pulmonology may help with airway clearance strategies such as chest physiotherapy to allow for expulsion of secretions form the respiratory tract. Gastroenterologist may focus on treatment of gastrointestinal reflux or motility issues that decrease pharyngoesophageal transit. Immunology may be involved in patients who are immunocompromised, and Infectious Disease can help in cases of rare or resistant pathogens.

If other potential causes of lung disease are addressed without improvement, this may suggest chronic aspiration of saliva as a contributing factor. Families should be counseled that for patients with drooling as assessed on physical examination or subjective scales, saliva reduction strategies may improve symptoms associated with aspiration of saliva. In patients with signs of aspiration of saliva without obvious drooling, endoscopic and radiographic assessments, as previously outlined, should be completed before offering drooling procedures.

Unfortunately, studies on drooling control and chronic aspiration lack consistent outcome measurements for chronic aspiration of saliva, which makes expectation management and shared decision-making key to determining a treatment strategy. Botulinum toxin injections may decrease respiratory hospitalizations, symptoms of coughing and choking, hospitalization days, and intensive care unit days.[52,53] Drooling procedures such as 4-duct ligation and SMGE + PDL may also have a positive effect on chronic aspiration, with some studies suggesting a greater effect following SMGE.[48,54]

Refractory Drooling

Failure rates for drooling procedures are wide ranging[28,42,55]; this owes in large part to the various measures of success including drooling severity and frequency scales, drooling quotient, unstimulated saliva flow rate, VAS, Drooling Impact Scale, parents' perceptions, reduction in anticholinergic medications, and frequency of respiratory events in the case of saliva aspiration. First, the surgeon must review the attainability of the family's goals. In some children, it may be unreasonable to eliminate anticholinergic medication use.[56] It may also be less reasonable to pursue a temporary treatment such as botulinum toxin injections, as it may not be realistic for the patient to have continued anesthetics/injections in the long run. In addition, a response to botulinum toxin does not predict surgical success.[27,37]

Refractory drooling after duct procedures requires an investigation for duct recanalization. Physical examination showing secretion of saliva through a previously ligated duct can be seen. Scintigraphy showing saliva flow of a ligated gland is diagnostic. In this study, technetium-99 pertechnetate is intravenously administered, and the radiotracer is absorbed by the major salivary glands. The salivary glands are stimulated with oral administration of lemon. The radiotracer will remain in salivary glands when the ligation is intact and will "washout" into the oral cavity when there is recanalization. In cases of recanalization, repeat duct ligation is not widely described. Botulinum toxin can be injected into gland with a recanalized duct. SMGE can be performed for recanalized SMGs. It may be pertinent to review operative and pathology reports in patients who have had SMGEs to confirm that salivary gland tissue was removed. Physical examination and ultrasound may aid in the identification of persistent SMGs. Anticholinergics can be used in patients postsurgery.

Continued respiratory morbidity after a drooling procedure requires multidisciplinary coordination. If no other drooling surgeries can be offered, then optimization in pharyngeal and esophageal clearance and pulmonary toilet is needed. The presence of laryngeal clefts or TEFs needs to be ruled out. Patients with cricopharyngeal dysfunction or achalasia may present with excessive oral secretions and can be managed with botulinum toxin injections and endoscopic or open cricopharyngeal myotomy.[57] Tracheostomy placement may be necessary to assist with pulmonary toilet, whereas laryngotracheal separation or diversion is an effective surgery for life-threatening chronic aspiration.[58] Review of goals of care is of utmost importance, especially in patients with progressive neuromuscular disease.

SUMMARY

Surgeons performing drooling surgery should use a drooling scale to track outcomes and assess patients for aspiration of saliva. Knowledge of the anticholinergics prescribed for drooling will allow for improved decision-making for drooling procedures. Botulinum toxin injections to the salivary glands can be an effected saliva reduction strategy. Bilateral submandibular gland excision is the most effective drooling procedure, and the addition of parotid duct procedures to it is controversial. Patients with drooling and aspiration of saliva with recurrent respiratory infections may need involvement of Pulmonology, Gastroenterology, Infectious Disease, and/or Immunology.

CLINICS CARE POINTS

- Validated rating scales for drooling include the Drooling Rating Scale, Drooling Severity and Frequency Scale, Drooling Impact Scale, Teaching Drooling Scale, and Drooling Quotient.
- Assessments for aspiration of saliva include the Murray Secretion Scale, FEES, and radionuclide salivagram.
- Glycopyrrolate is the most effective anticholinergic medication for saliva reduction but has side effects including xerostomia, constipation, and urinary retention.
- Botulinum toxin injection to the salivary glands is a widely accepted treatment of drooling.
- Several drooling procedures exist including duct ligation and duct rerouting, but bilateral submandibular gland excision (BSMGE) is the most effective. The addition of parotid duct procedures to BSMGE is controversial.

DISCLOSURE

The authors have no relevant financial disclosures related to this work.

REFERENCES

1. Reid SM, McCutcheon J, Reddihough DS, et al. Prevalence and predictors of drooling in 7- to 14-year-old children with cerebral palsy: a population study. Dev Med Child Neurol 2012;54(11):1032–6.
2. Tahmassebi JF, Curzon ME. The cause of drooling in children with cerebral palsy – hypersalivation or swallowing defect? Int J Paediatr Dent 2003;13(2):106–11.
3. Senner JE, Logemann J, Zecker S, et al. Drooling, saliva production, and swallowing in cerebral palsy. Dev Med Child Neurol 2004;46(12):801–6.
4. Chang SC, Lin CK, Tung LC, et al. The association of drooling and health-related quality of life in children with cerebral palsy. Neuropsychiatr Dis Treat 2012;8: 599–604.
5. Donzelli J, Brady S, Wesling M, et al. Simultaneous modified Evans blue dye procedure and video nasal endoscopic evaluation of the swallow. Laryngoscope 2001;111(10):1746–50.
6. Simons JP, Rubinstein EN, Mandell DL. Clinical predictors of aspiration on radionuclide salivagrams in children. Arch Otolaryngol Head Neck Surg 2008;134(9): 941–4.
7. Nascimento D, Carmona J, Mestre T, et al. Drooling rating scales in Parkinson's disease: a systematic review. Parkinsonism Relat Disord Oct 2021;91:173–80.
8. van Hulst K, Lindeboom R, van der Burg J, et al. Accurate assessment of drooling severity with the 5-minute drooling quotient in children with developmental disabilities. Dev Med Child Neurol Dec 2012;54(12):1121–6.
9. Westbom L, Bergstrand L, Wagner P, et al. Survival at 19 years of age in a total population of children and young people with cerebral palsy. Dev Med Child Neurol 2011;53(9):808–14.
10. Shoval HA, Antelis E, Hillman A, et al. Onabotulinum Toxin a injections into the salivary glands for spinal muscle atrophy Type I: a prospective case series of 4 patients. Am J Phys Med Rehabil 2018;97(12):873–8.
11. Kuo CW, Allen CT, Huang CC, et al. Murray secretion scale and fiberoptic endoscopic evaluation of swallowing in predicting aspiration in dysphagic patients. Eur Arch Otorhinolaryngol 2017;274(6):2513–9.
12. Camp-Bruno JA, Winsberg BG, Green-Parsons AR, et al. Efficacy of benztropine therapy for drooling. Dev Med Child Neurol 1989;31(3):309–19.
13. Van der Burg JJ, Didden R, Jongerius PH, et al. A descriptive analysis of studies on behavioural treatment of drooling (1970-2005). Dev Med Child Neurol 2007; 49(5):390–4.
14. Arvedson J, Clark H, Lazarus C, et al. The effects of oral-motor exercises on swallowing in children: an evidence-based systematic review. Dev Med Child Neurol 2010;52(11):1000–13.
15. Mier RJ, Bachrach SJ, Lakin RC, et al. Treatment of sialorrhea with glycopyrrolate: A double-blind, dose-ranging study. Arch Pediatr Adolesc Med 2000;154(12): 1214–8.
16. Parr JR, Todhunter E, Pennington L, et al. Drooling Reduction Intervention randomised trial (DRI): comparing the efficacy and acceptability of hyoscine patches and glycopyrronium liquid on drooling in children with neurodisability. Arch Dis Child 2018;103(4):371–6.

17. Thomsen TR, Galpern WR, Asante A, et al. Ipratropium bromide spray as treatment for sialorrhea in Parkinson's disease. Mov Disord 2007;22(15):2268–73.
18. Gerlinger I, Szalai G, Hollody K, et al. Ultrasound-guided, intraglandular injection of botulinum toxin A in children suffering from excessive salivation. J Laryngol Otol 2007;121(10):947–51.
19. Rodwell K, Edwards P, Ware RS, et al. Salivary gland botulinum toxin injections for drooling in children with cerebral palsy and neurodevelopmental disability: a systematic review. Dev Med Child Neurol 2012;54(11):977–87.
20. Moller E, Karlsborg M, Bardow A, et al. Treatment of severe drooling with botulinum toxin in amyotrophic lateral sclerosis and Parkinson's disease: efficacy and possible mechanisms. Acta Odontol Scand 2011;69(3):151–7.
21. Suskind DL, Tilton A. Clinical study of botulinum-A toxin in the treatment of sialorrhea in children with cerebral palsy. Laryngoscope 2002;112(1):73–81.
22. Reid SM, Johnstone BR, Westbury C, et al. Randomized trial of botulinum toxin injections into the salivary glands to reduce drooling in children with neurological disorders. Dev Med Child Neurol 2008;50(2):123–8.
23. Jongerius PH, van den Hoogen FJ, van Limbeek J, et al. Effect of botulinum toxin in the treatment of drooling: a controlled clinical trial. Pediatrics 2004;114(3):620–7.
24. Hassin-Baer S, Scheuer E, Buchman AS, et al. Botulinum toxin injections for children with excessive drooling. J Child Neurol 2005;20(2):120–3.
25. Jongerius PH, Joosten F, Hoogen FJ, et al. The treatment of drooling by ultrasound-guided intraglandular injections of botulinum toxin type A into the salivary glands. Laryngoscope 2003;113(1):107–11.
26. van Hulst K, Kouwenberg CV, Jongerius PH, et al. Negative effects of submandibular botulinum neurotoxin A injections on oral motor function in children with drooling due to central nervous system disorders. Dev Med Child Neurol 2017;59(5):531–7.
27. Bekkers S, Pruijn IMJ, Van Hulst K, et al. Submandibular duct ligation after botulinum neurotoxin A treatment of drooling in children with cerebral palsy. Dev Med Child Neurol 2020;62(7):861–7.
28. Reed J, Mans CK, Brietzke SE. Surgical management of drooling: a meta-analysis. Arch Otolaryngol Head Neck Surg 2009;135(9):924–31.
29. Martin TJ, Conley SF. Long-term efficacy of intra-oral surgery for sialorrhea. Otolaryngol Head Neck Surg 2007;137(1):54–8.
30. Khan WU, Islam A, Fu A, et al. Four-duct ligation for the treatment of sialorrhea in children. JAMA Otolaryngol Head Neck Surg 2016;142(3):278–83.
31. Kaplan I. Results of the Wilke operation to stop drooling in cerebral palsy. Plast Reconstr Surg 1977;59(5):646–8.
32. Stamataki S, Behar P, Brodsky L. Surgical management of drooling: clinical and caregiver satisfaction outcomes. Int J Pediatr Otorhinolaryngol 2008;72(12):1801–5.
33. Noonan K, Prunty S, Ha JF, et al. Surgical management of chronic salivary aspiration. Int J Pediatr Otorhinolaryngol 2014;78(12):2079–82.
34. Delsing CP, Viergever T, Honings J, et al. Bilateral transcervical submandibular gland excision for drooling: A study of the mature scar and long-term effects. Eur J Paediatr Neurol 2016;20(5):738–44.
35. Cooper MS, Levi E, Desai M, et al. Making decisions about surgical intervention for drooling in children with neurodisability. Dev Med Child Neurol 2021;63(9):1127–8.

36. De M, Adair R, Golchin K, et al. Outcomes of submandibular duct relocation: a 15-year experience. J Laryngol Otol 2003;117(10):821–3.
37. Kok SE, van Valenberg H, van Hulst K, et al. Submandibular gland botulinum neurotoxin A injection for predicting the outcome of submandibular duct relocation in drooling: a retrospective cohort study. Dev Med Child Neurol 2019;61(11): 1323–8.
38. Glynn F, O'Dwyer TP. Does the addition of sublingual gland excision to submandibular duct relocation give better overall results in drooling control? Clin Otolaryngol Apr 2007;32(2):103–7. https://doi.org/10.1111/j.1365-2273.2007.01388.x.
39. Correa LB, Basso MB, Sousa-Pinto B, et al. Oral health effects of botulinum toxin treatment for drooling: a systematic review. Med Oral Patol Oral Cir Bucal 2021; 26(2):e172–80.
40. Gutierrez GM, Siqueira VL, Loyola-Rodriguez JP, et al. Effects of treatments for drooling on caries risk in children and adolescents with cerebral palsy. Med Oral Patol Oral Cir Bucal 2019;24(2):204–10.
41. Thangirala A, Zhu H, Lambert EM. Submandibular excision with and without parotid duct ligation for sialorrhoea. Br J Oral Maxillofac Surg 2021. https://doi.org/10.1016/j.bjoms.2021.06.015.
42. Schild SD, Timashpolsky A, Ballard DP, et al. Surgical Management of Sialorrhea: A Systematic Review and Meta-analysis. Otolaryngol Head Neck Surg 2021; 165(4):507–18.
43. Becmeur F, Schneider A, Flaum V, et al. Which surgery for drooling in patients with cerebral palsy? J Pediatr Surg 2013;48(10):2171–4.
44. Bekkers S, van Hulst K, Erasmus CE, et al. An evaluation of predictors for success of two-duct ligation for drooling in neurodisabilities. J Neurol 2020;267(5): 1508–15.
45. Chanu NP, Sahni JK, Aneja S, et al. Four-duct ligation in children with drooling. Am J Otolaryngol 2012;33(5):604–7.
46. Manrique D, do Brasil Ode O, Ramos H. Drooling: analysis and evaluation of 31 children who underwent bilateral submandibular gland excision and parotid duct ligation. Braz J Otorhinolaryngol 2007;73(1):40–4.
47. Stern Y, Feinmesser R, Collins M, et al. Bilateral submandibular gland excision with parotid duct ligation for treatment of sialorrhea in children: long-term results. Arch Otolaryngol Head Neck Surg 2002;128(7):801–3.
48. Gerber ME, Gaugler MD, Myer CM 3rd, et al. Chronic aspiration in children. When are bilateral submandibular gland excision and parotid duct ligation indicated? Arch Otolaryngol Head Neck Surg 1996;122(12):1368–71.
49. O'Dwyer TP, Conlon BJ. The surgical management of drooling–a 15 year follow-up. Clin Otolaryngol Allied Sci 1997;22(3):284–7.
50. Hotaling AJ, Madgy DN, Kuhns LR, et al. Postoperative technetium scanning in patients with submandibular duct diversion. Arch Otolaryngol Head Neck Surg 1992;118(12):1331–3.
51. Proesmans M, Vreys M, Huenaerts E, et al. Respiratory morbidity in children with profound intellectual and multiple disability. Pediatr Pulmonol 2015;50(10): 1033–8.
52. Faria J, Harb J, Hilton A, et al. Salivary botulinum toxin injection may reduce aspiration pneumonia in neurologically impaired children. Int J Pediatr Otorhinolaryngol 2015;79(12):2124–8.
53. Pena AH, Cahill AM, Gonzalez L, et al. Botulinum toxin A injection of salivary glands in children with drooling and chronic aspiration. J Vasc Interv Radiol 2009;20(3):368–73.

54. Klem C, Mair EA. Four-duct ligation: a simple and effective treatment for chronic aspiration from sialorrhea. Arch Otolaryngol Head Neck Surg 1999;125(7): 796–800.
55. Hung SA, Liao CL, Lin WP, et al. Botulinum Toxin Injections for Treatment of Drooling in Children with Cerebral Palsy: A Systematic Review and Meta-Analysis. Child (Basel) 2021;25(12):8. https://doi.org/10.3390/children8121089.
56. Dohar JE. Sialorrhea & aspiration control - A minimally invasive strategy uncomplicated by anticholinergic drug tolerance or tachyphylaxis. Int J Pediatr Otorhinolaryngol 2019;116:97–101.
57. Huoh KC, Messner AH. Cricopharyngeal achalasia in children: indications for treatment and management options. Curr Opin Otolaryngol Head Neck Surg 2013;21(6):576–80.
58. Gelfand YM, Duncan NO, Albright JT, et al. Laryngotracheal separation surgery for intractable aspiration: our experience with 12 patients. Int J Pediatr Otorhinolaryngol 2011;75(7):931–4.

Multidisciplinary Pediatric Tracheostomy Teams

Yann-Fuu Kou, MD[a,b,*], Stephen R. Chorney, MD, MPH[b,c],
Romaine F. Johnson, MD, MPH[b,c]

KEYWORDS

- Tracheostomy • Multidisciplinary team • Patient safety • Quality improvement

KEY POINTS

- Pediatric tracheostomy patients are medically complex and at high risk for adverse outcomes.
- Multidisciplinary tracheostomy care involves physicians, respiratory therapists, speech language pathologists, nurses, and social workers.
- Establishment of a multidisciplinary pediatric tracheostomy team offers a valuable patient safety and quality improvement initiative.

INTRODUCTION

Tracheostomy is one of the oldest surgical procedures with descriptions found on ancient Egyptian tablets dating back to 3600 BC.[1] The objective is to create an opening into the trachea and place a tube as an artificial airway. In children, tracheostomy was historically indicated for acute airway obstruction from infectious or inflammatory causes. The introduction of childhood vaccination programs along with the advances in neonatology and pediatric cardiology has drastically shifted surgical indications.[2] Currently, pediatric tracheostomies are primarily placed for chronic respiratory failure in critically ill children with significant cardiopulmonary comorbidities.[3–5]

Children with tracheostomies are among the most vulnerable and medically fragile patients in our health-care system.[6] Severity of comorbidities, which often necessitate tracheostomy placement, result in significant morbidity burden and mortality risk. Furthermore, complications of having a tracheostomy, challenges with ongoing management, and variability in caregiver expertise contribute to poor outcomes among

[a] Department of Otolaryngology, University of Texas Southwestern Medical Center, 2001 Inwood Road 6th Floor, Dallas, TX 75390, USA; [b] Division of Pediatric Otolaryngology, Children's Medical Center Dallas, 2350 North Stemmons Freeway, Dallas, TX 75207, USA; [c] Children's Health Airway Management Program, Department of Pediatric Otolaryngology, Children's Medical Center Dallas, Dallas, TX, USA

* Corresponding author. Division of Pediatric Otolaryngology, Children's Medical Center Dallas, 2350 North Stemmons Freeway, Dallas, TX 75207.
E-mail address: yann-fuu.kou@utsouthwestern.edu

Otolaryngol Clin N Am 55 (2022) 1195–1203
https://doi.org/10.1016/j.otc.2022.07.005
0030-6665/22/© 2022 Elsevier Inc. All rights reserved.

oto.theclinics.com

tracheostomy-dependent children. Multidisciplinary tracheostomy (MDT) teams have been shown to improve safety and quality of care for these pediatric patients.[1,7,8] The following review describes MDT, offers recent updates on how these teams improve pediatric tracheostomy outcomes, and provides considerations for the future of MDT.

DISCUSSION

Tracheostomies occur in less than 1% of pediatric admissions but account for up to 4% of total pediatric hospital costs. Inpatient complication rates can approach 30% with a mortality rate of 8% on index hospitalization and 15% overall.[8–10] Tracheostomy-related complications account for half of airway-related deaths and hypoxic brain injuries in intensive care units.[1] Tracheostomy-related adverse events (TRAEs) are common due to a complex patient population, inadequate staff experience, or tracheostomy equipment issues.[11] As a means to address patient safety concerns, multiple hospitals worldwide began to implement MDT teams with successful reductions in TRAE and morbidity. In 2012, an international group of experts in tracheostomy and quality-improvement met to review the state of tracheostomy care worldwide. At this meeting, the Global Tracheostomy Collaborative (GTC) was formed to provide an organizing structure for future quality improvement efforts.[1,12] The GTC identified 5 "key drivers" as the foundation for these efforts: standardization of care, improved staff education, patient and family involvement, use of prospective database to track outcomes, and implementation of an MDT.[1]

Early studies on MDT teams were described in adult tracheostomy patients.[13] The goals for adults with a tracheostomy are different from those for children because adults often require tracheostomies for shorter durations, and there is emphasis on early decannulation among some adult MDT teams.[14] Although the goals and anticipated duration with a tracheostomy may be different, the MDT team began to gain popularity in pediatrics in the last 10 to 20 years. There is no set definition of who should be included in an MDT. However, most studies agree that the integral members of the team include physicians (usually otolaryngologists), respiratory therapists (RTs), speech-language pathologists (SLPs), nursing/clinical nurse specialists, and social workers. It also requires strong collaboration from other services in the hospital including pulmonary and intensive care.[12,15,16] The overall goals of MDT teams are to improve patient safety and decrease costs and to help facilitate all the other "key drivers" identified by the GTC.

Standardization of Care

Standardization is a common practice that has been shown to improve quality in medical and nonmedical fields.[17] Standardization decreases variability, reduces inefficiencies, and provides a baseline for institutional quality improvement initiatives. MDT teams are essential in creating and implementing standardized protocols for pediatric tracheostomy patients, which may be unique across hospitals. For example, the timing of the first tracheostomy change in children is often left to the discretion of the surgeon and institutional preference. A clinical consensus statement on tracheostomy care by Mitchell and colleagues in 2013 recommended that initial tracheostomy change to be performed at 5 to 7 days after placement.[18] A survey of the American Society of Pediatric Otolaryngology in 2020 showed that 83% of participants followed this recommendation with recent interest in earlier changes.[19] Although the optimal time may not be known, an MDT team that will consistently approach this early decision can advance patient care in a timely manner and reduce unnecessary variability.

Postoperative skin care is another aspect of tracheostomy management that benefits from standardization. Postoperative complications related to skin breakdown and wound infections have been reported in up to 29% of children with tracheostomies.[20] Baker and Chorney performed a systematic review in 2020 showing decreased tracheostomy wound complications with protective barriers under the faceplate and ties and early wound identification.[21] In addition to using protective barriers, there has been a change in practice from using woven cotton (twill) ties to using Velcro (hook-and-loop fastener) ties. The twill ties maintain a fixed length despite manipulation and were thought to decrease rates of accidental decannulations. However, due to the narrow width and increased tension on the ties, there was concern they would lead to increased pressure and skin breakdown.[6] A retrospective study by Bitners and colleagues showed that twill ties had significantly more skin breakdown.[22] A prospective study by Hart and colleagues comparing twill ties and Velcro ties showed no significant differences in skin breakdown or accidental decannulations.[23] Standardization of practices at an institution can facilitate earlier detection of skin/wound issues and help to minimize these events.

Improved Staff Education

Education of hospital staff is crucial to ensuring safety and quality care for tracheostomy patients. Previous studies showed that many hospital providers seemed uncomfortable with tracheostomies and caring for them. As few as 2% of clinicians reported being comfortable handling tracheostomy emergencies.[1,12,24] Often, this lack of confidence and education comes from a lack of opportunities. Yelverton and colleagues found that even a simple intervention such as a 45-minute presentation led to significant increases in knowledge and confidence regarding tracheostomies. This improvement was maintained even after 6 months.[24]

The next movement in staff education will be high-fidelity simulation. This will allow trainees to experience routine and emergency tracheostomy situations in a safe learning environment. Uyan and colleagues did a study with health-care providers without formal training in tracheostomy care. They found significant improvements in knowledge and comfort after the simulation course.[25] MDT teams caring for tracheostomy-dependent children will be crucial in not only designing this training but incorporating it into their programs. Health-care providers will benefit from training experience that will help them respond to tracheostomy emergencies in a timely and effective manner.

Patient and Family Involvement

Hospital staff is important for the immediate perioperative period. However, a major barrier to timely discharge and long-term safety is family involvement and education. Key aspects of education are not only the daily care but also management of tracheostomy emergencies and making sure that families have all necessary emergency equipment.[6,26] Another important aspect is standardizing the tracheostomy education curriculum for all caretakers. Recent studies have highlighted the role of MDT teams and the positive effect they have on family education. McKeon and colleagues described their MDT significantly decreasing TRAE and increasing caregiver preparedness.[27] Gaudreau and colleagues found that standardized tracheostomy education and wound care with a tracheostomy nurse significantly decreased the incidence of postoperative wounds at home.[28]

Learning to adjust their lives around a child with a tracheostomy can be challenging for some caretakers. The education process for caretakers should begin even before the actual surgery. This allows for careful setting of expectations as well as expediting the learning process.[8] In addition to traditional education, Ng and colleagues in the

United Kingdom has found that strategic use of technology and social media can be an effective method for disseminating educational materials.[29]

As with medical providers, simulation has been shown to be an effective tool for educating caregivers. Dorton and colleagues found that a 30-minute lecture followed by a 90-minute simulation session significant improved caregivers' knowledge as well as comfort levels. One of the specific deficiencies identified during the simulation was delayed recognition of a plugged or dislodged tracheostomy tube.[30] Future efforts and advances with caretaker education will likely center around simulation for not only routine tracheostomy care but also with emergency situations.

Tracking Outcomes

Standardization and process improvement lead to quality improvement. However, it is important to track outcomes overtime to assess these standards and processes to continue improving. The GTC recommended hospitals to track patient-level data in a prospective manner to allow the MDT to benchmark their outcomes over time and assess the impact of their initiatives.[1] At our institution, Children's Medical Center Dallas, we have instituted a "balanced scorecard" to track performance measures and ensure quality. This links performance to outcomes by tracking 4 perspectives: clinical excellence, operation excellence, exceptional experience, and financial strength. Performance is monitored monthly and adjustments in response to these perspectives allow us to continuously provide quality care for our patients.

Improving Outcomes

Improving patient safety is a broad term, and it is defined differently by every institution. As encouraged by the GTC, the preferred method of doing this is to create a prospective registry of tracheostomy patients. That registry is maintained in a prospective manner as events occur, and then retrospective analysis allows for tracking of outcomes. There are many studies that discuss the positive effects of their institution's MDT but outcome measures vary. Common outcome measures include reduction of TRAE, reduction of morbidity, improved staff and caregiver education, reduction of subsequent emergency room visits and admissions, and costs.

Chorney and colleagues retrospectively reviewed a prospective registry. They identified 239 patients who underwent tracheostomy during this time. They compared process and outcome measures from before and after implementation of an MDT team. The mean time to first education class for families was significantly improved from 13.7 to 1.9 days, and the rate of SLP consultations significantly improved from 68% to 95%. The average length of stay (LOS) was significant improved from 133 to 96 days, and costs were significantly less for hospital stays less than 90 days. Cost and LOS were also significantly affected by patient complexity (sepsis, major cardiac surgery, or need for total parenteral nutrition).[8]

McKeon and colleagues also had a prospective registry and had 700 patients. They implemented an MDT, and the main outcomes were reduction of TRAEs and standardization of tracheostomy supplies with distribution of tracheostomy "go-bags." As part of the MDT, they had monthly multidisciplinary meetings and outpatient clinic. They held twice-monthly inpatient tracheostomy rounds. Reported TRAEs were decreased by 43%, and they found that caretakers were more likely to have the correct tracheostomy supplies when traveling with their "go-bags."[27]

Abode and colleagues identified 123 patients with tracheostomies in their airway center. Their main goals were to decrease postoperative LOS, improve communication between caretakers and providers, and improve successful decannulation rate. They found that enhanced caretaker and hospital staff education and weekly care

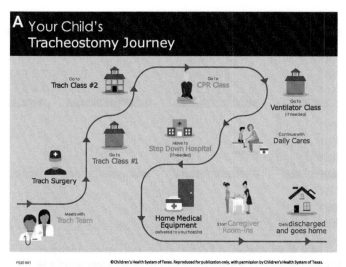

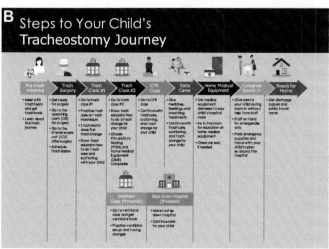

Fig. 1. (A) Tracheostomy journey map showing each step in a child's journey from tracheostomy to discharge. (B) More detailed information on each step in the above journey map. © Children's Health System of Texas. Reproduced for publication only, with permission by Children's Health System of Texas.

conferences were able to decrease average postoperative LOS from 37 to 26 days. Institutional protocols were implemented to standardize airway surveillance and the decannulation process. Adherence to these protocols improved successful decannulation rate from 68% to 86%.[7]

To date, most of the pediatric studies have been limited to single-institution experiences. In addition, every institution's implementation of an MDT may vary slightly, and the outcome measures they look for may vary as well. As more institutions publish their findings, systematic reviews and meta-analyses will be helpful in determining what outcome measures and quality improvement initiatives are positively impacted by the implementation of an MDT.

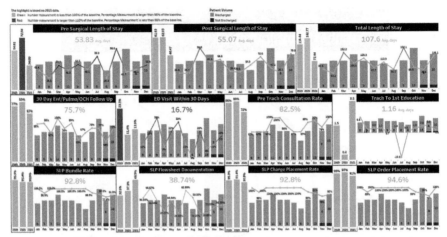

Fig. 2. An example of the Children's Health Airway Management Program balanced scorecard. Multiple clinical metrics are shown with the colored bar graphs to the left of each metric showing year-to-year averages. The line graph details month-to-month averages across a 12-month period.

In addition to individual institutions, the GTC has an ongoing patient database for all participating institutions. The goal is to increase the volume of patients to further power studies and quality improvement initiatives. There was some initial concern from multiple institutions regarding the burden of participating and the perceived benefit to their institution. Lavin and colleagues showed that database entry was straightforward and took less than 5 minutes per patient.[31]

Our Experience

The Children's Medical Center of Dallas formally started an MDT in 2018. The team now consists of 3 otolaryngologists, a nurse specialist, 2 RTs, 2 SLPs, 1 RN, a medical assistant, and a program coordinator. The overall goals of the group have been to improve safety while decreasing costs for these complex children. In the first year of implementation, we showed a significantly decreased LOS (from 133 to 96 days) and decreased total costs for admissions less than 90 days. One of the key components to this has been improved caregiver education and streamlining of the tracheostomy process to facilitate discharge from the hospital after tracheostomy. A journey map was created for caregivers, which can be found in **Fig. 1**.

Another driver for improvement for our team is a scorecard to track our clinical and financial metrics. This can be sorted by year and is compared with a baseline, which was set in 2015. This allows us to look back throughout the year to see if there are opportunities for improvement in our processes. An example of the scorecard can be found in **Fig. 2**.

SUMMARY

Advances in neonatal and pediatric cardiac care have evolved indications for pediatric tracheostomy. This has created a population of medically complex children with tracheostomies. These children are at high risk of adverse events due to their underlying comorbidities, inherent risks of tracheostomy, incomplete caretaker and hospital staff education, and lack of equipment. The Global Tracheostomy Collective was formed in

2012 to provide an international organizing structure for quality improvement initiatives. They proposed 5 key action items with one being implementation of an MDT team. Multiple single-institution studies have shown improvement in process and clinical outcomes after implementation of a multidisciplinary tracheostomy team in children. As more institutions publish their findings, future meta-analysis and systematic reviews should be done to further evaluate the benefit of MDT teams.

CLINICS CARE POINTS

- Children with tracheostomy are a vulnerable population for several reasons and are at a higher risk for adverse events.
- Multidisciplinary tracheostomy teams are a valuable resource that can improve the quality of care for children with tracheostomies by increasing patient safety and decreasing overall costs.
- Expertise and skills from multiple disciplines and allied health professionals is crucial in the care of children with tracheostomies.

DISCLOSURE

The authors have no financial disclosures or conflicts of interest. No additional sources of funding.

REFERENCES

1. Brenner MJ, Pandian V, Milliren CE, et al. Global Tracheostomy Collaborative: data-driven improvements in patient safety through multidisciplinary teamwork, standardisation, education, and patient partnership. Br J Anaesth 2020;125(1): e104–18.
2. Swift AC, Rogers JH. The changing indications for tracheostomy in children. J Laryngol Otol 1987;101(12):1258–62.
3. Gergin O, Adil EA, Kawai K, et al. Indications of pediatric tracheostomy over the last 30 years: Has anything changed? Int J Pediatr Otorhinolaryngol 2016;87: 144–7.
4. Ozmen S, Ozmen OA, Unal OF. Pediatric tracheotomies: a 37-year experience in 282 children. Int J Pediatr Otorhinolaryngol 2009;73(7):959–61.
5. Zenk J, Fyrmpas G, Zimmermann T, et al. Tracheostomy in young patients: indications and long-term outcome. Eur Arch Otorhinolaryngol 2009;266(5):705–11.
6. Smith MM, Benscoter D, Hart CK. Pediatric tracheostomy care updates. Curr Opin Otolaryngol Head Neck Surg 2020;28(6):425–9.
7. Abode KA, Drake AF, Zdanski CJ, et al. A Multidisciplinary Children's Airway Center: Impact on the Care of Patients With Tracheostomy. Pediatrics 2016;137(2): e20150455.
8. Chorney SR, Brown AF, Brooks RL, et al. Pediatric Tracheostomy Outcomes After Development of a Multidisciplinary Airway Team: A Quality Improvement Initiative. OTO Open 2021;5(3). 2473974X211045615.
9. Brown C, Shah GB, Mitchell RB, et al. The Incidence of Pediatric Tracheostomy and Its Association Among Black Children. Otolaryngol Head Neck Surg 2021; 164(1):206–11.

10. Muller RG, Mamidala MP, Smith SH, et al. Incidence, Epidemiology, and Outcomes of Pediatric Tracheostomy in the United States from 2000 to 2012. Otolaryngol Head Neck Surg 2019;160(2):332–8.

11. McGrath BA, Thomas AN. Patient safety incidents associated with tracheostomies occurring in hospital wards: a review of reports to the UK National Patient Safety Agency. Postgrad Med J 2010;86(1019):522–5.

12. Bedwell JR, Pandian V, Roberson DW, et al. Multidisciplinary Tracheostomy Care: How Collaboratives Drive Quality Improvement. Otolaryngol Clin North Am 2019; 52(1):135–47.

13. Mirski MA, Pandian V, Bhatti N, et al. Safety, efficiency, and cost-effectiveness of a multidisciplinary percutaneous tracheostomy program. Crit Care Med 2012; 40(6):1827–34.

14. Cetto R, Arora A, Hettige R, et al. Improving tracheostomy care: a prospective study of the multidisciplinary approach. Clin Otolaryngol 2011;36(5):482–8.

15. Bonvento B, Wallace S, Lynch J, et al. Role of the multidisciplinary team in the care of the tracheostomy patient. J Multidiscip Healthc 2017;10:391–8.

16. Crosbie R, Cairney J, Calder N. The tracheostomy clinical nurse specialist: an essential member of the multidisciplinary team. J Laryngol Otol 2014;128(2): 171–3.

17. Mĺkva M, Prajová V, Yakimovich B, et al. Standardization – One of the Tools of Continuous Improvement. Proced Eng 2016;149:329–32.

18. Mitchell RB, Hussey HM, Setzen G, et al. Clinical consensus statement: tracheostomy care. Otolaryngol Head Neck Surg 2013;148(1):6–20.

19. Chorney SR, Patel RC, Boyd AE, et al. Timing the First Pediatric Tracheostomy Tube Change: A Randomized Controlled Trial. Otolaryngol Head Neck Surg 2021;164(4):869–76.

20. Jaryszak EM, Shah RK, Amling J, et al. Pediatric tracheotomy wound complications: incidence and significance. Arch Otolaryngol Head Neck Surg 2011; 137(4):363–6.

21. Baker LR, Chorney SR. Reducing Pediatric Tracheostomy Wound Complications: An Evidence-Based Literature Review. Adv Skin Wound Care 2020;33(6):324–8.

22. Bitners AC, Burton WB, Yang CJ. Retrospective comparison of Velcro® and twill tie outcomes following pediatric tracheotomy. Int J Pediatr Otorhinolaryngol 2019; 116:192–5.

23. Hart CK, Tawfik KO, Meinzen-Derr J, et al. A randomized controlled trial of Velcro versus standard twill ties following pediatric tracheotomy. Laryngoscope 2017; 127(9):1996–2001.

24. Yelverton JC, Nguyen JH, Wan W, et al. Effectiveness of a standardized education process for tracheostomy care. Laryngoscope 2015;125(2):342–7.

25. Uyan ZS, Atag E, Ergenekon AP, et al. Efficacy of standardized tracheostomy training with a simulation model for healthcare providers: A study by ISPAT team. Pediatr Pulmonol 2022;57(2):418–26.

26. Kohn J, McKeon M, Munhall D, et al. Standardization of pediatric tracheostomy care with "Go-bags. Int J Pediatr Otorhinolaryngol 2019;121:154–6.

27. McKeon M, Kohn J, Munhall D, et al. Association of a Multidisciplinary Care Approach With the Quality of Care After Pediatric Tracheostomy. JAMA Otolaryngol Head Neck Surg 2019;145(11):1035–42.

28. Gaudreau PA, Greenlick H, Dong T, et al. Preventing Complications of Pediatric Tracheostomy Through Standardized Wound Care and Parent Education. JAMA Otolaryngol Head Neck Surg 2016;142(10):966–71.

29. Ng FK, Wallace S, Coe B, et al. From smartphone to bed-side: exploring the use of social media to disseminate recommendations from the National Tracheostomy Safety Project to front-line clinical staff. Anaesthesia 2020;75(2):227–33.
30. Dorton LH, Lintzenich CR, Evans AK. Simulation model for tracheotomy education for primary health-care providers. Ann Otol Rhinol Laryngol 2014; 123(1):11–8.
31. Lavin J, Shah R, Greenlick H, et al. The Global Tracheostomy Collaborative: one institution's experience with a new quality improvement initiative. Int J Pediatr Otorhinolaryngol 2016;80:106–8.

Complex Head and Neck Resection, Reconstruction, and Rehabilitation in Children

Amy L. Dimachkieh, MD*, Daniel C. Chelius, MD

KEYWORDS

- Pediatric • Head and neck • Tumor • Cancer • Ablation • Reconstruction
- Rehabilitation

KEY POINTS

- Pediatric head and neck tumors are uniquely challenging because of their complex 3-dimensional anatomy and the need to balance oncologic goals with functional morbidity.
- Multidisciplinary preoperative consultations include speech and language pathology for voice, swallowing, tracheostomy education, hearing, dental, and psychosocial assessments, in addition to ablative and reconstructive surgical teams.
- Intraoperative surgical planning considers airway interventions including short-term tracheostomy use as well as ventilating ear tube placement and nasolacrimal duct stenting.
- Reconstruction in pediatric patients should consider virtual surgical planning, future growth, nerve reconstruction, and dental restoration options.
- Free flap reconstruction can be used safely and effectively in children to restore craniofacial form and function.

INTRODUCTION

Pediatric head and neck tumors are uncommon but the consequences of radical resection are extensive. These tumors, benign and malignant, are uniquely challenging because of their proximity to critical functional and neurovascular structures and intimately affect speech, swallowing, voice, breathing, hearing, and vision. In addition, the psychosocial and emotional trauma from the cosmetic and functional consequences can be enduring. Their relative rarity limits surgeon experience and requires a focused effort to develop individual and programmatic expertise. A practiced

Disclosure: Dr A.L. Dimachkieh has no financial interests to disclose. Disclosure: D.C. Dr Chelius has a stipend and key leadership position with the American Academy of Otolaryngology Head and Neck Surgery as the Coordinator of the Annual Meeting.
Texas Children's Hospital – Pediatric Otolaryngology, Baylor College of Medicine – Otolaryngology, Head and Neck Surgery, 6701 Fannin Street, Suite 640, Houston, TX 77030, USA
* Corresponding author.
E-mail address: aldimach@texaschildrens.org

Otolaryngol Clin N Am 55 (2022) 1205–1214
https://doi.org/10.1016/j.otc.2022.07.018
0030-6665/22/© 2022 Elsevier Inc. All rights reserved.

oto.theclinics.com

multidisciplinary team can facilitate smooth preoperative evaluations, efficient coordinated operative procedures, comprehensive rehabilitation, and recovery, as well as optimal oncologic outcomes.

Primary considerations

There is an extensive range of tumors, benign and malignant, odontogenic and nonodontogenic, which cause swelling of the head and neck in children and young adults (**Table 1**). The treatments range from observation to medical management, curettage, and radical resection. The morbidity of aggressive treatment in children must be balanced with the risk of recurrence over the lifespan of our young patients. Though this list is far from complete, there are some pathologies that deserve special consideration.

Desmoid Tumors

Desmoid tumors are rare, benign, locally aggressive, and infiltrative tumors. They typically occur in children younger than 11 years and equally in male and female patients. Tumor genetics may reveal sporadic desmoid tumor with β-catenin mutation (*CTNNB1*) or familial adenomatous polyposis (FAP)-associated desmoids with a mutation in chromosome 5 associated with the APC gene.[1] Desmoid tumors of the head and neck typically appear as a painless mass adjacent to the mandible or cervical region but may also be found in the skull base or parapharyngeal regions. The diagnosis is challenging and either open biopsy or core needle biopsy is recommended. Open biopsy is preferred to perform tumor mutational analyses.[2] Historically, surgical treatment has been preferred with negative microscopic margins. However, this treatment plan is particularly difficult in the head and neck because of the extreme risk of cosmetic and/or functional deficits either from local tumor infiltration of critical head and neck structures or iatrogenic from aggressive surgical resection. More recent studies suggest that resection margins do not clearly correlate to prognosis and recurrence rates after surgical resection are high (20–70%).[3] Currently, the global Desmoid Tumor Working Group recommends an initial period of active surveillance with close-interval imaging and if aggressive tumor progression occurs, escalating treatment to medical treatment (conventional chemotherapy, antihormonal therapies, nonsteroidal anti-inflammatory drugs, or tyrosine kinase inhibitors) or surgical resection or radiation therapy.[2] Overall, there is a lack of evidence for a specific treatment algorithm and the current trend is shifting to a more conservative approach, with active surveillance and medical therapies when indicated.

Osteosarcoma, ewing sarcoma, and chondrosarcoma

Sarcomas are the most common primary bone tumor in children but rarely affect the head and neck. Owing to the low incidence, treatment paradigms often group these tumors with other pediatric head and neck malignancies or other subsite sarcomas. The incidence of bony sarcomas is increased in children with tumor predisposition syndromes or a history of head and neck radiation. Aggressive primary surgical resection with wide margins is preferred for maximum survival benefit but this is difficult in the pediatric head and neck because of the proximity of critical neurovascular structures, smaller pediatric anatomy, and cosmetic and functional morbidities.[4] Multimodality therapy is used in the treatment of bony sarcomas, but disease-specific survival is highest with surgery alone, reflecting the survival benefit of surgically resectable tumors.[5]

Rhabdomyosarcoma

Rhabdomyosarcoma is classified as a soft tissue sarcoma and is one of the most common tumors of childhood. The head and neck is a common site and tumors are

Table 1
Differential diagnosis of pediatric mandible and maxillary tumors

Benign	Malignant	Dental Tumors
Juvenile ossifying fibroma	Osteosarcoma[a]	Ameloblastoma
Osteoma	Chondrosarcoma[a]	Dentigerous cyst
Osteoblastoma	Malignant ameloblastoma	Keratocystic odotogenic tumor
Desmoid fibromatosis	Ewing sarcoma[a]	Adenomatoid odontogenic tumor
Desmoid tumor	Squamous cell carcinoma[a]	Calcifying epithelial odontogenic tumor
Desmoplastic fibroma	Rhabdomyosarcoma (invasion)[a]	Squamous odontogenic tumor
Fibromyxoma	Metastases[a]	Odontoma
Central Giant Cell Granuloma		Ameloblastic fibroma
Fibrous dysplasia		Ameloblastic fibrosarcoma[a]
Teratoma		Odontogenic myxoma
Lymphangioma		Cementoblastoma
Vascular tumor		Odontogenic fibroma
		Odontogenic fibromyxoma

[a] Malignancy.

bimodal in incidence, occurring most frequently in children younger than 5 years and adolescents aged 10 to 18 years.[6] Rhabdomyosarcoma is divided into the following categories: (1) embryonal, (2) alveolar, and (3) pleomorphic. This categorization is crucial for prognosis, with alveolar-type carrying the worst prognosis. Beyond histology, molecular diagnostics assessing for common tumor mutations also carry significant impact on prognosis, with the FOX-01 driver mutation leading to decreased survival and shortened disease-free intervals.[7] Treatment is multimodal and tumors are grouped based on resectability: group I is completely resected with clear microscopic margins, group II is gross tumor resection with residual microscopic disease, group III is gross residual disease or biopsy only, and group IV is distant metastases at presentation. Aggressive surgery is used in the head and neck for salvage when there is residual disease to reduce the radiation dose and long-term side effects, but often radiation therapy is necessary for group II patients or higher.[8]

Odontogenic Tumors
Many destructive masses of the mandible or maxilla are of odontogenic origin. Although MRI may help delineate the solid or cystic nature of the mass, a computed tomography scan is often equivocal or misleading. Cystic odontogenic cysts may be benign, such as odontogenic keratocyst, eruption cyst, and unicystic ameloblastoma. Odontogenic malignances include malignant ameloblastoma, ameloblastic fibroma, and odontogenic myxoma. Diagnosis typically requires open biopsy and treatment may range from observation to enucleation and curettage, to segmental resection.[9,10] Multidisciplinary care is necessary with experienced pathology, oral surgery, otolaryngology, and reconstructive surgery to ensure the care plan is neither overly conservative nor too aggressive.

PREOPERATIVE PLANNING

Multidisciplinary care relies on consistent and complete communication between services. Consultations with ablative and reconstruction teams include head and neck surgery, craniofacial and plastic surgery, oncology, neurosurgery, ophthalmology, dental surgery, anesthesia, speech and language pathology, child life, and social work. Clinical nursing and surgical coordinators are invaluable patient contacts to help coordinate visits when possible because of the extensive time burden of these consultations and associated imaging studies.

Surgical timing is very difficult in complex cases and is multifactorial. Early discussion between ablative and reconstruction teams initiates virtual surgical planning (VSP) when indicated, as these implants typically require 1-2 weeks for design and fabrication. In addition, many oncology patients require local control with surgical resection at a specific interval following induction chemotherapy treatments. Finally, coordinating multiple surgeons and surgical teams is always challenging. For this reason, we recommend a consistent team that is practiced and well-coordinated.

We employ a short preoperative planning session the week before the procedure with the entire intraoperative team: anesthesiology, nursing and scrub technician teams, and surgeons. The COVID-19 pandemic prompted us to switch to virtual meetings, which has allowed more regular and complete attendance. We find these meetings to be feasible and highly effective in ensuring a well-coordinated case. The team agrees and publishes a written plan that confirms the sequence of procedures, room setup, possibility of simultaneous tumor extirpation and free flap harvest, availability of all instruments and implants, specimen handoff with anticipation of frozen section analyses, perioperative disposition, and the need for staged procedures or adjuvant therapy. **Table 2** and **Fig. 1** are examples from the preoperative plan for surgical case 1.

SURGICAL CASES
Case 1: Maxilla

A 13-month-old infant boy was evaluated for a rapidly enlarging right facial mass. He underwent evaluation by oncology and otolaryngology and decision was made to proceed with sublabial biopsy which confirmed desmoid fibromatosis. Because of patient age and cosmetic risk of radical resection, decision was made for short-interval observation. Within 3 weeks, the tumor was noted to enlarge, and medical therapy with doxorubicin was initiated. The tumor improved minimally with 3 cycles of doxorubicin and decision was made to proceed with radical resection.

The patient underwent tracheostomy, right total maxillectomy, myringotomy and ventilation tube placement, right nasolacrimal duct stenting, and anterolateral thigh free tissue transfer. He tolerated the procedure well and was transferred to the intensive care unit for flap monitoring and fresh tracheostomy precautions. He did well postoperatively and was decannulated on postoperative day (POD) 15 and discharged home on day 16 with a soft diet. He is doing very well at 9 months after treatment with no evidence of recurrence (**Fig. 2**).

Case 2: Mandible

An 11-year-old girl was referred by the dental service for a rapidly enlarging right mandible tumor. Dental biopsy demonstrated ameloblastoma and pathology was confirmed with in-house pathologist. Decision was made to proceed with segmental resection with VSP. A temporary tracheostomy was placed at the time of the procedure for the perioperative period. Custom cutting guides and reconstruction plates were

Table 2
Example of preoperative planning session

Team	Procedure	Instruments and Equipment
Anesthesiology	Intubate, basic IV access	
Head and neck	Tracheostomy, myringotomy, and ventilating tube	5.0 Cuffed Tracheostomy
Anesthesia and nursing	Turn bed, padding/positioning, central lines, arterial line, and foley	U/S Probe cover
Head and neck Plastic Reconstruction	Tumor resection RIGHT lower ext. free flap preparation	Simultaneous: 2 tables, 2 set ups
	Marginal frozen section, timeout before reconstruction	
Dental, oculoplastics	Dental implant to fibula and/or nasolacrimal duct stenting	
Pathology	Frozen section confirmed	Clean set up
Plastic Reconstruction/ Craniofacial teams	Free flap inset Feeding tube insertion	
Anesthesia and nursing	Transfer to ICU	

designed and used for an osseous-only fibula free flap, which was harvested simultaneous to tumor resection. Dental implants were placed in the fibula before flap transfer and anastomosis to the facial vessels and flap inset. Also, nerve interposition graft was used to reinnervate the proximal inferior alveolar nerve and distal mental nerve segments.

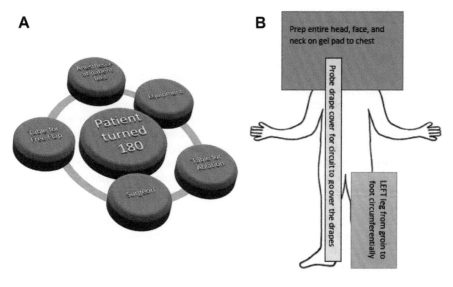

Table & Personnel arrangement   Draping plan

Fig. 1. Example of preoperative planning session figures. (*A*) Table and Personnel arrangement. (*B*) Draping plan.

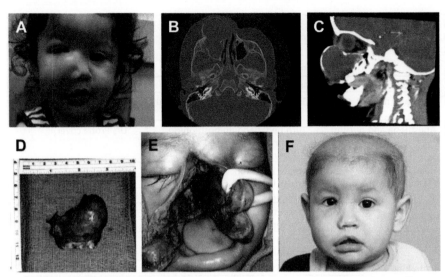

Fig. 2. Maxilla. (*A*) Preoperative photo. (*B*) Axial bone CT scan with large right maxillary tumor. (*C*) Sagittal soft tissue CT scan with large right maxillary tumor exerting inferior pressure on the globe. (*D*) Tumor extirpation. (*E*) Intraoperative surgical defect. (*F*) One-month postoperative photo.

The patient remained in the intensive care unit for recovery and fresh tracheostomy protocol. She was decannulated on POD 9 and discharged home on POD 10. She was tolerating full liquid oral diet at the time of discharge (**Fig. 3**).

Case 3: Neck/Skull Base, Lower Cranial Nerves

A 17-year-old male with a known history of type 1 neurofibromatosis (NF1) presented with a painful, enlarging left neck mass, dysphagia, and voice change. A PET scan showed FDG-avidity. Ultrasound-guided fine needle aspiration demonstrated concerning features for malignant peripheral nerve sheath tumor including high cellularity and loss of S100 IHC expression. He had normal vocal fold mobility on preoperative in-office laryngeal stroboscopy. In anticipation of voice and swallowing compromise following resection, the patient underwent radical neck dissection with transcervical radical tumor resection and sacrifice of the vagus nerve from the clavicle to skull base. Simultaneous recurrent laryngeal nerve (RLN) reinnervation was performed with direct anastomosis of the ipsilateral ansa cervicalis to the RLN, and intraoperative injection of the left vocal fold using carboxymethylcellulose. Final pathology revealed atypical neurofibroma with all lymph nodes demonstrating benign reactive follicular hyperplasia.

He was admitted to the pediatric intensive care unit and transferred to the floor on POD 3. Postoperative videofluoroscopic swallow study showed tracheal aspiration of thin and nectar-thick liquid barium with abundant residual in the piriform sinuses. A gastrostomy tube (G-tube) was placed on POD 17 and he was discharged home on POD 19. He continued to have aspiration of secretions and poor oral feeding. At 5 months postoperatively, he underwent in-office transcervical hyaluronic acid injection. At 6 months, he reported normal voice and was able to tolerate full oral diet without coughing (**Fig. 4**).

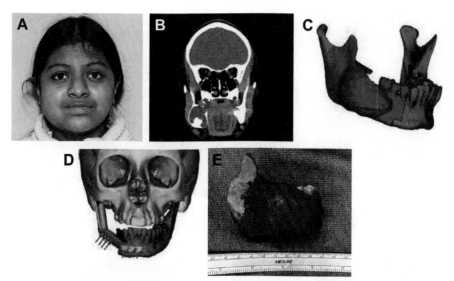

Fig. 3. Mandible. (*A*) Preoperative photo. (*B*) Soft tissue coronal CT scan demonstrating large cystic mass in right hemi mandible. (*C*) Virtual surgical planning images showing planned resection (*red*). (*D*) Virtual surgical planning with custom plate (*teal*), fibula segments (*yellow and green*), and dental implants (*blue posts*). (*E*) Tumor extirpation after segmental mandibulectomy, lateral view, with clear margins on frozen examination.

POSTOPERATIVE CONSIDERATIONS

Careful postoperative management is critical to successful reconstruction of the pediatric head and neck tumor patient. Patients are admitted to the acute care or critical care units with adequate analgesia to minimize risk to the reconstruction. Pediatric patients are often less likely to be compliant with immediate postoperative restrictions. Sedation is used for 24-72 hours if needed in the setting of a fresh free flap anastomosis and fresh tracheostomy. Short-term tracheostomy decannulation protocol may be used to rapidly wean airway support. Daily transtracheal pressure monitoring can be used to guide tracheostomy downsizing and capping trials to ensure safe and timely decannulation before discharge.[11] Experienced pediatric speech and language pathologists are critical for guiding decannulation as well as advancing swallow evaluations and oral feeding and in a concurrent fashion. This optimizes the patient's success for decannulation and full oral diet at the time of discharge. Patients typically spend 5-7 days in the critical care unit and another 5-7 days in the acute care setting.

Other pearls for the care of the pediatric patient are incorporating child life specialists and dedicated occupational and physical therapists in the immediate postoperative period. Children rehabilitate quickly when the patient and caregivers are actively engaged in their recovery. Patients rarely need sustained physical and occupational therapy in the outpatient setting after discharge.

LONG-TERM SURGICAL OUTCOMES AND REHABILITATION

Head and neck tumors in pediatric patients are particularly challenging because of the pathologic variability and rarity of any single pathology. In addition, reconstruction of surgical defects in the growing craniofacial skeleton and the restoration of form and function is more difficult in smaller patients with fewer donor site options, smaller

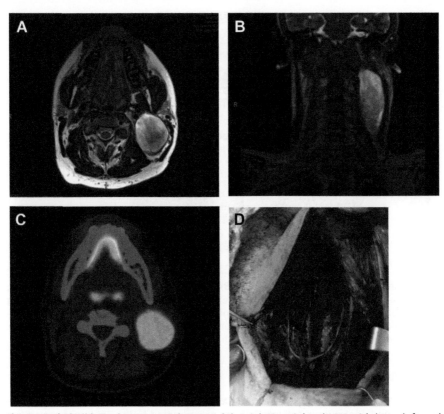

Fig. 4. Neck/skull base, lower cranial nerves. (*A*) Axial T2 weighted MRI with large left neck mass. (*B*) Coronal T2 weighted MRI demonstrating left neck mass extending along carotid space to skull base. (*C*) FDG PET with PET-avid lesion in left neck. (*D*) Intraoperative photo of left ansa-cervicalis post-tumor resection before RLN-ansa anastomoses.

anastomoses, and unpredictable postoperative compliance.[12,13] On the other hand, many pediatric head and neck tumors are benign, and our patients are less likely to have received preoperative chemotherapy and radiation therapy than adult head and neck patients. Overall, there are excellent options and outcomes for reconstruction including free tissue transfers in pediatrics for maxillary, mandibular, and other craniofacial defects.

Free flap reconstruction can be used safely and effectively for pediatric maxillary and mandibular defects with few complications.[10,12,14–19] In one multi-institutional study of pediatric free fibula reconstruction, minor short-term and long-term complications included minor wound dehiscence (7.8%) and cellulitis (4.5%) and lower incidence of major complications of wound infection (6.7%), dehiscence (2.2%), or flap failure (1.1%). Longer-term severe speech deficit was uncommon (6.5%). There were few complications to the donor site as well and no patients required orthopedic intervention as gait and limb length were normal. When compared to adult patients, there were fewer short-term and long-term complications[14] Another study reported an overall success rate of 95.6% for free tissue reconstruction of pediatric head and neck defects.[19] Complications were significantly increased in patients aged 5-9 years, which may be attributed to the smaller vessel size, but this conclusion is limited by the very rare incidence of flap failure.[19]

A primary concern for pediatric mandible and maxilla reconstruction is disruption of the growth of the craniofacial skeleton. Several studies have reported that most free flaps continue to grow in the recipient area.[19–22] Neo-growth of free fibula mandibular reconstruction is greatest when the condyle is preserved, mandible epiphyseal growth plate is preserved, and a younger age, hence greater growth potential of the donor fibula.[20] The growth of the mandibular reconstruction impacts long-term craniofacial development and mandibular symmetry, which is also significantly impacted by dental restoration. Proper dental occlusion encourages symmetric mandibular growth and when done concurrently, patients with dental rehabilitation at the time of free fibula reconstruction do not have long-term craniofacial abnormalities[14] Unfortunately, dental restoration is expensive and financial barriers lead most patients to undergo delayed dental implants.

Additional considerations should be given to peripheral sensory nerve restoration to improve quality of life after radical mandible resection. There is a growing trend and convincing evidence that immediate inferior alveolar nerve allograft reconstruction results in complete functional sensory recovery in pediatric patients.[23]

SUMMARY

Pediatric head and neck tumors are uniquely challenging because of the diagnostic diversity, small patient anatomy, and potential risks to their long-term growth and development. Although most tumors of the pediatric head and neck are benign, all head and neck tumors deserve detailed attention. Longitudinal experience within a focused team will allow a more accurate understanding of true morbidity to inform comprehensive oncologic planning discussions. Multidisciplinary care with oncology, otolaryngology, reconstructive surgery, and oral surgery affords the greatest opportunity for the best oncologic, cosmetic, and functional outcomes.

CLINICS CARE POINTS

- Pediatric head and neck tumors are diagnostically diverse and require thoughtful multidisciplinary evaluation and treatment.
- Complex pediatric head and neck resection and reconstruction can be safe and effective with detailed consideration to oncologic, cosmetic and functional outcomes.

REFERENCES

1. Zhao C, Domborwski N, Perez-Atayde A, et al. Desmoid tumors of the head and neck in the pediatric population: Has anything changed? Int J Pediatr Otorhinolaryngol 2021;140:110511.
2. Alman B, Attia S, Baumgarten C, et al. Desmoid Tumor Working Group. The management of desmoid tumors: a joint global consensus-based guideline approach for adult and paediatric patients. Eur J Cancer 2020;127:96–107.
3. Paul A, Blouin M, Minard-Colin V, et al. Desmoid-type fibromatosis of the head and neck in children: a changing situation. Int J Pediatr Otorhinolaryngol 2019; 123:33–7.
4. Brady J, Chung S, Marchiano E, et al. Pediatric head and neck bone sarcomas: an analysis of 204 cases. Int J Pediatr Otorhinolaryngol 2017;100:71–6.
5. Peng K, Grogan T, Wang M. Head and neck sarcomas: analysis of the SEER database. Otolaryngol Head Neck Surg 2014;151:627–33.

6. Qaisi M, Eid I. Pediatric head and neck malignancies. Oral Maxillofacial Surg Clin N Am 2016;29:11–9.

7. Rudzinski E, Anderson J, Chi Y, et al. Histology, fusion status, and outcome in metastatic rhabdomyosarcoma: a report from the Children's Oncology Group. Pediatr Blood Cancer 2017;64. https://doi.org/10.1002/pbc.26645.

8. Pappo A, Meza J, Donaldson S, et al. Treatment of localized nonorbital, nonparameningeal head and neck rhabdomyosarcoma: lessons learned from intergroup rhabdomyosarcoma studies III and IV. J Clin Oncol 2003;21:638–45.

9. Trosman S, Krakovitz P. Pediatric maxillary and mandibular tumors. Otolaryngol Clin North Am 2015;48:101–19.

10. George AP, Markiewicz M, Garzib S, et al. Adolescent and young adult oral maxillofacial tumors: a single-institution case series and literature review. J Adolesc Young Adult Oncol 2020;9:307–12.

11. You P, Dimachkieh A, Yu J, et al. Decannulation protocol for short term tracheostomy in pedatiric head and neck tumor patients. Int J Pediatr Otorhinolaryngol 2022;153:111012.

12. Dempsey R, Chelius D, Pederson W, et al. Pediatric craniofacial oncologic reconstruction. Clin Plast Surg 2019;46:261–73.

13. Hanasono M, Hofstede T. Craniofacial reconstruction following oncologic resection. Neurosurg Clin N Am 2013;24:111–24.

14. Slijepcevic A, Wax M, Hanasono M, et al. Post-operative outcomes in pediatric patients following facial reconstruction with fibula free flaps. Laryngoscope 2022. https://doi.org/10.1002/lary.30219. Online ahead of print.

15. Abramowicz S, Goudy S, Mitchell C, et al. A protocol for resection and immediate reconstruction of pediatric mandibles using microvascular free fibula flaps. J Oral Maxillofac Surg 2021;79:475–82.

16. Abrahams J, McCLure S. Pediatric odontogenic tumors. Oral Maxillofacial Surg Clin N Am 2016;28:45–58.

17. Perry K, Tkaczuk A, Caccamese J, et al. Tumors of the pediatric maxillofacial skeleton: a 20-year clinical study. JAMA Otolaryngol Head Neck Surg 2015;141:40–4.

18. Abramowicz S, Goldwaser B, Troulis M, et al. Primary jaw tumors in children. J Oral Maxillofac Surg 2013;71:47–52.

19. Liu S, Zhang W, Yao Yu, et al. Free flap transfer for pediatric head and neck reconstruction: What factors influence flap survival? Laryngoscope 2019;129:1915021.

20. Mertens F, Dormaar J, Poorten V, et al. Objectifying growth of vascularized bone transfers after mandibular reconstruction in the pediatric population. J Plant Reconstr Aesthet Surg 2021;74:1973–83.

21. Phillips J, Rechner B, Tompson B. Mandibular growth following reconstruction using free fibula graft in the pediatric facial skeleton. Plast Reconstr Surg 2005;116:419–24.

22. Temiz G, Bilkay U, Tiftikcioglu Y, et al. The evaluation of flap growth and long-term results of pedaitric mandible reconsrucitons using free fibular flaps. Microsurgery 2015;35:253–61.

23. Miloro M, Zuniga J. Does immediate inferior alveolar nerve allograft reconstruction result in functional sensory recovery in pediatric patients? J Oral Maxillofac Surg 2020;78:2073–9.

Update on Vascular Anomalies of the Head and Neck

Tara L. Rosenberg, MD[a],*, James D. Phillips, MD[b]

KEYWORDS

- Vascular anomalies • Vascular tumor • Vascular malformation
- Congenital vascular lesion • Hemangioma • Lymphatic malformation
- Venous malformation • Arteriovenous malformation

KEY POINTS

- The most common vascular tumor is infantile hemangioma.
- Problematic and high-risk infantile hemangiomas should be treated early to help prevent/ treat complications.
- The management of complex vascular malformations is often multimodal, and patients should be referred to a multidisciplinary vascular anomalies center.
- More high-quality outcomes research is needed to help identify the best, most effective modality/modalities for each specific vascular malformation.
- The genetic understanding of vascular malformations is advancing, with effective targeted therapies becoming available for patients with known genetic mutations.

INTRODUCTION

Vascular anomalies have been classified as vascular tumors and vascular malformations since 1982, when a pivotal article written by Mulliken and Glowacki[1] was published. Infantile hemangiomas are the most common vascular tumor. Vascular malformations are less common and can involve capillaries, veins, lymphatic vessels, arteries, or a combination of these, and their "best" modality of treatment is highly variable depending on the lesion (size and location), expert opinions, and experience. High-quality outcomes data are not yet available. The field of vascular anomalies has continued to grow and evolve, with the most recent advances in the field of genetics and molecular biology.

---

[a] Texas Children's Hospital/Baylor College of Medicine, 6701 Fannin Street, Suite D.0640.00, Houston, TX 77030, USA; [b] Monroe Carell Jr Children's Hospital at Vanderbilt, 2200 Children's Way, DOT 7, Nashville, TN 37232, USA
* Corresponding author.
E-mail address: tlrosenb@texaschildrens.org

Otolaryngol Clin N Am 55 (2022) 1215–1231
https://doi.org/10.1016/j.otc.2022.07.019
0030-6665/22/© 2022 Elsevier Inc. All rights reserved.

oto.theclinics.com

VASCULAR TUMORS
Infantile Hemangioma

Infantile hemangioma is the most common vascular tumor and the most common tumor of infancy (4%–5% of infants). Approximately 60% occur on the head and neck. The diagnosis of infantile hemangiomas is usually established by history and physical examination. They can be deep, superficial, or compound (with both deep and superficial components). An abdominal ultrasound is recommended when a patient has 5 or more cutaneous hemangiomas owing to their increased risk of concomitant liver hemangioma.[2,3] The biomolecular marker GLUT1 is strongly expressed in infantile hemangiomas. Therefore, it is useful in pathologic analysis to distinguish infantile hemangiomas from other vascular anomalies.[4]

Infantile hemangiomas generally follow a clinical course of proliferation (active growth phase) and later involution (regression of tumor). However, there is variation in the duration, rate, and degree of growth and involution. During the first few weeks of life, proliferation begins, and most infantile hemangiomas are first noticed. Most rapid growth occurs from 1 to 3 months of age. Maximum size is typically reached by 5 months of age.[5,6] The time of onset of the slow, gradual involutionary phase is variable. After about 3 to 4 years of age, most infantile hemangiomas do not change significantly.[2,7,8] The appearance after involution varies considerably between patients. In many patients, involution results in the return to normal skin. However, up to 40% of patients have residual skin changes, such as telangiectasias, fibrofatty tissue, laxity, or scarring.[7] These patients may warrant consideration for treatment because of their continued deformity.

High-Risk Head and Neck Infantile Hemangiomas

High-risk areas for infantile hemangiomas include airway, facial segmental, ear, lip, nose, and periocular, and lesions in these locations should be evaluated and treated early to prevent complications as much as possible (eg, airway compromise, disfigurement, ulceration, visual loss). One may miss the opportunity to treat before the onset of complications if a clinical observation or a "wait-and-see" approach is followed.[2]

PHACE Syndrome and Beard Distribution Infantile Hemangiomas

Infants with large segmental infantile hemangiomas (typically >5 cm) of the face, scalp, or neck are about 30% at risk for having PHACE syndrome[2,9–11] (**Table 1**). As clinical experience is gathered, the consequences of PHACE as patients age are better understood. More than 50% of patients with PHACE syndrome have long-term neurologic sequelae, such as stroke, seizures, developmental delay, migraines, and/or hearing loss.[12]

Segmental hemangiomas (**Fig. 1**) undergo an extended proliferative phase, do not completely regress, and are at higher risk for ulceration and scarring.[10] When PHACE syndrome is suspected, referral should be made for an ophthalmology evaluation, echocardiogram, and an MRI with and without contrast and magnetic resonance angiography (MRA) of the head and neck (including the origin of the aortic arch). Diagnostic criteria and consensus statements for the care of patients with PHACE syndrome have been established.[13]

Infantile hemangiomas in a beard distribution involve the chin, jawline, and preauricular areas. About 65% of patients with beard distribution hemangiomas have airway involvement,[14] most commonly in the subglottic and/or supraglottic regions.

Nose, Lip, Ear, and Periocular Infantile Hemangiomas

Nearly 16% of facial hemangiomas involve the nose.[15] The nasal tip is a common location, and growth of the hemangioma here distorts nasal anatomy and affects the

Table 1
PHACE syndrome: list of constellations of anomalies

PHACE	Anomalies	Risk
Posterior fossa anomalies	Cerebellar anomalies (Dandy-Walker malformation)	Developmental delay Pituitary dysfunctions
Hemangioma	Large facial hemangioma >5 cm, large-bearded distribution, shoulder, neck, back	Disfigurement, airway lesion, ulceration
Arterial	Cerebrovascular anomalies of major vessels: dysplasia, stenosis/ occlusion, hypoplasia/aplasia, aberrant origin, saccular aneurysm Persistent embryonic arteries	Progressive arterial occlusion Stroke Other neurologic issues
Cardiac	Aortic arch anomalies, including coarctation of the aorta, aortic dysplasia, aberrant subclavian artery, right-sided aortic arch, ventricular septal defect, atrial septal defect	Congenital heart disease requiring surgical repair
Eye	Microphthalmos, retinal vascular abnormalities, persistent fetal retinal vessels, exophthalmos, coloboma, and optic nerve atrophy	Visual loss

From Adams DM, Ricci KW. Infantile Hemangiomas in the Head and Neck Region. Otolaryngol Clin North Am. 2018 Feb;51(1):77-87. https://doi.org/10.1016/j.otc.2017.09.009. PMID: 29217069.

alignment of the nasal cartilage. Multimodality treatment is often used: some combination of oral propranolol, systemic steroid, intralesional steroid injection, pulsed-dye laser (PDL) therapy, and/or surgery[16] involving a variety of surgical technique options.[17] Lip hemangiomas are more likely to ulcerate (can cause pain and difficulty feeding in infants) and typically involute slowly. They are more likely to result in skin changes and scarring. Disfigurement and ulceration with destruction of the auricle

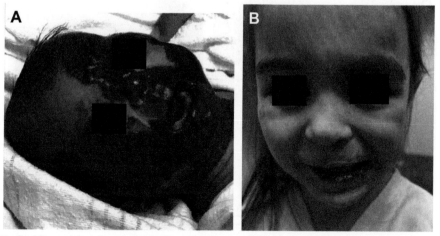

Fig. 1. Bilateral facial segmental infantile hemangioma. (*A*) At 4 weeks of age before treatment and (*B*) at 5 years of age after oral propranolol therapy and serial PDL treatments.

can occur in lesions of the pinna. If the external auditory canal is blocked, it can cause a conductive hearing loss.

Periocular hemangiomas (ie, upper eyelid, lower eyelid, or retrobulbar area) have the potential for ophthalmologic impairment that can quickly lead to amblyopia. Lesions greater than 1 cm in size, involve the upper eyelid, and cause globe displacement or ptosis are associated with higher risk of amblyopia.[18,19] Periocular infantile hemangiomas should have an early ophthalmology examination, and early treatment should be administered.[20]

Treatment of Infantile Hemangiomas

Many uncomplicated focal hemangiomas do not require intervention. However, rapidly proliferating lesions can be problematic and may cause a variety of complications: ulceration, bleeding, airway obstruction, and vision loss. Decisions for management should consider the patient age, rate of growth, location and size of the lesion, and any complications. Immediate treatment is necessary for large segmental hemangiomas, hemangiomas that affect function (ie, breathing or vision), and hemangiomas complicated by ulceration (most common complication). Early intervention is also indicated in those lesions that may leave permanent disfigurement. Complicated hemangiomas may require multimodal therapy. Major therapies currently include pharmacotherapy (eg, oral propranolol or topical timolol or systemic steroids), laser therapy, surgical excision, and intralesional steroid injection (**Fig. 2**). The effect of oral propranolol has been reported (first in 2008), and propranolol has replaced steroids as the first line in medical management.[2,21–23] It is safe and effective for most cutaneous and airway infantile hemangiomas.

The initiation and dosing of oral propranolol are variable, but the 2019 consensus statement on management of infantile hemangiomas is currently a good guide to follow. Some potential side effects of propranolol include hypoglycemia, hypotension, sleep disruption, bradycardia, and wheezing/bronchial reaction.[2]

Lasers (most commonly the PDL) are used in the management of infantile hemangiomas. The wavelength of the PDL targets the chromophore of oxygenated

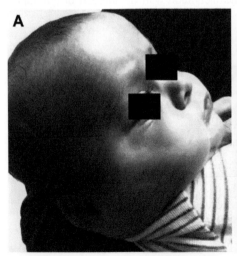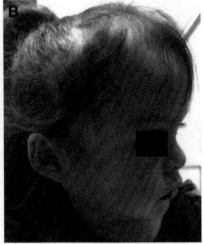

Fig. 2. Deep infantile hemangioma of right parotid. (*A*) At 5 months of age and (*B*) at 2.5 years of age after oral propranolol therapy and serial intralesional kenalog injections.

hemoglobin. Thus, it may be effectively used during involution to selectively remove the residual telangiectasias and during proliferation to promote wound healing of ulcerated hemangiomas that may be refractory to medical management.

Surgical excision of hemangiomas is beneficial in some cases. Hemangiomas that ulcerate, fail medical therapy, and can be excised completely are reasonable candidates for surgical excision. Periorbital hemangiomas that cause functional problems and/or are at high risk of causing amblyopia may be best treated expeditiously with excision, especially if they do not respond immediately to medical therapy. Pedunculated lesions that are unlikely to completely involute are also good candidates to excise. Last, hemangiomas that are disfiguring at a young age or those that result in permanent skin changes or fibrofatty mass around 3 to 4 years of age should be considered for excision. Although the timing for surgery can be controversial, surgical excision should be considered when it is judged that it would lead to a better result than the process of involution or medical therapy. The goal is to strive for the best overall outcome for the patient, including trying to prevent psychosocial distress by treating a disfiguring lesion early.[2]

Airway Hemangiomas

Airway hemangiomas are most identified in the subglottis but can occur in other subsites, such as the supraglottis. They may be focal or have a more diffuse, segmental distribution in the airway. Beard distribution hemangioma, anterior neck hemangiomas, and oral and/or pharyngeal mucosal lesions are at increased risk for airway involvement. Of note, although airway hemangiomas can occur in isolation, about 50% of patients with airway hemangiomas have concomitant cutaneous lesions.[24] Symptoms of airway hemangiomas (eg, progressive biphasic stridor and barky cough) typically begin within the first 2 to 3 months of life and may be mistaken for croup or reactive airway disease. This leads to delay in diagnosis (average age at diagnosis is 4 months).[2,25] When symptomatic, rigid bronchoscopy is typically performed for diagnosis. Subglottic hemangiomas are usually asymmetric, covered by smooth mucosa, and have a red/hypervascular appearance (**Fig. 3**). Subglottic hemangiomas may be treated with intralesional steroid injection at time of rigid bronchoscopy (avoid direct injection near the cricoid plate as cartilage resorption can occur) followed by short-term intubation (24 hours in most cases), initiation of oral propranolol therapy, and short postoperative course of systemic steroids. Open surgical techniques, which

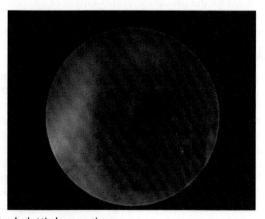

Fig. 3. Right-sided subglottic hemangioma.

would necessitate tracheal/cricoid split and submucosal excision of the hemangioma, are rarely needed. Laser ablation (carbon dioxide [CO_2] and KTP [potassium-titanyl-phosphate]) and microdebrider debulking have been used, but any technique that violates the mucosal barrier risks causing further subglottic stenosis from scarring.[24,25] Tracheotomy is rarely necessary but can be used in refractory cases. A reasonable algorithm (**Fig. 4**) for management of airway hemangiomas has been published and can be considered, although there are variations in management.[26]

Congenital Hemangiomas

Congenital hemangiomas (CHs) differ from infantile hemangiomas in that they are fully formed high-flow lesions at birth and are typically violaceous solitary lesions. They do not undergo postnatal growth. CHs are GLUT1 negative and represent only about 3% of hemangiomas diagnosed in infancy. CHs are divided into subgroups: rapidly involuting congenital hemangiomas (RICHs), noninvoluting congenital hemangiomas (NICHs), and partially involuting congenital hemangiomas (PICHs).[27] RICHs usually involute by about age 12 months and result in a patch of atrophic skin with prominent veins and minimal subcutaneous fat. PICHs undergo partial involution, and NICHs do not involute and may require surgical excision.

Kasabach-Merritt Phenomenon

Kasabach-Merritt phenomenon (KMP) is associated with 2 other vascular tumors: tufted angioma and kaposiform hemangioendothelioma (KHE) (**Fig. 5**). KMP is a rare but possibly life-threatening condition during which the vessels within the tumor entrap platelets. This causes severe functional thrombocytopenia and consumptive coagulopathy. Consensus-derived practice standards for treatment of KHE with or without KMP have been published.[28] More recently, sirolimus has been shown to be a promising treatment option for KHE.[29] If the tumor does not respond to drug treatment, embolization and/or surgical resection may be necessary. Blood products, such as platelets and packed red blood cells, are administered only if necessary, as in cases with active bleeding or before any invasive procedures.[28]

Vascular Malformations

Vascular malformations comprise abnormal blood vessels, and they typically have a slow, indolent course. They are present at birth and often insinuate themselves into normal tissue, making them difficult to eradicate completely. Often the best treatment strategy is management for the alleviation/improvement of symptoms and avoidance of complications. Vascular malformations are classified according to their predominant vessel type: capillary, venous, lymphatic, arterial, or a combination of these.

Diagnostic Considerations

On evaluation of a patient with a suspected vascular malformation, particular attention should be paid to certain elements of the history: the age at which the lesion became evident, rate of growth, fluctuations in color or size, and changes in the lesion temporally related to inflammatory episodes (eg, upper respiratory infection or local trauma). Important elements on physical examination include the extent and color of the lesion, temperature on palpation, presence of vascular markings of the epidermis, presence of pulsations, and compressibility. Fast-flow lesions may emit a bruit on auscultation. Venous malformations (VMs) may engorge and enlarge when in a dependent position.

Radiologic imaging is frequently the next step in diagnosis. Imaging modalities include ultrasound, cross-sectional imaging such as magnetic resonance and computed tomography (both typically with and without contrast), and more advanced

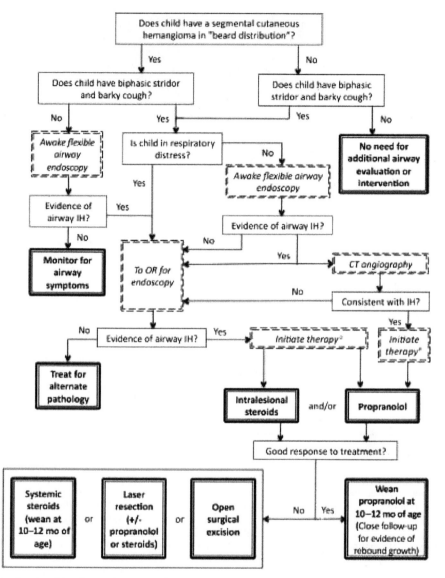

Fig. 4. Algorithm for evaluation and management of airway infantile hemangioma. [a] In rare cases in which expert medical or surgical management is not readily accessible and symptoms are severe, placement of a temporary tracheotomy may be most expedient. OR, operating room; IH, infantile hemangioma. (*From* Darrow DH. Management of Infantile Hemangiomas of the Airway. Otolaryngol Clin North Am. 2018 Feb;51(1):133-146. https://doi.org/10.1016/j.otc.2017.09.001. PMID: 29217058.)

imaging techniques, such as traditional arteriogram and lymphoscintigraphy (**Table 2**). It is often helpful to consult with a diagnostic radiologist or interventional radiologist familiar with vascular malformations to know the best diagnostic strategy. This is particularly important in children, who will often require sedation so as to maximize the diagnostic benefit of any anesthetic exposure.

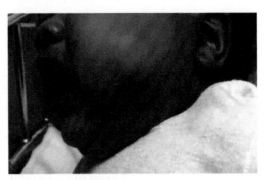

Fig. 5. A 5-month-old girl with left lower facial KHE.

Capillary Malformations

Capillary malformations (CMs) are the most common vascular malformation, consisting of a superficial collection of ectatic vessels in the dermis. Nevus simplex, also known as salmon patches, are pink macules on the forehead, eyelids, nose, and/or occipital region. They may be referred to as "angel kisses" or "stork bites" and generally fade during childhood. Nevus flammeus (also known as port-wine stain [PWS]), however, do not fade, and rather, they persist and gradually become raised, nodular, or darken to a deep red or purple color. PWS occur in 3:1000 newborns and frequently follow the divisions of the trigeminal nerve.[30]

Special consideration for Sturge-Weber syndrome must be made when a facial PWS is present, particularly in the ophthalmic division.[31] These patients must be evaluated for glaucoma and vascular eye abnormalities, as well as central nervous system

Table 2 Imaging characteristics of major vascular anomalies		
	Ultrasound	**MRI**
Hemangiomas (proliferative phase)	Noncompressible hypervascular soft tissue mass with large internal and draining vessels	Avid enhancement with contrast, moderate T2 hyperintensity
Lymphatic malformation (macrocystic)	Compressible, well-defined fluid filled cyst	Low T1, high T2 signal without contrast enhancement. May see fluid-fluid levels with history of hemorrhage into the cyst
Venous malformation	Compressible tubular vascular channels with low flow doppler signal. Enlargement with Valsalva	T2 hyperintense with contrast enhancement. Phleboliths are pathognomonic
Ateriovenous malformation	Ill-defined vascular channels (not a mass) with pulsatile fast flow on Doppler	Infiltrative ill-defined area of vascularity. Flow voids throughout tissue, mild contrast enhancement, and T2 hyperintensity reflective of edema

leptomeningeal involvement. Consultation with ophthalmology and an MRI are appropriate.

PWS may be treated with laser ablation to lighten the discoloration and ultimately to obviate progression to more darkly colored and nodular lesions. PDL, with a wavelength of 595 nm, is typically first line, as it is preferentially absorbed by oxyhemoglobin.[32]

Venous Malformations

VMs are made of localized or diffuse ectatic, abnormal veins. Because of engorgement and localized clotting secondary to turbulent flow, they may cause pain, disfigurement, or compressive symptoms, particularly in the aerodigestive tract.[33] Superficial VMs present as a bluish skin coloration, which is compressible and enlarges when in a dependent position or with Valsalva maneuver. Phleboliths may be palpated as firm nodules or visualized on imaging and are pathognomonic for VMs.[34]

Treatment of VMs depends on the location and associated symptoms.[34] The source of pain within the malformation often arises from phleboliths, which precipitate a local inflammatory response and can thus be treated with nonsteroidal anti-inflammatory medications or anticoagulants. Medical grade compression garments may be prescribed for VMs in the extremities. Consistent usage improves symptoms, as static venous blood is squeezed out of the malformation and not allowed to pool.

Surgical excision may be a good option for focal, accessible lesions. Preoperative embolization with n-butyl cyanoacrylate (NBCA) glue can facilitate these cases by turning an amorphous, difficult-to-control bleeding lesion into a mass that can be manipulated with relative hemostasis.[35] More extensive lesions (**Fig. 6**) are not usually amenable to complete resection, and sclerotherapy is often performed.[36] The

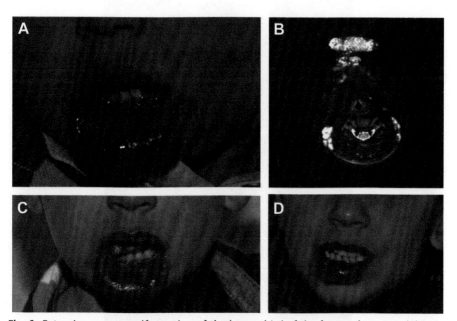

Fig. 6. Extensive venous malformation of the lower third of the face and tongue: (*A*) in infancy before treatment. (*B*) Axial T2-weighted MRI neck showing extensive VM of lip. (*C*) and (*D*) after multimodal therapy including sclerotherapy, Nd:Yag laser therapy and surgical debulking.

GentleYAG is an Nd:YAG laser, which protects the epidermis with a dynamic cooling spray and can be applied safely to cutaneous lesions.[37] The traditional fiber delivery mechanism can be used for mucosal lesions, either with direct visualization in the oral cavity or with endoscopic guidance distally. The fiber may also be passed through a 14-gauge needle to apply the Nd:YAG to interstitial tissue.

Lymphatic Malformations

Lymphatic malformations (LMs) (previously called "lymphangiomas" or "cystic hygromas") are formed from disturbances in the development of the lymphatic system. They may manifest in a wide variety of clinical presentations, but in the head and neck, they are mostly seen as cystic lesions. Common LMs may be categorized as macrocystic, microcystic, and mixed. Macrocystic is defined by cysts measuring 2 cm or more in diameter. In contrast, microcystic malformations (**Fig. 7**) present as clear (often mixed with dark purplish color), tiny vesicles that infiltrate into normal tissue.[38] Large cervicofacial LMs may be diagnosed in utero and may signal the need for advanced airway interventions at the time of delivery. Some may require an EXIT (ex utero intrapartum treatment) procedure.[39,40]

Treatment of LMs may be complex and challenging and involves 4 potential modalities: observation, surgical resection, sclerotherapy, and systemic medical treatment. Depending on the size/location of the malformation and extent of disease, treatment may be single or multimodal. Close clinical observation is a reasonable option for patients who do not have functional or symptomatic effects from the lesion.[41] Surgery remains a good choice of treatment for patients with macrocystic LMs who have

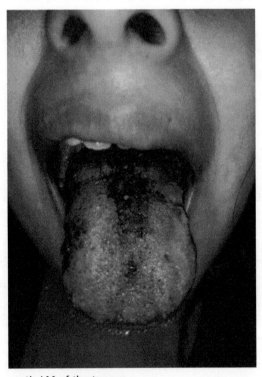

Fig. 7. Diffuse microcystic LM of the tongue.

lateral disease, which is safely exposed.[42] Laser therapy (commonly the CO_2 laser) may be useful for microcystic lesions with skin or mucosal involvement.

Sclerotherapy can be very effective at reducing the bulk and swelling of macrocystic LMs. Currently, bleomycin, doxycycline, and sodium tetradecyl sulfate are the most commonly used agents. Doxycycline is the most effective, although bleomycin is also beneficial.[43] Doxycycline tends to cause a more robust inflammatory response in comparison to bleomycin, and thus, bleomycin is preferentially used in closed compartments, such as the orbit. Bleomycin is also especially useful for interstitial/submucosal injection for mucosal tongue microcystic lesions. Potential adverse effects of sclerotherapy include swelling of the malformation/treatment area (which may cause airway symptoms), fever, and local inflammatory reaction with tenderness and erythema that gradually resolve over a couple weeks.

Systemic medical therapy is a useful option for many patients. Sirolimus, or rapamycin, affects the mTOR/PIK3CA pathway. It is particularly beneficial in microcystic disease of the head and neck and orbit, disease which may be reticent to other forms of treatment.[44,45] Possible adverse effects include mucositis, elevated triglycerides, and infections related to immunosuppression.[46]

Arteriovenous Malformations

Arteriovenous malformations (AVMs) are high-flow lesions that arise owing to abnormal connections between veins and arteries. They usually become evident in childhood or puberty, likely in response to hormonal changes. Rapid expansion can occur from trauma, incomplete resection, or pregnancy.[47] AVMs can be relentless, resistant to treatment, and potentially very dangerous. There are 2 groups of AVMs: focal and diffuse. Focal AVMs have 1 to 2 arteries feeding the lesion and have distinct borders on examination/imaging, which makes them more amenable to surgical resection and subsequent cure. Diffuse AVMs, on the other hand, are larger lesions that extensively infiltrate normal tissue and therefore have no distinct boundaries on examination/imaging. They are very difficult to treat and are prone to recidivism.

AVMs are noted on physical examination by warmth, a palpable thrill/pulsation, sometimes a bruit on auscultation, and overlying skin/mucosal erythema (**Fig. 8**). Imaging with MRI is used to determine the extent of soft tissue disease, and computed tomography scan helps show bone involvement. Computed tomographic angiography or MRA can also help determine the specific blood vessels involved and then plan management. The gold-standard imaging for diagnosis and evaluation of an AVM is conventional angiography, during which interventions, such as embolization, can be performed when indicated.[47]

The natural history of AVMs leads to pain, lesion enlargement, ulceration of soft tissue, and life-threatening bleeding. Therefore, early appropriately aggressive therapy is indicated to control AVMs and prevent catastrophic complications. Embolization can be performed with agents such as NCBA (glue), absolute ethanol, polyvinyl alcohol, and Onyx. However, embolization alone has a high recurrence rate of disease. Ideally, embolization is followed immediately by surgical resection, which gives the best chance for cure. When complete resection is not possible, which is common in diffuse lesions, this may be staged every 3 months to attempt to eliminate sections of the AVM at a time or to control the disease. Interstitial sclerotherapy with bleomycin can help control residual or diffuse disease not amenable to resection. Cutaneous involvement may be treated with combination of PDL and Nd:YAG lasers, and oral mucosal disease may be treated with Nd:YAG laser.[47] High rates of recurrence or residual disease leads to the importance of close clinical monitoring over time with examinations and imaging.

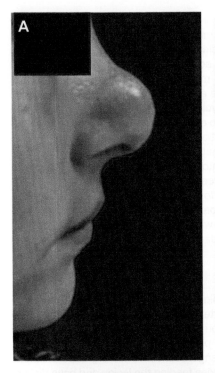

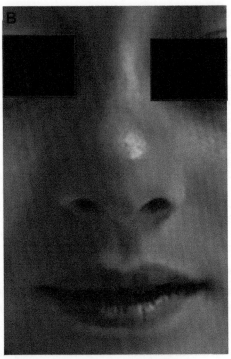

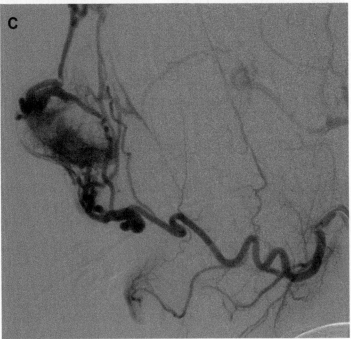

Fig. 8. A 7-year-old girl with AVM of the nose. (*A, B*) Note bulbous nasal tip. Was pulsatile and warm on examination, and patient was having severe epistaxis at time of presentation. (*C*) Angiogram showing nidus at the nasal tip.

Genetics of Vascular Anomalies

Genetic mutations have been identified in many vascular anomalies. Many of these are somatic as opposed to germline, indicating a chimeric mechanism for pathogenesis. This finding is also consistent with the observation that vascular malformations often do not follow a traceable, Mendelian pattern of inheritance. Because these mutations are somatic, sequencing must be performed on an involved piece of tissue (ie, biopsy) rather than a blood sample. Most mutations identified in vascular anomalies affect tyrosine kinase signaling (most commonly through RAS and PIK3CA pathways) (**Fig. 9**). This affects cellular proliferation, differentiation, and survival as well as angiogenesis and endothelial cell signaling.[48,49] PIK3CA mutations may lead to LMs and VMs, as well as lymphatic anomalies and associated overgrowth syndromes. Mutations in GNAQ have been found in patients with CMs.[48,50] Autosomal dominant inheritance is seen in

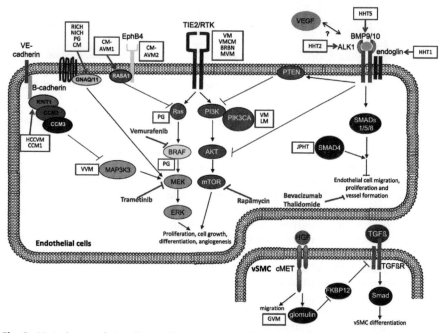

Fig. 9. Mutations and signaling pathways involved in vascular diseases and vascular tumors and hypothetical treatment options. Mutations in GNAQ/GNA11, RASA1, EPHB4, MAP3K3, and KRIT1 lead to constitutive activation of RAS/MEK/ERK signaling. Mutations in TIE2 and mutations in ALK1, BMP9, and endoglin lead to permanent activation of PI3K/AKT/mTOR pathway. In GVM, loss of glomulin may lead to the inhibition of TGF-ß signaling and thus to abnormal differentiated vSMCs. BMP, bone morphogenetic protein; BRBN, blue rubber bleb nevus syndrome; CCM, cerebral cavernous malformation; GVM, glomuvenous malformations; HCCVM, hyperkeratotic cutaneous capillary venous malformation; HGF, hepatocyte growth factor; HHT, hereditary hemorrhagic telangiectasia; JPHT, juvenile polyposis/HHT syndrome; MVM, multifocal venous malformation; TGF, transforming growth factor; VEGF, vascular endothelial growth factor; VMCM, cutaneomucosal venous malformations; vSMC, vascular smooth muscle cells; VVM, verrucous venous malformations. (*From* Queisser A, Boon LM, Vikkula M. Etiology and Genetics of Congenital Vascular Lesions. Otolaryngol Clin North Am. 2018 Feb;51(1):41-53. https://doi.org/10.1016/j.otc.2017.09.006. PMID: 29217067.)

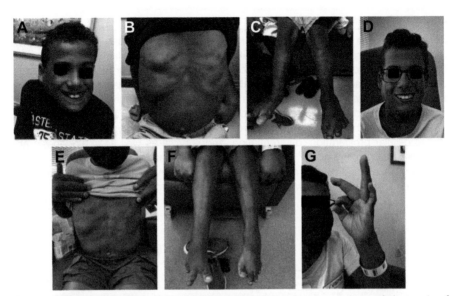

Fig. 10. Comparing facial, torso, and lower-extremity deformity at time of diagnosis of CLOVES (*A–C*) and 6 months into alpelisib therapy after patient had an identified PIK3CA mutation (*D–F*). Improved pincer grasp also demonstrated (*G*).

germline RASA1 mutations in CM-AVM1 syndrome. TIE2/TEK gene mutations seen in mucocutaneous VMs are also autosomal dominant transmission.[51,52]

With improved understanding of the molecular biology of vascular malformations, potential pharmacologic options targeting specific mutations have become available.[48] For example, biopsy of affected tissue in a patient with overgrowth of their face (hemihypertrophy) associated with overlying CM may show pathologic mutation in the PIK3CA gene. Early studies indicate this patient (**Fig. 10**) may be safely offered a PIK3CA inhibitor with the expectation of normalization of the tissue.[53]

Developments in this area are rapid and encouraging. As more about the pathogenesis of vascular anomalies is understood, terms to classify these lesions may change so that they are classified based on molecular genetic pathways associated with each vascular anomaly (eg, PIK3CA-related overgrowth syndrome). It is anticipated that the number of efficacious targeted medical therapies will increase over time, and, optimistically, alleviation or perhaps even cure may be anticipated for even some of the more deforming and impairing malformations.[48,54]

SUMMARY

The care of vascular anomalies of the head and neck is a rapidly evolving field. Pediatric otolaryngologists should be able to recognize the clinical presentation of various lesions as well as be familiar with both medical and surgical options for these patients. As the underlying molecular pathogenesis of vascular anomalies is better understood, genetically targeted treatments have become available. High-quality outcomes research as well as establishing clinical practice guidelines to help guide management are essential.

DISCLOSURE

No disclosures or conflicts of interest.

REFERENCES

1. Mulliken JB, Glowacki J. Classification of pediatric vascular lesions. Plast Reconstr Surg 1982;70(1):120–1.
2. Krowchuk DP, Frieden IJ, Mancini AJ, et al. Clinical practice guideline for the management of infantile hemangiomas. Pediatrics 2019;143(1).
3. Horii KA, Drolet BA, Frieden IJ, et al, Hemangioma Investigator Group. Prospective study of the frequency of hepatic hemangiomas in infants with multiple cutaneous infantile hemangiomas. Pediatr Dermatol 2011;28(3):245–53.
4. North PE, Waner M, Mizeracki A, et al. GLUT1: a newly discovered immunohistochemical marker for juvenile hemangiomas. Hum Pathol 2000;31(1):11–22.
5. Chang LC, Haggstrom AN, Drolet BA, et al, Hemangioma Investigator Group. Growth characteristics of infantile hemangiomas: implications for management. Pediatrics 2008;122(2):360–7.
6. Drolet BA, Esterly NB, Frieden IJ. Hemangiomas in children. N Engl J Med 1999; 341(3):173–81.
7. Baselga E, Roe E, Coulie J, et al. Risk factors for degree and type of sequelae after involution of untreated hemangiomas of infancy. JAMA Dermatol 2016; 152(11):1239–43.
8. Couto RA, Maclellan RA, Zurakowski D, et al. Infantile hemangioma: clinical assessment of the involuting phase and implications for management. Plast Reconstr Surg 2012;130(3):619–24.
9. Haggstrom AN, Garzon MC, Baselga E, et al. Risk for PHACE syndrome in infants with large facial hemangiomas. Pediatrics 2010;126(2).
10. Metry DW, Garzon MC, Drolet BA, et al. PHACE syndrome: current knowledge, future directions. Pediatr Dermatol 2009;26(4):381–98.
11. Adams DM, Ricci KW. Infantile hemangiomas in the head and neck region. Otolaryngol Clin North Am 2018;51:77–87.
12. Burrows PE, Robertson RL, Mulliken JB, et al. Cerebral vasculopathy and neurologic sequelae in infants with cervicofacial hemangioma: report of eight patients. Radiology 1998;207(3):601–7.
13. Garzon MC, Epstein LG, Heyer GL, et al. PHACE syndrome: consensus-derived diagnosis and care recommendations. J Pediatr 2016;178:24–33.
14. Orlow SJ, Isakoff MS, Blei F. Increased risk of symptomatic hemangiomas of the airway in association with cutaneous hemangiomas in a "beard" distribution. J Pediatr 1997;131(4):643–6.
15. Waner M, North PE, Scherer KA, et al. The nonrandom distribution of facial hemangiomas. Arch Dermatol 2003;139(7):869–75.
16. Hochman M, Mascareno A. Management of nasal hemangiomas. Arch Facial Plast Surg 2005;7(5):295–300.
17. Waner M, Kastenbaum J, Scherer K. Hemangiomas of the nose: surgical management using a modified subunit approach. Arch Facial Plast Surg 2008; 10(5):329–34.
18. Schwartz SR, Blei F, Ceisler E, et al. Risk factors for amblyopia in children with capillary hemangiomas of the eyelids and orbit. J AAPOS 2006;10(3):262–8.
19. Frank RC, Cowan BJ, Harrop AR, et al. Visual development in infants: visual complications of periocular haemangiomas. J Plast Reconstr Aesthet Surg 2010; 63(1):1–8.
20. Waner M. The surgical management of infantile hemangiomas. Otolaryngol Clin N Am 2018;51:125–31.

21. Leaute-Labreze C, Dumas de la Roque E, Hubiche T, et al. Propranolol for severe hemangiomas of infancy. N Engl J Med 2008;358(24):2649–51.
22. Buckmiller L, Dyamenahalli U, Richter GT. Propranolol for airway hemangiomas: case report of novel treatment. Laryngoscope 2009;119(10):2051–4.
23. Denoyelle F, Leboulanger N, Enjolras O, et al. Role of Propranolol in the therapeutic strategy of infantile laryngotracheal hemangioma. Int J Pediatr Otorhinolaryngol 2009;73(8):1168–72.
24. Rahbar R, Nicollas R, Roger G, et al. The biology and management of subglottic hemangioma: past, present, future. Laryngoscope 2004;114(11):1880–91.
25. Bitar MA, Moukarbel RV, Zalzal GH. Management of congenital subglottic hemangioma: trends and success over the past 17 years. Otolaryngol Head Neck Surg 2005;132(2):226–31.
26. Darrow DH. Management of infantile hemangiomas of the airway. Otolaryngol Clin N Am 2018;51:133–46.
27. Berenguer B, Mulliken JB, Enjolras O, et al. Rapidly involuting congenital hemangioma: clinical and histopathologic features. Pediatr Dev Pathol 2003;6(6):495–510.
28. Drolet BA, Trenor CC, Brandao LR, et al. Consensus-derived practice standards plan for complicated kaposiform hemangioendothelioma. J Pediatr 2013;163(1):285–91.
29. Adams DM, Trenor CC, Hammill AM, et al. Efficacy and safety of sirolimus in the treatment of complicated vascular anomalies. Pediatrics 2016;137(2).
30. Barsky SH, Rosen S, Geer DE, et al. The nature and evolution of port wine stains: a computer-assisted study. J Invest Dermatol 1980;74(3):154–7.
31. Comi AM, Mehta P, Hatfield LA, et al. Sturge-Weber syndrome associated with other abnormalities: a medical record and literature review. Arch Neurol 2005;62(12):1924–7.
32. Anderson RR, Parrish JA. Selective photothermolysis: precise microsurgery by selective absorption of pulsed radiation. Science 1983;220(4596):524–7.
33. Glade RS, Richter GT, James CJ, et al. Diagnosis and management of pediatric cervicofacial venous malformations: retrospective review from a vascular anomalies center. Laryngoscope 2010;120(2):229–35.
34. Richter GT, Braswell L. Management of venous malformations. Facial Plast Surg 2012;28(6):603–10.
35. Tieu DD, Ghodke BV, Vo NJ, et al. Single-stage excision of localized head and neck venous malformations using preoperative glue embolization. Otolaryngol Head Neck Surg 2013;148(4):678–84.
36. Burrows PE, Mason KP. Percutaneous treatment of low flow vascular malformations. J Vasc Interv Radiol 2004;15(5):431–45.
37. Ulrich H, Baumler W, Hohenleutner U, et al. Neodymium-YAG laser for hemangiomas and vascular malformations—long term results. J Dtsh Dermatol Ges 2005;3(6):436–40.
38. Available at: https://www.issva.org/classification. Accessed February 16, 2021.
39. Shamshirsaz AA, Stewart KA, Erfani H, et al. Cervical lymphatic malformations: prenatal characteristics and ex utero intrapartum treatment. Prent Diagn 2019;39(4):287–92.
40. Cash H, Bly R, Masco V, et al. Prenatal imaging findings predict obstructive fetal airways requiring EXIT. Laryngoscope 2021;131(4):E1357–62.
41. Bonilla-Velez J, Whitlock KB, Ganti S, et al. Active observation as an alternative to invasive treatments for pediatric head and neck lymphatic malformations. Laryngoscope 2021;131(6):1392–7.

42. Bonilla-Velez J, Moore BP, Cleves MA, et al. Surgical resection of macrocystic lymphatic malformations of the head and neck: short- and long-term outcomes. Int J Pediatr Otorhonlaryngol 2020;134:110013.

43. De Mari L, De Sanctis P, Balakrishnan K, et al. Sclerotherapy for lymphatic malformations of head and neck: systematic review and meta-analysis. J Vasc Surg Venous Lymphat Disord 2020;8(1):154–64.

44. Strychoswky JE, Rahbar R, O'Hare MJ, et al. Sirolimus as treatment for 19 patients with refractory cervicofacial lymphatic malformation. Laryngoscope 2018; 128(1):269–76.

45. Shoji MK, Shishido S, Freitag SK. The use of sirolimus for treatment of orbital lymphatic malformations: a systematic review. Ophthalmic Plast Reconstr Surg 2020;36(3):215–21.

46. Rossler J, Baelga E, Davila V, et al. Severe adverse events during sirolimus "off-label" therapy for vascular anomalies. Pediatr Blood Cancer 2021;68:e28936.

47. Rosenberg TL, Suen JY, Richter GT. Arteriovenous malformations of the head and neck. Otolaryngol Clin North Am 2018;51(1):185–95.

48. Blatt J, Powell CM, Burkhart CN. Genetics of hemangiomas, vascular malformations, and primary lymphedema. J Pediatr Hematol Oncol 2014;36(8):587–93.

49. Greene AK, Goss JA. Vascular anomalies: from a clinicohistologic to a genetic framework. Plast Reconstr Surg 2018;141(5):709e–17e.

50. Pang C, Lim CS, Brookes J, et al. Emerging importance of molecular pathogenesis of vascular malformations in clinical practice and classifications. Vasc Med 2020;25(4):364–77.

51. Queisser A, Boon LM, Vikkula M. Etiology and genetics of congenital vascular lesions. Otolaryngol Clin N Am 2018;51:41–53.

52. Yadav P, De Castro DK, Waner M, et al. Vascular anomalies of the head and neck: a review of genetics. Semin Ophthalmol 2013;28(5–6):257–66.

53. Venot Q, Blanc T, Rabia SH, et al. Targeted therapy in patients with PIK3CA-related overgrowth syndrome. Nature 2018;558(7711):540–6.

54. Frigerio A, Stevenson DA, Grimmer JF. The genetics of vascular anomalies. Curr Opin Otolaryngol Head Neck Surg 2012;20(6):527–32.

Aerodigestive Approach to Pediatric Chronic Cough

Zi Yang Jiang, MD[a],*, Chelsea Gatcliffe, MD[b], Tu Mai, MD[c], Zhen Huang, MD[a]

KEYWORDS

- Chronic cough • Aerodigestive • Nonspecific cough • Specific cough
- Psychogenic cough • Upper airway cough syndrome • Laryngeal cleft
- Protracted bacterial bronchitis

KEY POINTS

- Pediatric chronic cough is defined as a cough that has been ongoing for more than 4 weeks in children < 14 years old.
- Chronic cough can be grouped by diagnosis types, management strategies, or by presenting symptoms and characteristics. A common paradiagm is to classify cough as normal (expected), specific (with cough pointers), and nonspecific types.
- An aerodigestive team evaluation allows for a comprehensive evaluation with more efficient care and decrease the chance fo specialty availability bias.

INTRODUCTION

Cough is among the top 10 most common reasons for visits to the physician's office in the United States. It is more common than hypertension, anxiety, or diabetes.[1] It represents a confluence of integrated diseases with multiple causes with diagnostic and management challenges. Prevalence estimates vary from 4.7% to 23% of all visits in primary care settings.[2] In this article, the authors focus on the diagnostic pathway for outpatient encounters for children with chronic cough, as the clinical dilemma for cough in pediatrics is in the diverse causes and often with overlapping signs and symptoms. Details of treatment of specific causes are available in the literature for the reader to explore further.

When a child starts coughing from an acute respiratory tract infection, 50% of children recover by 10 days, 90% by 3 weeks, and only 10% of children may have cough in the third and fourth week.[3,4] Therefore, chronic cough in children is generally considered a cough that has been ongoing for more than 4 weeks in patients aged

No financial disclosures to report.
[a] Department of Otorhinolaryngology - Head and Neck Surgery, University of Texas Health Science Center at Houston, 6431 Fannin MSB 5.036, Houston, TX 77030, USA; [b] Division of Pulmonary Medicine, Department of Pediatrics, University of Texas Health Science Center at Houston; [c] Division of Gastroenterology, Department of Pediatrics, University of Texas Health Science Center at Houston
* Corresponding author. 6431 Fannin Street MSB 5.036, Houston, TX 77030.
E-mail address: zi.yang.jiang@uth.tmc.edu

14 years or older.[5,6] In children younger than 6 years, a recent study suggested several predictors that suggest the child's cough will turn into a chronic cough: age less than 12 months, wheezing in the past 12 months, gestational age less than 37 weeks, child-care attendance, and presence of other medical conditions such as recurrent tonsillitis, chronic ear disease, congenital birth defects, heart disease, neurological diseases, diabetes, and kidney diseases. In children who attend childcare, a history of intermittent itchy rash in the past 12 months and pets at home were also positive associations for the development of chronic cough.[7]

The classification of chronic cough can be grouped by diagnosis types, management strategies, or by presenting symptoms/characteristics.[8,9] The ACCP Guidelines for evaluating chronic cough in pediatrics popularized the approach to classify cough into normal (expected), specific, and nonspecific cough types with overlap in some patients.[9]

Normal children with no known pathophysiology may cough 1 to 34 times every 24-hour period (with the average school-aged child coughing 11 times per day).[10] Factors such as passive second-hand smoke and presence of furry pets at home do not seem to affect frequency in normal children.[10] Furthermore, nocturnal coughing is unusual. Even in patients who have an aerodigestive pathology causing cough, coughing at night is usually suppressed.[11] Coughing severity is very subjective, and parental reports are often not reliable. Interestingly, children's report of cough severity best correlates with objective measures of severity.[12]

Specific coughs are a constellation of pathophysiologies that have "cough pointers." These pointers have been classified into systemic and pulmonary pathologies,[5] with further pointers from related fields of otolaryngology and gastroenterology.[13,14] These pointers have specific associated causes that warrant investigation and confirmation before treatment (**Table 1**).

AERODIGESTIVE TEAM EVALUATION

Aerodigestive programs have historically evaluated patients with a host of issues related to feeding and breathing, which may include chronic cough, failure to thrive, noisy breathing, recurrent upper respiratory tract infection, tracheostomy dependence, stridor and/or recurrent croup, and wheezing, among other conditions.[15] In a recent consensus statement, essential core members of the aerodigestive team include a care coordinator, gastroenterology, nursing, otolaryngology, pulmonology, and speech-language pathology.[15] Other specialists who provide input on a more limited basis for cough may include allergy/immunology, neurology, cardiology, infectious disease, and psychiatry.[16]

Availability bias can result in diagnostic errors in the clinical setting[17,18] both for individual members of the aerodigestive team in their clinics as well as the collective group. This bias can be illustrated by the reported prevalence of different diagnoses based on specialty and location.[8,19] Following a set protocol can decrease the propensity for bias and allow comparison of effectiveness and set priorities for future research and protocol change. When treatment follows a set protocol, there is evidence that more children have symptom resolution by day 56 of cough onset than when treatment is just by conventional practice (58% vs 40%).[20]

Key questions, for diagnosis and treatment, to ask include the following:[20,21]

1. Does the cough have specific pointers, classic features, or chest radiograph and spirometry abnormalities? If so, then consider treatments for diseases associated with specific pointers, if not, then continue down this list.

Table 1
Classification of cough pointers and possible causes

Classification	Pointer	Possible Causes
Systemic	Allergy/Atopy	Chronic rhinosinusitis/asthma
Pulmonary	Auscultatory findings	Wheeze-intrathoracic airway lesions (eg, tracheomalacia, asthma); crepitations, any airway lesions (from secretions), or parenchyma disease such as interstitial disease
Systemic	Cardiac abnormalities	Associated airway abnormalities, cardiac failure
Pulmonary	Chest pain	Arrhythmia, asthma
Pulmonary	Chest wall deformity	Airway or parenchymal disease
Otolaryngology	Chronic mouth breathing	Adenoid hypertrophy, upper airway cough syndrome (postnasal drip)
Pulmonary	Daily moist or productive cough	Suppurative lung disease
Systemic	Digital clubbing	Suppurative lung disease
Otolaryngology	Dysphonia	Vocal cord paralysis/vocal cord dysfunction
Pulmonary	Dyspnea or tachypnea	Airway or parenchymal disease, ciliary dyskinesia
Systemic	Failure to thrive	Any serious systemic including pulmonary illness such as cystic fibrosis
Systemic	Feeding difficulties	Any serious systemic illness, aspiration, laryngeal cleft
Gastroenterology	Heartburn/Spit ups/Dystonic neck posturing	Reflux
Pulmonary	Hemoptysis	Suppurative lung disease, vascular abnormalities
Pulmonary	Hypoxia/cyanosis	Airway or parenchymal disease, cardiac disease
Systemic	Immune deficiency	Suppurative lung disease or atypical infection
Otolaryngology	Intubation history	Subglottic stenosis
Systemic	Neurodevelopmental abnormality	Aspiration
Otolaryngology	Recurrent croup	Tracheomalacia/Subglottic stenosis/Immune deficiency
Pulmonary	Recurrent pneumonia	Immunodeficiency, atypical infections, suppurative lung disease, congenital lung abnormalities, missed foreign body, H-type tracheoesophageal fistulas

(continued on next page)

Table 1 (continued)		
Classification	**Pointer**	**Possible Causes**
Pulmonary	Spirometry	Obstructive/Restrictive lung disease
Otolaryngology	Stridor	Glottic/subglottic/tracheal stenosis or tracheomalacia

Data from Chang, A. B., R. G. Newman, J. B. Carlin, P. D. Phelan, and C. F. Robertson. 1998. "Subjective Scoring of Cough in Children: Parent-Completed vs Child-Completed Diary Cards vs an Objective Method." The European Respiratory Journal: Official Journal of the European Society for Clinical Respiratory Physiology 11 (2): 462–66; Greifer, Melanie, Maria T. Santiago, Kalliope Tsirilakis, Jeffrey C. Cheng, and Lee P. Smith. 2015. "Pediatric Patients with Chronic Cough and Recurrent Croup: The Case for a Multidisciplinary Approach." International Journal of Pediatric Otorhinolaryngology 79 (5): 749–52; Weinberger, Miles, and Manju Hurvitz. 2020. "Diagnosis and Management of Chronic Cough: Similarities and Differences between Children and Adults." F1000Research 9 (July).

   a. Classic coughs include the croupy/barking cough of tracheomalacia, the staccato cough for chlamydia, cough with casts, and the whoop for pertussis.
   b. Assess risk factors for foreign body inhalation and contributions from rhinosinusitis and reflux.
2. Is the cough wet? If so, consider treatment of protracted bacterial bronchitis.
   a. Consider checking immune status, pertussis, and mycoplasma.
3. Is the cough dry? If so, consider inhaled corticosteroids for 2 weeks for asthma/asthmalike illnesses.

Chronic cough makes up a substantial percentage of reasons for evaluation in a multidisciplinary setting (up to 44%).[22] Typically, patients have already seen their primary care physician as well as one member of the aerodigestive team before referral. Children receive a thorough history and physical examination followed by consideration for immediate fiberoptic laryngoscopy and pulmonary function testing. Diagnostic interventions include the triple endoscopy, multichannel intraluminal impedance/pH probe testing, immune evaluation, sweat chloride testing, and cilia biopsy.[22]

The triple endoscopy represents the collaborative efforts of otolaryngology, pulmonology, and gastroenterology to evaluate the entire aerodigestive tract that has possible implications in cough pathogenesis: rigid laryngoscopy/bronchoscopy, flexible bronchoscopy and lavage, and esophagogastroduodenoscopy with guided biopsies. In a series of 243 pediatric patients with chronic cough, 83.5% of patients had at least one positive finding. Fifty percent of patients had more than one specialty diagnosis. The most common diagnosis was tracheomalacia (48.6%), followed by a positive bronchoalveolar lavage (42%), gastroesophageal reflux (26%), and laryngeal cleft (22%). Other less frequent findings include subglottic stenosis, vocal cord paralysis, adenoid hypertrophy, laryngomalacia, and eosinophilic esophagitis.[23] Age less than 3 years may increase likelihood of airway pathology in those who present with recurrent croup.[24]

SPECIFIC CAUSES
Adenoid Hypertrophy, Rhinosinusitis, Postnasal Drip, and Upper Airway Cough Syndrome

Enlarged adenoids, rhinosinusitis, and related postnasal drip have long been considered a possible cause of chronic cough in children. Conceptually, these pathologies have been grouped under upper airway cough syndrome (UACS) due to uncertainty over whether the secretions cause cough in the upper airway or merely a marker for other pathology for which cough is a symptom.[25] Postulated mechanisms include possible nidus of infection and dripping of secretions inferiorly and irritation of laryngeal cough receptors and/or stimulation of oropharyngeal cough receptions.[26,27] Signs and symptoms include sensation of something dripping down the throat, frequent throat clearing, "cobblestone" mucosa, secretions in oropharynx, nasal discharge, and inflammation on ear, nose, and throat examination.[26] Nevertheless, most patients with postnasal drip symptoms do not have a cough.[28] The proportion of chronic cough attributed to UACS varies from 3% to 38%.[29–31] Variability likely reflects local prevalence of disease as well as selection bias (pulmonary versus allergy/immunology practice groups).

Protracted Bacterial Bronchitis

In the pulmonary literature, protracted bacterial bronchitis (PBB) is one of the most common causes of cough in children. Current European Respiratory Society (ERS) guidelines define PBB as a mostly clinical diagnosis of presence of chronic (>4 weeks' duration) wet or productive cough, absence of symptoms or signs (i.e., specific cough pointers) that suggest other causes of wet or productive cough, and cough resolution following a 2- to 4-week course of an appropriate oral antibiotic.[32] Treatment pathways include antibiotics for up to 4 weeks based on common respiratory bacteria and local antibiotic sensitivities.[5,31] The current ERS guidelines suggest 2-week trial of amoxicillin-clavulanate if there are no specific cough pointers. The aforementioned pathway excludes infants and neonates, as tachypnea, dyspnea, and/or hypoxia are the more common manifestations of respiratory infections in infants and neonates rather than cough.[31]

Gastroesophageal Reflux Disease/Laryngopharyngeal Reflux Disease

Reflux has been postulated as a possible trigger to cough. Theories regarding the pathophysiology include microaspiration of gastric contents casting airway irritation, vagal-mediated bronchospasms, and increased airway hyperresponsiveness due to irritation receptions in the distal esophagus.[33] A study with an acoustic cough monitor and simultaneous impedance/pH recording demonstrated that 70% of patients have temporal associations between cough and reflux, similar proportions for cough preceded by reflux or cough followed by reflux.[34]

However, recent research in pediatric cough has demonstrated that reflux-related cough may be uncommon in children. In one cohort, the common causes of cough in adults: asthma, gastroesophageal reflux disease, and upper airway cough syndrome (postnasal drip) together make up less than 10% of the underlying reason for cough in children.[31] The routine use of antireflux medication is not recommended without specific signs or symptoms that suggest reflux.[31,33] Such symptoms should be recurrent regurgitation, dystonic neck posturing in infants, or heartburn/epigastric pain in older children.[35] In infants, behavioral changes should be instituted first (such as avoidance of overfeeding, thickening feeds, and encouragement to continue breastfeeding, if possible). If there is no improvement, then consider 2 to 4 weeks of a protein hydrolysate or amino acid–based formula or eliminate cow's milk in the maternal diet for breastfeeding infants. Gastroenterology referral should be considered before a trial of acid suppression. In older children, if lifestyle and dietary modifications fail to change symptoms, acid suppression can be considered for 4 to 8 weeks. If symptoms persist or recur after weaning, gastroenterology evaluation and endoscopy should be considered.[36]

Eosinophilic Esophagitis

Eosinophilic esophagitis (EOE) is defined as a "chronic, immune-mediated or antigen-mediated esophageal disease characterized clinically by symptoms related to esophageal dysfunction and histologically by eosinophil-predominant inflammation."[37] Symptoms of EOE in children may vary, depending on the age of diagnosis: feeding difficulties are seen more frequently in infants and toddlers, whereas vomiting and pain present more frequently in older children.[38,39] Histologically, EOE shows high eosinophil counts in the esophagus (>15 eosinophils/high-power field [hpf]), without the involvement of other parts of the gastrointestinal tract.[40]

A subset presents with concurrent respiratory disease.[41] Cough is the most common respiratory symptom, with hoarseness, throat clearing, and burping also present.[42] There is a high prevalence in the past medical history of environmental allergies (up to 70%), asthma, food allergies, allergic rhinitis, and recurrent croup.[42]

Laryngeal Cleft

Cough in patients with laryngeal cleft is more common in higher cleft levels (classified by the Benjamin-Inglis classification). In one series, cough was present in 3% of patients with a type 1 cleft but 11% of patients in type II and III.[43] Many patients with aspiration, including those with laryngeal cleft type 1, have asymptomatic, silent aspirations, or laryngeal penetration, and by definition, cough is absent.[44,45] There is limited evidence that for type 1 clefts injection laryngoplasty may help coughing symptoms even if it does not help dysphagia symptoms overall.[46]

Psychogenic Cough

Cough due to psychological causes is a form of a conversion disorder. It may exist with already diagnosed conversion disorder or present with mixed anxiety and depressive disorders.[47] In a large series of 1636 patients with chronic cough (adults and children), 32 (1.3%) were diagnosed with psychogenic cough.[47] Psychogenic cough seems to be more common in children than adults.[48] In another series of 33 children with psychogenic cough, the average age for psychogenic cough was 9.6 years (range 5–14 years).[49] The typical profile is an unusually loud (croupy, barky, and explosive) cough. The patient may have a chin-on chest posture with a hand held to the neck while coughing.[49] Diagnosis can only be made after tic disorders and Tourette syndrome have been evaluated and the cough improves with specific therapy such as behavior modification or psychiatric therapy. Until the improvement, the cough should be classified as "unexplained cough."[48]

Rare Causes

Other rare causes have been reported in the literature including tonsils or the uvula impinging on the epiglottis.[50] Foreign body in the ear has been reported due to stimulation of Arnold nerve.[51] Other rare causes can be foreign body aspiration or swallowing with eventual erosion into the mediastinum.[52]

OUTCOMES WHEN DIAGNOSIS IS UNCERTAIN

Prognostically, in a prospective cohort, more than 50% of children with chronic wet cough younger than 3 years were symptom free by age 7 years.[53] In the aerodigestive setting, cough may also spontaneously improve. In a study of 226 patients in an aerodigestive clinic for cough, 77% of patients with a diagnosis (144/188) improved, whereas 44% of patients without a diagnosis had symptomatic improvement (16/36).[23] In another study, 23/58 (40%) of patients in a control arm (where there was no intervention by investigators) had cough resolution by day 56 compared with 33/57 (58%) of children in the intervention group that followed a standard protocol for treatment.[20] The number needed to treat has been reported to be between 3 and 5.[5,20] Evidence suggests that even when a specific diagnosis is unknown, certain types of cough are subjected to the period effect of spontaneous resolution.

SUMMARY

Chronic cough is defined as cough lasting more than 4 weeks in children aged 14 years or older. Normal children, without pathophysiology, can cough up to more than 30 times a day. When cough occurs pathologically, it is often more often and can be divided into specific and nonspecific cough types. Specific cough pointers can lead to identification of causes in the aerodigestive tract and can be identified by clinical history, physical examination, fiberoptic laryngoscopy, chest radiographs, pulmonary function, and other specific serologic and genetic tests. Protracted bacterial bronchitis may be suspected in children with a nonspecific wet cough that responds to oral antibiotics. Asthma may be suspected in children with a nonspecific dry cough that responds to inhaled corticosteroids. Inputs from otolaryngology, pulmonary medicine, and gastroenterology, along with other specialties in an aerodigestive team setting, allow a team approach to consider a wide variety of causes of cough and coordinate diagnostic procedures with treatment.

CLINICS CARE POINTS

- Does the cough have specific pointers, classic features, or chest radiograph and spirometry abnormalities?

- Is the cough wet? If so, consider treatment of protracted bacterial bronchitis.

- Is the cough dry? If so, consider inhaled corticosteroids for 2 weeks for asthma/asthmalike illnesses.Specific cough pointers can lead to identification of causes in the aerodigestive tract and can be identified by clinical history, physical examination, fiberoptic laryngoscopy, chest radiographs, pulmonary function, and other specific serologic and genetic tests.Inputs from otolaryngology, pulmonary medicine, and gastroenterology, along with other specialties in an aerodigestive team setting, allow a team approach to consider a wide variety of causes of cough and coordinate diagnostic procedures with treatment.

REFERENCES

1. NAMCS 2018 Data. Available at: https://www.cdc.gov/nchs/data/ahcd/namcs_summary/2018-namcs-web-tables-508.pdf. Accessed from CDC on 02/10/2022.
2. Bergmann M, Haasenritter J, Beidatsch D, et al. Coughing children in family practice and primary care: a systematic review of prevalence, aetiology and prognosis. BMC Pediatr 2021;21(1):260.
3. Thompson M, Vodicka TA, Blair PS, et al, TARGET Programme Team. Duration of symptoms of respiratory tract infections in children: systematic review. BMJ 2013; 347(December):f7027.
4. Hay AD, Wilson AD. The natural history of acute cough in children aged 0 to 4 years in primary care: a systematic review. Br J Gen Pract J R Coll Gen Pract 2002;52(478):401–9.
5. Chang AB, Oppenheimer JJ, Weinberger M, et al. Children with chronic wet or productive cough–treatment and investigations: a systematic review. Chest 2016;149(1):120–42.

6. Morice AH, Millqvist E, Bieksiene K, et al. ERS guidelines on the diagnosis and treatment of chronic cough in adults and children. Eur Respir J 2020;55(1).

7. Au-Yeung, Yin T, Chang AB, et al. Risk Factors for Chronic Cough in Young Children: A Cohort Study. Front Pediatr 2020;8(August):444.

8. Cash H, Trosman S, Abelson T, et al. Chronic cough in children. JAMA Otolaryngology– Head Neck Surg 2015;141(5):417–23.

9. Chang AB, Glomb WB. Guidelines for evaluating chronic cough in pediatrics: ACCP evidence-based clinical practice guidelines. Chest 2006;129(1 Suppl):260S–83S.

10. Munyard P, Bush A. How much coughing is normal? Arch Dis Child 1996;74(6):531–4.

11. Chang AB, Phelan PD, Robertson CF, et al. Frequency and perception of cough severity. J Paediatr Child Health 2001;37(2):142–5.

12. Chang AB, Newman RG, Carlin JB, et al. Subjective scoring of cough in children: parent-completed vs child-completed diary cards vs an objective method. Eur Respir J 1998;11(2):462–6.

13. Greifer M, Santiago MT, Tsirilakis K, et al. Pediatric patients with chronic cough and recurrent croup: the case for a multidisciplinary approach. Int J Pediatr Otorhinolaryngol 2015;79(5):749–52.

14. Weinberger M, Hurvitz M. Diagnosis and management of chronic cough: similarities and differences between children and adults. F1000Research 2020;9:1–10.

15. Boesch RP, Balakrishnan K, Acra S, Benscoter DT, et al. Structure and functions of pediatric aerodigestive programs: a consensus statement. Pediatrics 2018;141(3).

16. Altman KW, Irwin RS. Cough: a new frontier in otolaryngology." otolaryngology– head and neck surgery. Official J Am Acad Otolaryngology-Head Neck Surg 2011;144(3):348–52.

17. Li P, Cheng ZY, Liu Gui Lin. Availability bias causes misdiagnoses by physicians: direct evidence from a randomized controlled trial. Intern Med 2020;59(24):3141–6.

18. Mannion R, Thompson C. Systematic biases in group decision-making: implications for patient safety. Int J Qual Health Care J Int Soc Qual Health Care/ISQua 2014;26(6):606–12.

19. Chang AB, Robertson CF, Van Asperen PP, et al. A multicenter study on chronic cough in children : burden and etiologies based on a standardized management pathway. Chest 2012;142(4):943–50.

20. O'Grady KF, Grimwood K, Torzillo PJ, et al. Effectiveness of a chronic cough management algorithm at the transitional stage from acute to chronic cough in children: a multicenter, nested, single-blind, randomised controlled trial.". Lancet Child Adolesc Health 2019;3(12):889–98.

21. Kennedy AA, Anne S, Hart CK. Otolaryngologic management of chronic cough in school-aged children: a review. JAMA Otolaryngology– Head Neck Surg 2020. https://doi.org/10.1001/jamaoto.2020.2945.

22. Rotsides JM, Krakovsky GM, Pillai DK, et al. Is a multidisciplinary aerodigestive clinic more effective at treating recalcitrant aerodigestive complaints than a single specialist? Ann Otol Rhinol Laryngol 2017;126(7):537–43.

23. Fracchia M, Shannon GD, Cook A, et al. The diagnostic role of triple endoscopy in pediatric patients with chronic cough. Int J Pediatr Otorhinolaryngol 2019;116(January):58–61.

24. Chun R, Preciado DA, Zalzal GH, et al. Utility of bronchoscopy for recurrent croup. Ann Otol Rhinol Laryngol 2009;118(7):495–9.

25. Pratter MR. Chronic Upper Airway Cough Syndrome Secondary to Rhinosinus Diseases (previously Referred to as Postnasal Drip Syndrome): ACCP evidence-based clinical practice guidelines. Chest 2006;129(1 Suppl):63S–71S.

26. Kemp A. Does post-nasal drip cause cough in childhood? Paediatr Respir Rev 2006;7(1):31–5.

27. Gao F, Gu Q-L, Jiang Z-D. Upper airway cough syndrome in 103 children. Chin Med J 2019;132(6):653–8.

28. O'Hara J, Jones NS. 'Post-nasal drip syndrome': most patients with purulent nasal secretions do not complain of chronic cough. Rhinology 2006;44(4):270–3.

29. Guc U, Belgin, Asilsoy S, et al. The assessment and management of chronic cough in children according to the british thoracic society guidelines: descriptive, prospective, clinical trial. Clin Respir J 2014;8(3):330–7.

30. Asilsoy S, Bayram E, Agin H, et al. Evaluation of chronic cough in children. Chest 2008;134(6):1122–8.

31. Marchant JM, Brent Masters I, Taylor SM, et al. Evaluation and outcome of young children with chronic cough. Chest 2006;129(5):1132–41.

32. Kantar A, Chang AB, Shields MD, et al. ERS statement on protracted bacterial bronchitis in children. Eur Respir J 2017;50:1602139.

33. Benedictis F M de, Bush A. Respiratory manifestations of gastro-oesophageal reflux in children. Arch Dis Child 2018;103(3):292–6.

34. Smith JA, Decalmer S, Kelsall A, et al. Acoustic cough-reflux associations in chronic cough: potential triggers and mechanisms. Gastroenterology 2010; 139(3):754–62.

35. Chang AB, Oppenheimer JJ, Kahrilas PJ, et al, CHEST Expert Cough Panel. Chronic cough and gastroesophageal reflux in children: CHEST guideline and expert panel report. Chest 2019;156(1):131–40.

36. Rosen R, Vandenplas Y, Singendonk M, et al. Pediatric Gastroesophageal Reflux Clinical Practice Guidelines: Joint Recommendations of the North American Society for Pediatric Gastroenterology, Hepatology, and Nutrition and the European Society for Pediatric Gastroenterology, Hepatology, and Nutrition. J Pediatr Gastroenterol Nutr 2018;66(3):516–54.

37. Liacouras CA, Furuta GT, Hirano, et al. Eosinophilic esophagitis: updated consensus recommendations for children and adults. J Allergy Clin Immunol 2011;128(e6):3–20.

38. Aceves SS, Newbury RO, Dohil MA, et al. A symptom scoring tool for identifying pediatric patients with eosinophilic esophagitis and correlating symptoms with inflammation. Ann Allergy Asthma Immunol 2009;103(5):401–6.

39. Mukkada VA, Haas A, Maune NC, et al. Feeding dysfunction in children with eosinophilic gastrointestinal diseases. Pediatrics 2010;126:e672–7.

40. Blanchard C, Wang N, Marc ER. Eosinophilic esophagitis: pathogenesis, genetics, and therapy. J Allergy Clin Immunol 2006;118(5):1054–9.

41. Orenstein SR, Shalaby TM, Di Lorenzo C, et al. The spectrum of pediatric eosinophilic esophagitis beyond infancy: a clinical series of 30 children. Am J Gastroenterol 2000;95(6):1422–30.

42. Otteson TD, Mantle BA, Casselbrant ML, et al. The otolaryngologic manifestations in children with eosinophilic esophagitis. Int J Pediatr Otorhinolaryngol 2012; 76(1):116–9.

43. Martha VV, Vontela S, Alyssa N, et al. Laryngeal cleft: a literature review. Am J Otolaryngol 2021;42(6):'.

44. Strychowsky JE, Dodrill P, Moritz E, et al. Swallowing dysfunction among patients with laryngeal cleft: more than just aspiration? Int J Pediatr Otorhinolaryngol 2016; 82(March):38–42.

45. Velayutham P, Irace AL, Kawai K, et al. Silent aspiration: who is at risk? Laryngoscope 2018;128(8):1952–7.

46. Miglani A, Scott S, Clarke PY, et al. An aerodigestive approach to laryngeal clefts and dysphagia using injection laryngoplasty in young children. Curr Gastroenterol Rep 2017;19(12):60.

47. Bhatia MS, Chandra R, Vaid L. Psychogenic cough: a profile of 32 cases. Int J Psychiatry Med 2002;32(4):353–60.

48. Irwin RS, Glomb WB, Chang AB. Habit cough, tic cough, and psychogenic cough in adult and pediatric populations: ACCP evidence-based clinical practice guidelines. Chest 2006;129(1 Suppl):174S–9S.

49. Cohlan SQ, Stone SM. The cough and the bedsheet. Pediatrics 1984;74(1):11–5.

50. Gurgel RK, Brookes JT, Weinberger MM, et al. Chronic cough and tonsillar hypertrophy: a case series. Pediatr Pulmonol 2008;43(11):1147–9.

51. Ryan NM, Gibson PG, Birring SS. Arnold's nerve cough reflex: evidence for chronic cough as a sensory vagal neuropathy. J Thorac Dis 2014;6(Suppl 7): S748–52.

52. Łoś-Rycharska E, Wasielewska Z, Nadolska K, et al. A foreign body in the mediastinum as a cause of chronic cough in a 10-year-old child with asthma. J Asthma 2021;58(2):276–80.

53. Sørensen KG, Bruun Mikalsen I, Neven A, et al. Half of children with recurrent or chronic wet cough before three years of age were symptom-free by age seven. Acta Paediatr 2020;109(12):2664–70.

Three-dimensional Printing in Pediatric Otolaryngology

Peng You, MD, FRCSC[a],*, Michael Bartellas, MSc (Med), MD[b]

KEYWORDS

- 3D printing • Rapid prototyping • Innovation • Pediatric • Otolaryngology
- Head and neck surgery • Bioprinting

KEY POINTS

- Increased access to three-dimensional printing (3Dp) has helped improve adoption within pediatric otolaryngology. This technology complements the shift toward personalized medicine.
- 3Dp has been increasingly used in surgical planning ranging from aiding preoperative discussions, helping surgeons improve understanding of patient-specific anatomy, and serving as intraoperative implants and surgical guides.
- Educations using 3Dp can create accurate models to help trainees acquire procedural skills, explore unique patient anatomy/pathology, and improve the multidisciplinary approach.
- Improvements in biocompatibility and further high-quality clinical studies will support more generalized uptake of tissue engineering and bioprinting in Otolaryngology.

INTRODUCTION

Three-dimensional printing (3Dp) describes an additive manufacturing process whereby objects are formed by gradually layering materials.[1,2] Although 3Dp has been well recognized within manufacturing sectors, its application in medicine has also rapidly expanded in recent years.

The versatility of 3Dp lies in its flexibility and precision. Shapes can be designed and formed to a great degree of accuracy. The customized objects are not limited by the complexity of their shape. They can be created using a myriad of materials, which can be rigid or flexible plastic or even metal.[2] Furthermore, the 3Dp process is much faster than the arduous traditional manufacturing process with 3Dp models taking hours to print. Concurrently, the growing interest and adoption of 3Dp in the commercial space have also reduced the barriers to entry. The 3D printers are now affordable, and the

[a] Department of Otolaryngology-Head & Neck Surgery, Western University, B3-451 800 Commissioner Road East, London, Ontario N6A 5W9, Canada; [b] Department of Otolaryngology-Head & Neck Surgery, University of Ottawa, Otolaryngology-Head and Neck Surgery. S3, 501 Smyth Road, Ottawa, Ontario K1H 8L6, Canada
* Corresponding author.
E-mail address: peng.you@lhsc.on.ca

Otolaryngol Clin N Am 55 (2022) 1243–1251
https://doi.org/10.1016/j.otc.2022.07.013
0030-6665/22/© 2022 Elsevier Inc. All rights reserved.
oto.theclinics.com

software that accompanies them is designed with the average consumer in mind. A consumer 3D printer, and its various key components, is illustrated in **Fig. 1**. The growing familiarity and experience with 3Dp have opened new opportunities to expand its applications.

Medicine has seen the increased availability of 3Dp, which expanded the possibility for personalized medicine and high fidelity simulation. This article describes the advances and capabilities of this emerging technology by itemizing the various 3Dp innovations within pediatric otolaryngology. Understanding this growing technology can help clinicians take advantage of its various applications and see how it may be applied to address their clinical questions.

Clinical Applications

Otolaryngology involves complex anatomy. Within pediatric otolaryngology, clinicians often face unique problems with critical functional implications. A key advantage of 3Dp is the ability to produce objects of various shapes or complexity. In turn, the printed models help with the precise understanding of intricate anatomy and provide an avenue to personalized solutions.

The early adoption of 3Dp in pediatric otolaryngology was most notable around the treatment of complex airways.[3,4] Zopf and Green were the first to describe the feasibility in creating a 3Dp bioresorbable airway splint, which was successfully used under emergency approval for a pediatric patient with severe tracheobronchomalacia (TBM).[3] A follow-up study by Morrison and colleagues[5] described external airway splints implanted in 3 patients with previous TBM. After some time, these patients showed no life-threatening pulmonary or extrapulmonary manifestations of their once critical TBM. In a 2021 systematic review, Sood and colleagues[6] reported 29 bioresorbable 3Dp airway splints used for 15 severe TBM patients. Their results showed 12 long-term survivors, with only a single patient still requiring hospitalization. A recent animal study explored using 3Dp bioresorbable polycaprolactone scaffolding for a posterior cricoid graft for glottic stenosis and subglottic stenosis.[7]

These pioneering cases helped to energize the use of 3Dp within the clinical setting. In addition to intraoperative scaffolding, 3Dp also helped preoperative planning in pediatric airway surgeries. Stramiello and colleagues[8] conducted a systematic review, which showed that presurgical printing of patient airways improved surgical approach,

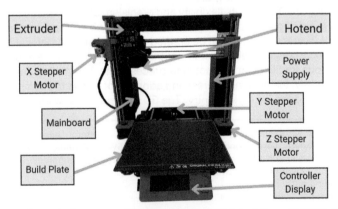

Fig. 1. Image of a typical consumer/hobby 3D printer (Original Prusa i3 MK3). Key components are labeled. (*Courtesy of* Michael Bartellas, MSc (Med)., MD, PolyUnity Tech Inc, Ottawa, Ontario Canada.)

selection of medical device customizations (stents), and patient/family discussions. For example, in the case of open laryngotracheal surgeries, one group noted that the 3D models were important for preoperative planning with the potential in the future for this process to be a "common practice."[9] Additionally, antenatal 3Dp has specifically allowed teams to simulate and plan ex utero intrapartum treatment of babies with upper congenital high airway obstruction.[10] In a case described by VanKoevering and colleagues,[11] 3Dp was performed of the aberrant facial anatomy base on fetal imaging. In doing so, the model helped the team better appreciate the airway and gave them the confidence to proceed with a successful delivery without a planned ex utero intrapartum treatment procedure.

The skull base is another area that can benefit from patient-specific preoperative planning/simulation and intraoperative guidance.[12,13] 3Dp models simulated the procedure preoperatively and served as intraoperative reference guides. Takahashi described a unique case in whch a sterilized 3Dp model facilitated the removal of congenital cholesteatoma and a foreign body (tip of round knife in-situ from previous surgery).[13] In this challenging clinical scenario, a supra-cochlear approach was selected after 3D surgical simulation, and the intraoperative model assisted the surgeon in avoiding critical surrounding structures. Ahmed described using 3D printed preoperative models to practice repairing tegmen defects in adults.[14] The authors used the 3D printed model to help shape the Silastic sheets later sterilized and used as a template for the dural replacement graft. Although this was an adult cohort, the principles can be adapted to pediatric patients with tegmen defects and recalcitrant cerebrospinal fluid leak. An example of 3Dp application in pediatric anterior skull base involves a 2-year old with craniopharyngioma.[15] Both virtual reality and 3Dp allowed surgeons to be confident that an endoscopic endonasal approach would be feasible despite absences of sinus pneumatization and a narrowed nasal cavity. Ultimately, the augmented preoperative planning allowed for a successful surgery. In general, the added preoperative preparations are thought to improve surgical outcomes by familiarizing the surgical team and, in turn, reducing the operating time and the duration of the anesthetic.

The soft tissue aspect of facial plastic reconstruction is another domain that is well suited for 3Dp. The intricate and personalized anatomic considerations and the overarching goal of achieving symmetry have prompted many to explore the feasibility of adopting 3Dp. In a systematic review by Hong and colleagues,[16] microtia was one of the most common disease entities in which 3Dp was used. Authors have described various approaches to applying 3Dp in creating intraoperative templates to best replicate the complex geometry of the ear.[17-23] Jeon and colleagues[22] created molds of the normal ear using alginate impression material, and the cast was then scanned with a laser scanner. Other authors have generated 3D models from existing computed tomographic images.[3] Optical surface scanning has also been applied to capture, digitally mirror, then print the patient's normal ear to serve as an intraoperative reference.[17]

As interest in 3Dp grows, improved access to ancillary technology such as 3D scanning has also improved. The ability to capture any object can be helpful in clinical applications. Although dedicated three-dimensional stereo-photogrammetry systems exist, such as the 3dMD (3dMD, Atlanta, GA, USA),[24] more recently, consumer technology has improved access to 3D scanning. Light detection and ranging sensor have become commonplace in modern-day smartphones, and the TrueDepth camera found on an Apple iPhone (Apple, Inc.; Cupertino, CA, USA) can be used by dedicated applications to perform detailed 3D scans.[17] Although primarily described in auricular reconstruction, the combined use of 3D optical scanning and 3Dp can be easily extrapolated to other aspects of facial plastics such as rhinoplasty.

Education

Beyond the operating room, 3Dp has the potential to improve the education of trainees and patients. This is because 3Dp allows for the rapid and affordable fabrication of anatomically accurate models.

For trainees, simulation provides an opportunity to amass experience to gain comfort and expertise. Educators can now produce high-fidelity simulators for common or challenging scenarios at a relatively low cost using 3Dp. The Pediatric Group from the University of Michigan has set up an exclusive 3Dp course where Pediatric Otolaryngology Fellows and Senior Residents can hone their skills in airway graft carving, microtia ear framework carving, and cleft lip/palate repair.[25] Similarly, Kovatch and colleagues[26] described a 3D printed task trainer to help promote multidisciplinary pediatric airway management. In this simulation, staff and residents in Anesthesia and Otolaryngology simulated emergency pediatric airway procedures while working in a realistic team.

In addition to preparing trainees for time-sensitive situations, 3D printed models can also help trainees practice fundamental procedural skills. Within rhinology, there exist published reports of 3D printed models aimed to improve septoplasty[27] and endoscopic sinus surgery skills.[28] Specifically to pediatrics, London and colleagues[29] studied the feasibility of a 3D printed pediatric anterior skull base model. The simulation allowed the participants to gain experience in an otherwise rare pathologic condition with unique anatomic challenges. The ability to represent anatomy accurately has attracted other studies in creating pediatric-specific task trainers for endoscopy, including bronchoscopy[30] and endoscopic ear surgery.[31,32]

A key part of an Otolaryngology training program involves understanding middle ear anatomy and developing the skill set to perform mastoidectomies safely. However, temporal bone laboratories can be costly to maintain, and the availability of cadaveric temporal bones varies between training programs. Therefore, many studies have utilized 3Dp as a supplemental tool in teaching middle ear anatomy and testing trainees' performance.[33–37] The American Academy of Otolaryngology-Head and Neck Surgery Foundation's 3D-Printed Temporal Bone Working Group recently released a study that evaluated several different materials types and examples of 3Dp temporal bones.[33] They supported a potential benefit in surgical training with standardized temporal bone models and provided preoperative patient-specific simulations. Studies are still needed to determine the impact of subsequent surgical performance.[37]

In addition to trainees, clinicians provide education to the patients. It can sometimes be hard to convey challenging clinical problems, even with two-dimensional illustrations. The use of a 3D model can help overcome the barriers in communication and visually represent the clinical problem and the proposed surgery better. In turn, the visual aid can help the patient appreciate the anticipated recovery and the postoperative expectations. For example, Lee and colleagues[38] informed parents of their surgical approach through 3Dp aids for a 7-year-old patient with a juvenile aggressive ossifying fibroma requiring aggressing resection. The authors found the 3D model to be impactful in the shared decision-making process and allowed the family to fully appreciate the functional and cosmetic implications of the ablative surgery. Similarly, literature in other domains has shown the positive influence of 3D models on patient understanding to facilitate decision-making.[39,40]

Future Directions and Challenges

Because 3Dp continues to gain popularity, the introduction of 3D printed patient-specific instruments may become more commonplace. Among adult otolaryngology patients, 3Dp models have allowed surgeons to preoperatively contour reconstruction plates for various applications such as the mandible[41–43] and orbital reconstruction.[44,45] Virtual surgical planning and intraoperative osseous cutting guides have also been well described.[46,47] The added precision from 3D printed surgical guides has been found to reduce complications, operating time, and the rate of radiographic nonunion.[47] It has been shown that 3D printed items can be adequately sterilized for intraoperative use without deformation following typical steam sterilization processes.[48] With the increased accessibility and decrease in cost of 3Dp, surgical instruments can now be conceptualized, printed, and tested in a short window.

Although 3Dp is becoming more commonplace, there are still aspects of 3Dp that, until recently, seemed to be excepted out of science fiction. Exciting developments in 3Dp in the upcoming years will likely include tissue engineering and the feasibility of bioprinting. Tissue engineering entails incorporating tissue with the 3Dp scaffold.[2,49] The added spatial framework created by the scaffold becomes a base onto which cells can theoretically grow.

Presently, a key limitation of 3Dp material is biocompatibility. Stramiello and colleagues[50] reported an overall complication rate of 21.7% among pediatric patients with intraluminal airway stents made with a bioresorbable material. To decrease the complication rate, a scaffold can be embedded with autologous tissue. Early experiments in creating tissue-engineered grafts have shown promise in animal studies.[51,52] Goldstein and colleagues[51] showing it is feasible to develop a tissue-engineered graft for airway reconstruction through in vitro and in vivo animal studies. The group seeded a 3D printed scaffold with mature chondrocytes and collagen gel and found good viability in rabbits. In studying auricular reconstruction, authors have successfully incorporated stem cells[52] or cartilage[53] with the printed constructs using animal models. Recently, an extension of this study has been completed by Zhou and colleagues,[54] whereby patient-specific ear-shaped cartilage was constructed out of biodegradable scaffold seeded with autologous chondrocytes. The authors reported their data on 5 patients with good success. These advances establish the feasibility for clinical application; however, more long-term data is necessary to determine its safety.

The next frontier of 3Dp would be bioprinting. In bioprinting, the cells are placed into their 3D constructs to create the desired tissue or organ and later incorporated into the patient.[2,49] Within otolaryngology, research has included efforts to replicate the tympanic membrane.[55] Although this remains very much in its infancy, bioprinting has the potential to influence the future of surgical practice significantly.

Because the 3Dp space presents possible applications, it is important to appreciate that many reports are small case series without objective comparative data.[16] Ultimately, large-scale clinical studies are required to understand the efficacy of this technology. Furthermore, although the cost of 3Dp has fallen over time, the investment for the initial setup and recruitment of capable personnel remains an obstacle for early adopters. Typical hobby 3D printers are relatively affordable, costing hundreds of dollars, and can print standard plastic material such as polylactic acid or acrylonitrile butadiene styrene. In comparison, industrial grade printers or 3D printers capable of bioprinting, may cost upward of hundreds of thousands, are specifically designed for certain material such as hydrogel, various metals (steel, bronze, gold, nickel, titanium, and aluminum), carbon fibers, graphene, and so forth. Choice of the printer and the associated cost would be contingent on the intended purpose of the final material, and this decision-making step would require some background understanding to the general limitations of various printers and materials. Moreover, the sweeping adoption of this technology in daily clinical activities by clinicians may not be feasible without a more defined model for reimbursement. Finally, before widespread clinical application within pediatric otolaryngology, there will need to be a continued emphasis on standardization and quality assurance protocols in line with local regulatory entities.[56]

SUMMARY

3Dp is an exciting and disruptive technology with various clinical and educational applications. The technology has become more accessible over time, and it is likely to be increasingly used in pediatric otolaryngology. 3Dp compliments the current shift toward personalized medicine and holds immense potential in bioprinting. Understanding the fundamentals of this technology and the current landscape will help otolaryngologists take advantage of its numerous applications.

CLINICS CARE POINTS

- Three dimensional printing technology has various clinical and educational applications within pediatric otolaryngology

DISCLOSURE

- P. You has no conflict of interest.
- M. Bartellas is a cofounder of a 3D printing health-care company, PolyUnity Tech Inc. There has been no conflict of interest or commercial/financial pursuits influenced or related to the creation of this article.

REFERENCES

1. VanKoevering KK, Hollister SJ, Green GE. Advances in 3-dimensional printing in otolaryngology: a review. JAMA Otolaryngol Head Neck Surg 2017;143(2): 178–83.
2. Zadpoor AA, Malda J. Additive manufacturing of biomaterials, tissues, and organs. Ann Biomed Eng 2017;45(1):1–11.
3. Zopf DA, Hollister SJ, Nelson ME, et al. Bioresorbable airway splint created with a three-dimensional printer. N Engl J Med 2013;368(21):2043–5.
4. Jain L. Three-dimensional printing and beyond: what lies ahead for pediatric otolaryngology. Clin Perinatol 2018;45(4):xv–xviii.
5. Morrison RJ, Hollister SJ, Niedner MF, et al. Mitigation of tracheobronchomalacia with 3D-printed personalized medical devices in pediatric patients. Sci Transl Med 2015;7(285):285ra64.
6. Sood V, Green GE, Les A, et al. Advanced therapies for severe tracheobronchomalacia: a review of the use of 3D-printed, patient-specific, externally implanted, bioresorbable airway splints. Semin Thorac Cardiovasc Surg Pediatr Card Surg Annu 2021;24:37–43.
7. Michaels R, Ramaraju H, Crotts SJ, et al. Early preclinical evaluation of a novel, computer aided designed, 3D printed, bioresorbable posterior cricoid scaffold. Int J Pediatr Otorhinolaryngol 2021;150:110892.
8. Stramiello JA, Saddawi-Konefka R, Ryan J, et al. The role of 3D printing in pediatric airway obstruction: a systematic review. Int J Pediatr Otorhinolaryngol 2020; 132:109923.
9. Wasserzug O, Fishman G, Carmel-Neiderman N, et al. Three dimensional printed models of the airway for preoperative planning of open Laryngotracheal surgery

in children: Surgeon's perception of utility. J Otolaryngol Head Neck Surg 2021; 50(1):47.

10. Shalev S, Ben-Sira L, Wasserzug O, et al. Utility of three-dimensional modeling of the fetal airway for ex utero intrapartum treatment. J Anesth 2021;35(4):595–8.

11. VanKoevering KK, Morrison RJ, Prabhu SP, et al. Antenatal three-dimensional printing of aberrant facial anatomy. Pediatrics 2015;136(5):e1382–5.

12. Rose AS, Webster CE, Harrysson OLA, et al. Pre-operative simulation of pediatric mastoid surgery with 3D-printed temporal bone models. Int J Pediatr Otorhinolaryngol 2015;79(5):740–4.

13. Takahashi K, Morita Y, Aizawa N, et al. Patient-specific 3D-printed model-assisted supracochlear approach to the petrous apex. Otol Neurotol 2020;41(8):e1041–5.

14. Ahmed S, VanKoevering KK, Kline S, et al. Middle cranial fossa approach to repair tegmen defects assisted by three-dimensionally printed temporal bone models. Laryngoscope 2017;127(10):2347–51.

15. Fernandez-Miranda JC, Hwang P, Grant G. Endoscopic endonasal surgery for resection of giant craniopharyngioma in a toddler-multimodal presurgical planning, surgical technique, and management of complications: 2-dimensional operative video. Oper Neurosurg (Hagerstown, Md) 2020;19(1):E68–9.

16. Hong CJ, Giannopoulos AA, Hong BY, et al. Clinical applications of three-dimensional printing in otolaryngology-head and neck surgery: A systematic review. Laryngoscope 2019;129(9):2045–52.

17. You P, Liu Y-CC, Silva RC. Fabrication of 3D models for microtia reconstruction using smartphone-based technology. Ann Otol Rhinol Laryngol 2022;131(4): 373–8.

18. Hatamleh MM, Watson J. Construction of an implant-retained auricular prosthesis with the aid of contemporary digital technologies: a clinical report. J Prosthodont 2013;22(2):132–6.

19. Zhu P, Chen S. Clinical outcomes following ear reconstruction with adjuvant 3D template model. Acta Otolaryngol 2016;136(12):1236–41.

20. Liacouras P, Garnes J, Roman N, et al. Designing and manufacturing an auricular prosthesis using computed tomography, 3-dimensional photographic imaging, and additive manufacturing: a clinical report. J Prosthet Dent 2011;105(2):78–82.

21. Chen K, Fu Y, Yang L, et al. A new three-dimensional template for the fabrication and localization of an autogenous cartilage framework during microtia reconstruction. ORL J Otorhinolaryngol Relat Spec 2015;77(3):150–4.

22. Jeon B, Lee C, Kim M, et al. Fabrication of three-dimensional scan-to-print ear model for microtia reconstruction. J Surg Res 2016;206(2):490–7.

23. Zeng W, Lin F, Shi T, et al. Fused deposition modelling of an auricle framework for microtia reconstruction based on CT images. Rapid Prototyp J 2008;14(5):280–4.

24. Chen HY, Ng LS, Chang CS, et al. Pursuing mirror image reconstruction in unilateral microtia: customizing auricular framework by application of three-dimensional imaging and three-dimensional printing. Plast Reconstr Surg 2017; 139(6):1433–43.

25. Chang B, Powell A, Ellsperman S, et al. Multicenter advanced pediatric otolaryngology fellowship prep surgical simulation course with 3D printed high-fidelity models. Otolaryngol Head Neck Surg 2020;162(5):658–65.

26. Kovatch KJ, Powell AR, Green K, et al. Development and multidisciplinary preliminary validation of a 3-dimensional-printed pediatric airway model for emergency airway front-of-neck access procedures. Anesth Analg 2020;130(2):445–51.

27. AlReefi MA, Nguyen LHP, Mongeau LG, et al. Development and validation of a septoplasty training model using 3-dimensional printing technology. Int Forum Allergy Rhinol 2017;7(4):399–404.

28. Alrasheed AS, Nguyen LHP, Mongeau L, et al. Development and validation of a 3D-printed model of the ostiomeatal complex and frontal sinus for endoscopic sinus surgery training. Int Forum Allergy Rhinol 2017;7(8):837–41.

29. London NR, Rangel GG, VanKoevering K, et al. Simulation of pediatric anterior skull base anatomy using a 3D printed model. World Neurosurg 2021;147:e405–10.

30. Al-Ramahi J, Luo H, Fang R, et al. Development of an Innovative 3D Printed Rigid Bronchoscopy Training Model. Ann Otol Rhinol Laryngol 2016;125(12):965–9.

31. Jenks CM, Patel V, Bennett B, et al. Development of a 3-dimensional middle ear model to teach anatomy and endoscopic ear surgical skills. OTO Open 2021;5(4). 2473974X2110465.

32. Barber SR, Kozin ED, Dedmon M, et al. 3D-printed pediatric endoscopic ear surgery simulator for surgical training. Int J Pediatr Otorhinolaryngol 2016;90:113–8.

33. Mowry SE, Jabbour N, Rose AS, et al. Multi-institutional comparison of temporal bone models: a collaboration of the AAO-HNSF 3D-printed temporal bone working group. Otolaryngol Head Neck Surg 2021;164(5):1077–84.

34. Hochman JB, Rhodes C, Wong D, et al. Comparison of cadaveric and isomorphic three-dimensional printed models in temporal bone education. Laryngoscope 2015;125(10):2353–7.

35. Da Cruz MJ, Francis HW. Face and content validation of a novel three-dimensional printed temporal bone for surgical skills development. J Laryngol Otol 2015;129(Suppl):S23–9.

36. Rose AS, Kimbell JS, Webster CE, et al. Multi-material 3D models for temporal bone surgical simulation. Ann Otol Rhinol Laryngol 2015;124(7):528–36.

37. Frithioff A, Frendø M, Pedersen DB, et al. 3D-printed models for temporal bone surgical training: a systematic review. Otolaryngol Head Neck Surg 2021;165(5):617–25.

38. Lee AY, Patel NA, Kurtz K, et al. The use of 3D printing in shared decision making for a juvenile aggressive ossifying fibroma in a pediatric patient. Am J Otol 2019;40(5):779–82.

39. Eisenmenger LB, Wiggins RH, Fults DW, et al. Application of 3-dimensional printing in a case of osteogenesis imperfecta for patient education, anatomic understanding, preoperative planning, and intraoperative evaluation. World Neurosurg 2017;107:1049.e1–7.

40. Jones DB, Sung R, Weinberg C, et al. Three-dimensional modeling may improve surgical education and clinical practice. Surg Innov 2016;23(2):189–95.

41. Azuma M, Yanagawa T, Ishibashi-Kanno N, et al. Mandibular reconstruction using plates prebent to fit rapid prototyping 3-dimensional printing models ameliorates contour deformity. Head Face Med 2014;10:45.

42. Ro EY, Ridge JA, Topham NS. Using stereolithographic models to plan mandibular reconstruction for advanced oral cavity cancer. Laryngoscope 2007;117(4):759–61.

43. Prisman E, Haerle SK, Irish JC, et al. Value of preoperative mandibular plating in reconstruction of the mandible. Head Neck 2014;36(6):828–33.

44. Kozakiewicz M, Elgalal M, Loba P, et al. Clinical application of 3D pre-bent titanium implants for orbital floor fractures. J Craniomaxillofac Surg 2009;37(4):229–34.

45. Gander T, Essig H, Metzler P, et al. Patient specific implants (PSI) in reconstruction of orbital floor and wall fractures. J Craniomaxillofac Surg 2015;43(1):126–30.
46. Goodrum H, Breik O, Koria H, et al. Novel in-house design for fibula cutting guide with detachable connecting arm for head and neck reconstruction. J Oral Maxillofac Surg 2021;79(8):1769–78.
47. May MM, Howe BM, O'Byrne TJ, et al. Short and long-term outcomes of three-dimensional printed surgical guides and virtual surgical planning versus conventional methods for fibula free flap reconstruction of the mandible: decreased nonunion and complication rates. Head Neck 2021;43(8):2342–52.
48. Aguado-Maestro I, De Frutos-Serna M, González-Nava A, et al. Are the common sterilization methods completely effective for our in-house 3D printed biomodels and surgical guides? Injury 2020;xxxx:1–5.
49. Ozbolat IT, Yu Y. Bioprinting toward organ fabrication: challenges and future trends. IEEE Trans Biomed Eng 2013;60(3):691–9.
50. Stramiello JA, Mohammadzadeh A, Ryan J, et al. The role of bioresorbable intraluminal airway stents in pediatric tracheobronchial obstruction: a systematic review. Int J Pediatr Otorhinolaryngol 2020;139:110405.
51. Goldstein TA, Smith BD, Zeltsman D, et al. Introducing a 3-dimensionally printed, tissue-engineered graft for airway reconstruction: a pilot study. Otolaryngol Head Neck Surg 2015;153(6):1001–6.
52. Sterodimas A, de Faria J. Human auricular tissue engineering in an immunocompetent animal model. Aesthet Surg J 2013;33(2):283–9.
53. Chang B, Cornett A, Nourmohammadi Z, et al. Hybrid three-dimensional-printed ear tissue scaffold with autologous cartilage mitigates soft tissue complications. Laryngoscope 2021;131(5):1008–15.
54. Zhou G, Jiang H, Yin Z, et al. In Vitro regeneration of patient-specific ear-shaped cartilage and its first clinical application for auricular reconstruction. EBioMedicine 2018;28:287–302.
55. Kozin ED, Black NL, Cheng JT, et al. Design, fabrication, and in vitro testing of novel three-dimensionally printed tympanic membrane grafts. Hear Res 2016; 340:191–203.
56. Morrison RJ, Kashlan KN, Flanangan CL, et al. Regulatory considerations in the design and manufacturing of implantable 3D-printed medical devices. Clin Transl Sci 2015;8(5):594–600.

Slide Tracheoplasty
Complete Tracheal Rings and Beyond

Clare M. Richardson, MD[a,b], Catherine K. Hart, MD, MS[c,d],
Kaalan E. Johnson, MD[a,b], Mark E. Gerber, MD[e,*]

KEYWORDS

- Tracheal stenosis • Complete tracheal rings • Slide tracheoplasty • Management
- Surgical technique • Surgical planning • Pediatric airway

KEY POINTS

- Slide tracheoplasty is the preferred surgical treatment for symptomatic congenital tracheal stenosis and can be applied to a variety of other pathologies.
- Before undergoing slide tracheoplasty, thorough workup is essential and includes computed tomography imaging, bronchoscopy, and multidisciplinary input.
- Concurrent cardiopulmonary pathology is common in patients undergoing slide tracheoplasty and may increase surgical complexity and perioperative risk.
- Advanced surgical planning can be helpful to tailor the procedure to the individual patient and may include adjuncts such as three-dimensional models and simulation sessions.
- Postoperative protocols and active multidisciplinary care are crucial following slide tracheoplasty to reduce complications and maximize clinical outcomes.

INTRODUCTION

Congenital tracheal stenosis (CTS) is a rare but potentially life-threatening condition. Any degree of narrowing in the infant airway can cause significant consequences, as a reduction of only 1 mm can decrease luminal cross-sectional area by over 40%.[1] Incidence of CTS is estimated to be 1 in 64,500 births, and accounts for only 0.1% to 0.3% of all types of laryngotracheal stenosis.[1,2] The most common cause of CTS is complete tracheal rings, which were first identified in 1899.[3] Complete

[a] Division of Pediatric Otolaryngology–Head and Neck Surgery, Seattle Children's Hospital, MS OA.9.220, PO Box 5371, Seattle, WA 98145, USA; [b] Department of Otolaryngology–Head and Neck Surgery, University of Washington; [c] Division of Pediatric Otolaryngology–Head and Neck Surgery, Cincinnati Children's Hospital Medical Center, 3333 Burnet Avenue, MLC 2018, Cincinnati, OH 45229, USA; [d] Department of Otolaryngology–Head and Neck Surgery, University of Cincinnati College of Medicine; [e] Division of Pediatric Otolaryngology–Head and Neck Surgery, Phoenix Children's Hospital, 1920 East Cambridge Avenue, Suite 201, Phoenix, AZ 85006, USA
* Corresponding author.
E-mail address: mgerber1@phoenixchildrens.com

Otolaryngol Clin N Am 55 (2022) 1253–1270
https://doi.org/10.1016/j.otc.2022.07.014
0030-6665/22/© 2022 Elsevier Inc. All rights reserved.

tracheal rings occur when the posterior membranous trachea fails to develop during the 8 week of gestation (**Fig. 1**).[4] Subcategories of CTS include short segment stenosis, funnel-shaped stenosis (of varying length), and long segment stenosis, which occurs when it involves >50% of the trachea.[4,5] Long-segment tracheal stenosis (LSTS) is the most challenging to manage, and before modern surgical options, had mortality rates between 43% and 100%.[6–8]

The most common presenting symptom of CTS is biphasic stridor. This is sometimes referred to as "washing machine" stridor due to the wet, rattling sound that can occur due to secretions passing through the stenosis.[5] Stridor often presents in infancy, and may be accompanied by increased work of breathing, retractions, nonproductive cough, and intermittent cyanotic events.[1,5] Symptoms can sometimes be unmasked by a respiratory infection, when additional mucosal inflammation narrows the tracheal lumen. This can lead to rapid respiratory decline and may be fatal if immediate medical care is not pursued.[1] Patients with more mild stenosis may be diagnosed incidentally (eg, on imaging or when being intubated for another procedure) or later in life with dyspnea on exertion or asthma-like symptoms.[9]

Cardiac and pulmonary comorbidities are common in patients with CTS. The most common associated cardiac anomaly is pulmonary artery sling, which occurs when the left pulmonary artery arises anomalously from the right pulmonary artery and courses posterior to the trachea. Pulmonary artery sling is present in approximately 30% of patients with CTS, and up to 66% of patients with a pulmonary artery sling will have CTS.[3,10] This frequent association is sometimes called the "ring-sling" complex. Other common comorbidities include tetralogy of Fallot, atrial and/or ventricular septal defect, pulmonary atresia, and tracheobronchomalacia.[11] Patients with an underlying diagnosis of Trisomy 21 or VACTERL association (vertebral, anorectal, cardiac, tracheoesophageal fistula, esophageal atresia, renal, and limb anomalies) are at an increased risk of CTS.[9]

History of Slide Tracheoplasty

The first open surgical treatment described for CTS was tracheal resection performed by Cantrell and Guild in 1964.[12] For the next two decades, CTS remained a predominantly lethal diagnosis as resection length was limited to 25% to 30% of total tracheal length.[1,3] In 1982, the first surgical technique for the treatment of LSTS was introduced with the cartilage tracheoplasty, and was followed by other techniques including

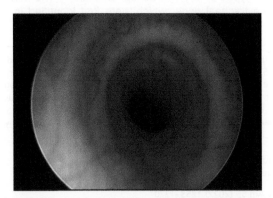

Fig. 1. Congenital tracheal stenosis caused by complete tracheal rings as seen on rigid bronchoscopy.

pericardial patch tracheoplasty, slide tracheoplasty (ST), homograft tracheoplasty, and tracheal autograft.[13–17] Of these, ST has emerged as the preferred surgical treatment for CTS, especially LSTS, due to improved efficiency, lower rates of postoperative and long-term complications, reduced perioperative cost, and lower mortality compared with other procedures.[4,5,18,19]

The first account of surgical technique for ST was by Tsang and Goldstraw.[15] Grillo adapted, promoted, and studied this technique throughout 1990s, which contributed significantly to its popularization.[3,20] Both descriptions used a straight (90°) tracheal transection incision and the same basic surgical steps, but with opposite placement of the proximal and distal segment longitudinal incisions. Tsang originally reported placing the proximal longitudinal incision anteriorly and the distal incision posteriorly, ending the anterior anastomosis at the proximal trachea, whereas Grillo[20] described the opposite.[15,20] Regardless of direction, ST doubles the tracheal diameter and increases lumen of the stenotic trachea by fourfold. The next significant change in ST surgical technique was described by de Alarcon and Rutter in 2012, when they introduced the concept of a beveled tracheal transection incision as opposed to a straight incision.[21] Recent research has shown that this incision type provides an additional benefit of increased postoperative tracheal length and volume over the traditional description.[22]

Applications of Slide Tracheoplasty Beyond Complete Tracheal Rings

ST has subsequently been adapted past its initial use for complete tracheal rings. In a broad sense, technique can now be divided into cervical ST, which is performed through a neck incision, and cervicothoracic ST, which is performed via a sternotomy incision with the patient on cardiopulmonary bypass (CPB).[21]

Cervical ST is ideal for high tracheal or laryngotracheal lesions. It is frequently used to address iatrogenic problems such as acquired stenosis and tracheal A-frame deformity due to prior tracheostomy placement but can also be applied to other pathology such as tracheal tumors, tracheal trauma injuries, and tracheoesophageal fistulas (TEFs).[21,23] Surgical technique is similar to cervicothoracic ST with resulting increase in the anastomotic caliber and may involve including the cricoid cartilage in the slide. Cervical ST is an excellent option in select patients as an alternative to tracheal resection.

Cervicothoracic ST has been modified and applied to many types of intrathoracic pathology. Multiple iterations have been described for tracheal bronchus with distal complete tracheal rings (also sometimes called bridging bronchus), which consists of a combination tracheal or tracheobronchial stenosis and abnormal bronchial arborization (**Fig. 2**).[24–29] ST has also successfully been used to treat TEFs, both for primary repair as well as for treatment of large or recurrent fistulas that fail traditional

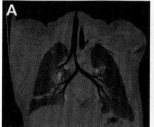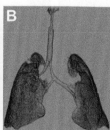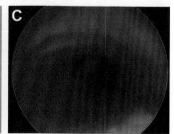

Fig. 2. Tracheal bronchus with distal complete tracheal rings as seen on (*A*) CT image, (*B*) three-dimensional rendering, and (*C*) rigid bronchoscopy.

endoscopic or thoracotomy approaches (**Fig. 3**).[30–33] Provezano and colleagues[32] described a modified ST technique to use the resected tracheal rings as an additional layer for closure of complex TEFs. Other ST applications include revision tracheoplasty,[34,35] combination subglottic and tracheal stenosis,[36,37] tracheal bronchus without associated stenosis (bronchus suis),[25] isolated bronchial stenosis,[9,25] congenital absence of tracheal rings,[9,38] carinal stenosis,[39] tracheal tumors,[9] and tracheocartilaginous sleeve.[9,40,41]

Despite its many applications, ST is still, by far, most commonly performed for CTS because of complete tracheal rings.[42]

Surgical Decision-making

Most children with complete tracheal rings require surgical intervention because of the small diameter of the airway and/or the severity of symptoms. There is a small subset of patients that can be managed expectantly and may not require surgical intervention.[43,44] As previously mentioned, this group of patients tends to present at a later age with mild symptoms such as dyspnea on exertion or asthma-like symptoms. A review of 149 patients with complete rings found that nearly 17% were able to be conservatively managed without operative intervention.[44] Patients with unrepaired complete tracheal rings were diagnosed outside of infancy and they typically had short segment complete rings with minimal airway symptoms. This cohort showed median airway growth of 0.37 mm per year.[44] Non-operative management is reasonable in patients with minimal or mild airway symptoms as long as the airway diameter is not critically small. In patients being managed conservatively, interval airway endoscopy should be performed until the child reaches puberty to ensure the continued growth of the segment of complete rings. Strict documentation of an airway plan (especially endotracheal tube [ETT] size) should be maintained in case of acute respiratory compromise. Operative intervention with ST should be considered if airway symptoms worsen over time or if the airway fails to grow.

For most of the patients who do require repair, the timing of surgical intervention is dictated by the severity of airway compromise. In patients with severe symptoms, ST should be undertaken as quickly as possible once the necessary preoperative evaluation is complete (see below). If necessary, use of steroids (topical and/or systemic), humidification, and intubation can be used as temporizing measures in symptomatic patients until definitive repair can be performed. In some instances, extracorporeal membrane oxygenation (ECMO) can be used to bridge unstable patients to definitive repair.

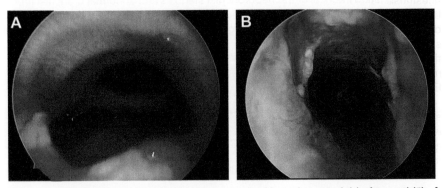

Fig. 3. Large tracheoesophageal fistula as seen on rigid bronchoscopy (A) before and (B) after slide tracheoplasty.

In most patients, cardiac and airway repair should be performed at the same time to avoid the risk of revision sternotomy and increased bypass time.[19,35] Individual patient factors should be considered by a multi-disciplinary team to determine appropriateness of concurrent repair.

Preoperative Workup

Although urgent surgical intervention is required in many patients, there are components of the preoperative evaluation that are necessary before proceeding with ST. Airway endoscopy is essential to determine the location, length, and caliber of the stenosis, as well as to assess for concurrent airway problems. When possible, an ETT should be used to measure the diameter of the stenosis. This is accomplished by placing an uncuffed ETT under endoscopic visualization to ensure that the narrowest portion of the stenosis is measured. Leak test is then performed, and airway size is determined by taking the outer diameter (in millimeters) of the largest ETT with a leak at less than 20 cm of water.[44] In older children, this often requires modifying an ETT in order to reach the distal airway (**Fig. 4**). In some instances, the stenosis is too narrow to accommodate an ETT in which case the diameter of the endoscope can be used to estimate the size of the airway. Great care must be taken during bronchoscopy to avoid converting a compromised airway to a critical airway by forcing a bronchoscope or ETT through a tight stenosis. Medications such as steroids or racemic epinephrine can be used to limit postoperative mucosal swelling.

Once bronchoscopy has confirmed the presence of tracheal stenosis, high-resolution contrasted computed tomography (CT) of the chest using vascular imaging protocols should be completed to further define the anatomic relationships between the airway and vascular structures. In patients with complex anatomy, presurgical three-dimensional (3D) modeling can facilitate planning of repair to optimize outcomes (see the section "Simulation and New Frontiers"). An echocardiogram is also necessary to assess for any concurrent cardiac abnormalities. Consultation with cardiology and cardiothoracic surgery should be obtained. Multidisciplinary evaluation is essential to providing optimal care of patients with CTS. Medical management for concurrent pulmonary disease and gastroesophageal reflux disease should be optimized. Additional engagement of critical care, pediatric surgery, genetics, and pulmonology should be considered.

Surgical Technique

Initial steps and tracheal exposure are similar across most applications of ST. General anesthesia is induced with spontaneous ventilation. Microlaryngoscopy and rigid bronchoscopy are performed to confirm the pathology, including the proximal and distal extent and lumen caliber. If respiratory culture has not yet been obtained, it should be done during this step before administering perioperative antibiotics. The patient is then intubated with an appropriately sized ETT, taking care to minimize mucosal trauma. Recurrent laryngeal nerve monitoring should be considered via ETT sensor or external probe placement.

Median sternotomy is performed, and the thymus is divided to expose the great vessels and trachea. Depending on the proximal extent of the anticipated ST, the thyroid isthmus may need to be divided to expose the cricoid. The innominate vessels and aorta are mobilized and retracted. Surrounding lymphatics and soft tissue are then freed from the trachea, taking care to avoid trauma to the recurrent laryngeal nerve. Lateral attachments should be left where possible to preserve tracheal blood supply. The carina is freed, and the main-stem bronchi are dissected deep to the pulmonary arteries to facilitate later mobilization of the distal tracheal segment. Careful dissection

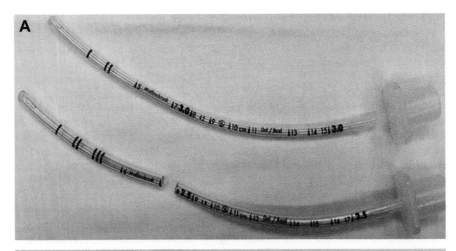

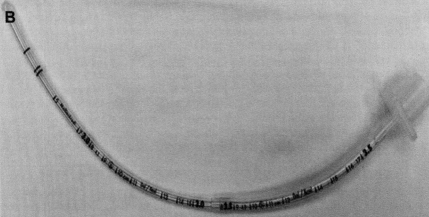

Fig. 4. Creation of a modified ETT for measuring airway stenosis. (*A*) A 3.5 ETT is divided, and the adapter is removed from the 3.0 ETT. (*B*) The proximal portion of the 3.5 ETT is slide over the top of the 3.0 ETT to create a longer ETT.

is performed to separate the trachea from the esophagus along its length. Dissection is kept directly against the trachea to avoid esophageal injury. Performing as much tissue mobilization as is safe before entering the airway reduces the time needed on CPB. Cannulation is then performed, and the patient is placed on CPB. If cardiac repair is required, this is performed before entering the trachea.

Complete Tracheal Rings

The length of tracheal stenosis is measured, and the midpoint is identified. Sometimes repeat bronchoscopy is performed during this step while a needle is passed through the anterior tracheal wall to confirm the superior and inferior extent of the stenosis. The trachea is then transected at the midpoint (**Fig. 5**A). Although historically this has been performed with a straight (90°) incision, it is preferable to use a beveled incision of approximately 45° to preserve tracheal length.[21,22] Tissue mobilization is completed to fully free the proximal and distal tracheal segments and opposing longitudinal incisions are made in each segment. The direction of the bevel will dictate the placement

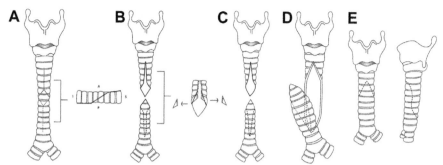

Fig. 5. Technique for slide tracheoplasty for complete tracheal rings. (*A*) Tracheal transecion incision is made at the midpoint of the stenosis with bevel. (*B*) Opposing longitudinal incisions are made in the proximal and distal tracheal segments. (*C*) Small triangles of cartilage are removed from the corners of the proximal and distal trachal segments to round the edges. (*D,E*) Anastamosis is performed in a running fashion beginning inferiorly to yield the final reconstructed trachea. (*From* Chen H, Shi G, Zhu L, et al. Intermediate-term outcomes of slide tracheoplasty in pediatric patients with ring-sling complex. Ann Thorac Surg 2020;109(3):820-27.)

of these incisions anteriorly or posteriorly and will therefore dictate the direction of the slide. Although both directions can be used successfully with similar caliber improvements, an anterior-superior to posterior–inferior bevel to end the anastomosis anteriorly on the proximal segment may be slightly preferable. It allows for the incorporation of the cricoid or tracheostomy stoma into the incision when needed and also allows for easier extension and adjustment compared with the opposite direction which had limited flexibility because of terminating near the carina.

Small triangles of cartilage are removed from the corners of the proximal and distal tracheal segments to round the edges (**Fig. 5**B). Anastomosis is then performed in a running fashion beginning inferiorly. This is done with a double-armed, absorbable monofilament suture, typically a 5 to 0 or 6 to 0. Nonabsorbable suture is discouraged as any intraluminal component can cause increased granulation tissue formation and risk of re-stenosis. Using a double-armed suture allows for symmetric repair as the anastomosis proceeds superiorly (**Fig. 5**C). In addition, using a running horizontal mattress technique can aid eversion of the edges to help minimize figure of 8 deformity.[45] Before completing the anastomosis, the airway is cleared of secretions and ETT is positioned so the tip lies in the middle of the repair. This can also be done under direct visualization with bronchoscopy, if needed. Small metallic clips may be placed at the superior and inferior ends of the anastomosis anteriorly in the pretracheal soft tissue to allow for postoperative radiographic confirmation of proper ETT position. The mediastinum is then filled with saline and a leak test is performed up to 30 mm Hg. Any identified leaks should be repaired with interrupted sutures. Fibrin glue can be placed along the anastomosis if desired. The patient is then weaned from CPB. Mediastinal drain(s) are placed, and the chest is closed in the usual fashion.

Tracheal Bronchus with Distal Complete Tracheal Rings

ST for tracheal bronchus with distal complete rings is performed in a similar fashion to ST for complete tracheal rings, with several important modifications. Incision placement will depend on the length of the stenotic segment as well as any involvement of the true mainstem bronchi. In the absence of bronchial involvement, the incision can be placed at the midpoint or superior aspect of the stenosis (**Fig. 6**A). If the

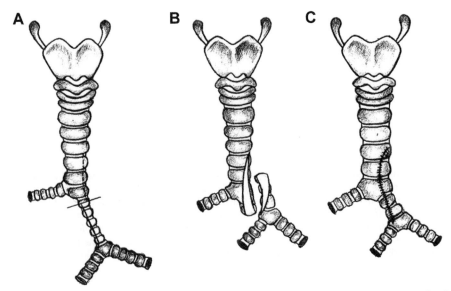

Fig. 6. Technique for slide tracheoplasty for tracheal bronchus with distal complete tracheal rings. (*A*) Tracheal transection incision is made at the midpoint or superior aspect of the stenosis. The bevel and longitudinal incisions should be placed laterally. (*B*) The incision should always extend partially into normal trachea to prevent stenosis at the superior aspect of the anastomosis. (*C*) Final repair yields a wider stenotic segment and a tracheal bronchus that is closer to the true carina. (*From* Chen H, Shi G, Zhu L, et al. Intermediate-term outcomes of slide tracheoplasty in pediatric patients with ring-sling complex. Ann Thorac Surg 2020;109(3):820-827.)

stenosis does include one of the bronchi, the inferior incision can be carried into the bronchus to incorporate it into the slide. The bevel should have its apex laterally as opposed to anteriorly to avoid the tracheal bronchus. The incision should always extend partially into normal trachea to prevent stenosis at the superior aspect of the anastomosis (**Fig. 6**B). Final repair yields a wider stenotic segment and a tracheal bronchus that is closer to the true carina (**Fig. 6**C). If the tracheal bronchus is located more distal to begin with, it may create a trifid appearing carina.

Tracheoesophageal Fistula

ST can be modified to include interposition flaps for repair of recurrent or complex TEFs. The initial approach is similar to ST for complete tracheal rings, with the exception of the preoperative microlaryngoscopy and bronchoscopy. In addition to these steps, esophagoscopy is performed and an esophageal bougie is placed. The length of the TEF should be measured as accurately as possible during this step. The size and location of the fistula will also dictate how much dissection is needed to mobilize the proximal and distal tracheal segments. before tracheal incision, repeat bronchoscopy should be performed and a needle passed through the anterior tracheal wall to identify the exact location of the TEF. The trachea is then divided superiorly and inferiorly to the fistula, leaving a segment of trachea attached to the tract (**Fig. 7**A). This is then divided anteriorly to allow for access to the fistula (**Fig. 7**B). The trachealis is separated from the esophageal mucosa and esophageal repair is performed. The tracheal mucosa is removed from the cartilage, infolded, and used to reinforce repair. The cartilage segments can be left attached for additional support. A sternal

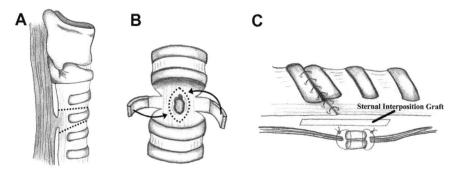

Fig. 7. Technique for slide tracheoplasty for tracheoesophageal fistula. (*A*) The trachea is divided superiorly and inferiorly to the fistula, leaving a segment of trachea attached to the tract. (*B*) The tracheal mucosa is removed from the cartilage, infolded, and used to reinforce esophageal repair. If needed, the cartilage segments can be left attached for additional support. (*C*) A sternal interposition graft is then placed over the cartilage, and the tracheal repair is performed in a running oblique fashion. (*From* Provenzano MJ, Rutter MJ, von Allmen D, et al. Slide tracheoplasty for the treatment of tracheoesophogeal fistulas. J Pediatr Surg. 2014 Jun;49(6):910-4.)

interposition graft is then placed over the cartilage, and the tracheal repair is performed (**Fig. 7**C). Tracheal closure includes a running oblique running anastomosis.

Postoperative Care

Following surgery, patients should be intubated with an appropriately sized ETT under direct visualization. Care should be taken to choose an ETT that will not put excess pressure on suture lines. Extubation should ideally be performed within 24 to 48 h, if possible, with observation in the intensive care unit (ICU) until time of first postoperative bronchoscopy. Younger patients and those with concurrent cardiac or pulmonary co-morbidities may require longer use of mechanical ventilation and longer ICU stays.[46,47] Immediate post-extubation respiratory support should not exceed the positive pressure of that performed during intraoperative leak test (generally around 30 mm Hg). High-flow oxygen cannula and Heliox can be good support options. If needed, repeat intubation should ideally be performed by the otolaryngology team under direct bronchoscopic visualization.

Meticulous pulmonary hygiene is critical following ST as clearance may be compromised in these patients due to impaired mucociliary function across the anastomosis, perioperative sedation, pulmonary comorbidities, and overall increase in secretion burden. Continuous humidification and routine suctioning should be provided while the patient is mechanically ventilated, as well as post-extubation with humidified oxygen or facemask. Some reports advocate for use of nebulized steroids/antibiotic drops (such as Ciprodex), but no randomized trials have shown benefit over non-medicated humidification.[48] The risk of using postoperative steroids (either enteral or topical) on wound healing should be considered and weighed with the potential benefit of reducing inflammation and granulation tissue.[46] Pulmonary toilet should be tailored to each individual patient with input from the surgical team, pulmonology, and respiratory therapy. Routine chest X-ray should be performed while the patient is in the ICU to monitor for postoperative atelectasis and direct pulmonary hygiene. Additional imaging with CT is generally not needed.

Antibiotic therapy past standard perioperative administration should be directed by the surgical team. A culture of tracheal secretions obtained at the time of preoperative bronchoscopy can be helpful to direct antibiotic choice, and additional treatment may be indicated if methicillin-resistant *Staphylococcus aureus* (MRSA) or Pseudomonas are identified.[49] There is no standardized length of time antibiotics are recommended before or after ST, but generally do not extend past 1 to 2 weeks. An exception to this is in cases of anastomotic dehiscence, in which broad-spectrum antibiotics should be administered/continued to prevent mediastinitis.

Postoperative bronchoscopies should be initially performed one to 2 weeks after ST to assess healing, inspect the anastomosis, and monitor for granulation tissue formation (**Fig. 8**B and C). Results from these bronchoscopies combined with overall clinical picture can help direct factors such as transition from ICU to floor status, need for further bronchoscopies, and estimated discharge date. If healing progresses uneventfully, outpatient surveillance bronchoscopy is generally performed at increasing intervals following inpatient postoperative bronchoscopies. A large cohort study showed that ST patients require an average of 10 postop bronchoscopies.[9] Most of the patients showed an average post-repair tracheal growth of 0.42 mm per year, which is commensurate to the growth of children with normal tracheas.[9]

Complications

Overall, ST is a successful procedure that has significantly improved outcomes compared with other tracheoplasty techniques.[4,18,19] Mortality rates are low overall, between 5% and 7%, but may be higher in patients with associated cardiopulmonary comorbidities.[19,46,50]

There are several early postoperative changes in the trachea that are, to an extent, expected, but can become pathologic if severe or untreated. These include things like figure 8 deformity, mucosal edema and sloughing, and granulation tissue formation. figure 8 deformity occurs due to the natural memory of the cartilage rings and relaxes over time as the trachea continues to heal (see **Fig. 8**). Symptomatic figure 8 deformity occurs in <3% of patients with ST, and only requires intervention if severe and obstructive or if synechiae form between shelves.[46] Mucosal edema and sloughing can contribute to overall secretion burden and cause mucous plugging, but this can be mitigated by strict adherence to postoperative humidification and pulmonary toilet protocols. Granulation tissue forms as a normal reactive part of the healing process along the anastomosis, but if excessive, can lead to airway obstruction. Factors that may contribute to granulation formation include exposed suture, excessive anastomotic tension, and indwelling airway devices (stents or tracheostomy tubes).[1] When necessary, granulation can be treated with excision and topical/inhaled steroid medication.[46,51]

Respiratory complications can also occur after ST and are often commensurate with co-existing cardiac or pulmonary comorbidities. Early extubation is ideal after ST and can be achieved in >50% of cases.[52] Patients who required mechanical ventilation before ST or had extended intraoperative CPB time are more likely to require prolonged postoperative intubation and mechanical ventilation.[42,52] There also appears to be an inverse relationship between intubation time and patient age/weight, indicating that younger ST patients may also need protracted respiratory support.[42] Up to 12% of ST patients may require postoperative tracheostomy placement, with higher rates in patients with concurrent cardiopulmonary issues.[42,46] Tracheomalacia can also present a perioperative challenge, and increase the likelihood of post-ST tracheostomy or stent placement.[50] If diagnosed preoperatively, procedure such as tracheopexy or aortopexy can be combined with ST to reduce this risk.[50,53]

Infectious complications after ST are rare but can be devastating when they do occur. MRSA may be more prevalent in ST patients as they have a history of

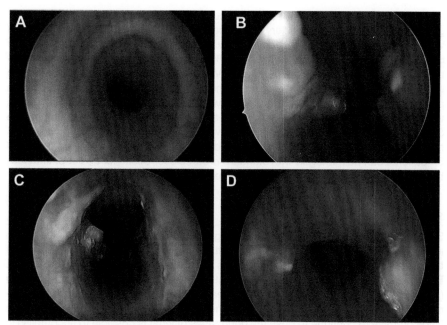

Fig. 8. Bronchoscopy images of a patient with CTS (*A*) before repair, (*B*) immediately following repair, (*C*) 1-week postoperative, and (*D*) 3 months postoperative. Note figure 8 deformity relaxing over time as the trachea heals, evidenced in the difference between image b and c with image d.

prematurity, prior hospitalizations, prior exposure to antibiotics, and invasive airway device placement such as tracheostomy.[54] Screening for MRSA and *Pseudomonas aeruginosa* should be undertaken preoperatively to determine if perioperative pathogen-specific antibiotics are indicated. Infection after ST can lead to compromise of the tracheal cartilage, tissue loss, and resultant anastomotic dehiscence. In addition to infectious etiologies, anastomotic dehiscence can also occur because of excess tissue tension or vascular compromise. If observed, it should be closely followed with serial bronchoscopy to assess for progression. Some patients may benefit from support on ECMO to allow for extubation and airway rest.[55] Although some patients with dehiscence can be treated with intravenous antibiotic therapy and watchful waiting, others will require revision surgery.

Many patients will require endoscopic interventions following ST, including granulation excision, steroid injection, and balloon dilation.[9,56] It is important to counsel families and multidisciplinary teams about this potential need to set expectations and to keep an open dialogue about number and timing of postoperative bronchoscopies. Recurrent stenosis can occur in ST patients in up to 12%.[46,50] If minimally invasive interventions fail, these patients sometimes require placement of endoluminal stents. Although these can be successful in the short term and facilitate patient growth, risks and benefits must be thoroughly considered because of the risk of excessive granulation formation, erosion, and migration.[56] Revision ST is also a treatment option for recurrent stenosis, with good outcomes achieved and similar morbidity and mortality risks when compared with primary ST.[35]

ST can also affect functional outcomes including voice and swallowing. Rates of recurrent laryngeal nerve injury and subsequent vocal cord immobility (VCI) are reported to be between 3% and 29%, although may be up to 47% in patients undergoing concurrent pulmonary artery sling repair.[57,58] These are comparable to rates of VCI reported for congenital cardiac surgery and can be expected to follow a similar trajectory with a recovery rate of 77% to 79%.[57] Dysphagia is also common in ST patients, and may be present independent of VCI. An estimated 20% of patients will go into ST with preexisting swallowing concerns, but up to 70% will develop dysphagia postoperatively.[58] Comprehensive workup with clinical swallow evaluation and often video fluoroscopic swallow study should be an expected component of postoperative ST care. A subset of these patients (20%) will have silent, asymptomatic aspiration, reinforcing the need for close monitoring and follow-up.[58] Dysphagia in postoperative ST patients can be managed with standard protocols for thickener and supplementation, and have a high likelihood (>80%) of resolution within a year of surgery.[58]

Simulation and New Frontiers

Surgical techniques for ST have only undergone minor modifications since their original description, but the technology and institutional infrastructure available to support the surgeons performing these procedures have changed dramatically since 1989. Enhanced imaging modalities, use of simulation and advanced surgical planning (ASP), and perioperative multidisciplinary team management have continued to support steady improvements in patient outcomes. Additional advances in these growing fields promise to continue to push the boundaries of what is possible to accomplish in the care of these singularly complex airway patients.

CT scans were initially performed on test subjects in 1971 by Godfrey Hounsfield and original images were grainy and difficult to interpret. Recent advances in imaging technology have moved far beyond this, and include higher slice systems, iterative reconstruction, and spectral CT imaging. These advances allow for lower radiation exposures, faster image acquisition, dynamic imaging, and improved resolution. They have allowed surgical teams to create 3D reconstructions of airway anatomy, dynamic image sequences to evaluate how structures move over time, and layered rendering of images to enhance realism and clinical utility for addressing specific clinical questions (**Fig. 9**). Dual-energy and photon-counting detector technology hold potential to even further improve the resolution and differentiation of the images obtained as we move into the future of imaging capabilities.[59]

The ability to create realistic digital 3D reconstructions of airway images has also allowed for adaptation into files that can be 3D printed for simulation of airway procedures. This is a form of advanced surgical planning (ASP), which has been applied to many forms of robotic surgery, simulation, and surgical planning.[41,60] ASP and 3D printing have been used to aid in planning of complex tracheal surgeries including ST, and there has been a steady evolution of techniques in recent years.[41,61,62] These 3D printed models provide the potential to improve many aspects of the surgical care process from patient and family communication, surgical technique planning, and team preparation. They also provide a unique opportunity to perform the actual surgery (including various alternatives for approaches) on the 3D printed before entering the OR. Using models for teaching these surgical techniques at airway courses and during training of future airway surgeons also now has the potential to be completely personalized to the specifically desired airway pathology and techniques (**Fig. 10**). Lastly, utilization of 3D printed models can be extended to explore research aims. Volumetric analyses of 3D printed surgical specimens have shown anatomic benefits of different surgical techniques, such as beveled tracheal incisions resulting in a lesser reduction in tracheal length with preserved volume expansion.[22] Potential clinical

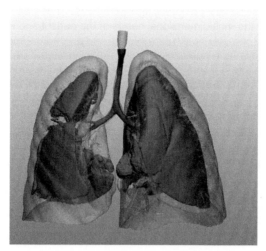

Fig. 9. Advances in CT imaging has allowed for visualization of complex structures and decision-making in ST. This image shows overlayered 3D reconstructions of CT scans of a patient with CTS obtained 15 months apart, showing that although the patient had grown in size and lung volume, their tracheal diameter did not increase significantly.

implications of such research lie in identifying the optimal surgical approach to maintain airway benefit while lowering anastomotic tension and risk of dehiscence.

Multidisciplinary team formation to support airway surgery has gradually become the standard of care in recent decades. We have moved away from the singular surgeon who is expected to cover every need for the patient and toward a complex

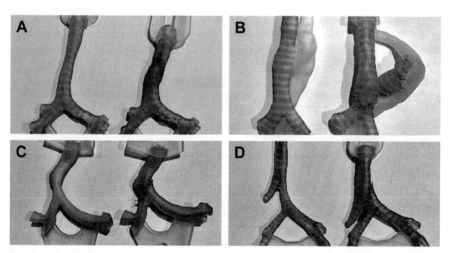

Fig. 10. Advanced surgical planning with 3D modeling for slide tracheoplasty has been used for a variety of tracheal pathologies such as (*A*) complete tracheal rings, (*B*) tracheoesophageal fistula tracheal bronchus with distal complete tracheal rings, (*C*) tracheocartilaginous sleeve with tracheobronchial stenosis, and (*D*) tracheal bronchus with distal complete tracheal rings. Images show the preoperative appearance of 3D-printed model on left and postoperative model on right).

network of inter-disciplinary providers and resources. These can be carefully constructed to support the multidimensional needs of the patient and family as they navigate an increasingly complex health care system and procedural sequences. This care model has been shown to reduce cost, improve efficiency, and decrease patient risk. Further expansion and development of team-based care holds promise to continue to improve patient outcomes and the patient and family experience moving forward.[63,64]

SUMMARY

ST has evolved to address a wide range of pathologies and provides excellent outcomes for conditions that were previously fatal. Multidisciplinary collaboration is crucial for the treatment of these complex patients, and can reduce costs, maximize efficiency, and improve outcomes. Recent advances in technology with advanced imaging and 3D modeling provide more exciting opportunities to further outcomes gains, personalize care, and improve the patient and family experience.

CLINICS CARE POINTS

- The most common cause of congenital tracheal stenosis is complete tracheal rings, and the most common symptom biphasic stridor that presents in infancy. Patients with more mild stenosis may be diagnosed incidentally at a later age.

- Up to 66% of patients with a pulmonary artery sling will have tracheal stenosis, therefore investigation for tracheal stenosis/complete trachea rings should be undertaken in all patients with this diagnosis.

- Up to 17% of patients with congenital tracheal stenosis can be observed, but operative intervention should be considered if airway symptoms worsen over time or if the airway fails to grow.

- Slide tracheoplasty is the preferred surgical treatment for symptomatic congenital tracheal stenosis and can also be used to treat many other pathologies. Approach can be cervical for proximal tracheal pathology, or cervicothoracic on cardiopulmonary bypass for long segment or distal tracheal pathology.

- A beveled tracheal transection incision is preferred over a straight incision to preserve tracheal length.

- Postoperative care of slide tracheoplasty patients includes early extubation (when possible), meticulous pulmonary hygiene, and rigid bronchoscopy within one to 2 weeks to monitor the anastomosis.

- Perioperative multidisciplinary collaboration is imperative in slide tracheoplasty patients to provide high-quality care.

FUNDING AND CONFLICTS OF INTEREST

This research did not receive funding in public, commercial, or not-for-profit-sectors. The authors have no conflicts of interest.

REFERENCES

1. Ho AS, Koltai PJ. Pediatric tracheal stenosis. Otolaryngol Clin North Am 2008; 41(5):999–1021.
2. Herrera P, Caldarone C, Forte V, et al. The current state of congenital tracheal stenosis. Pediatr Surg Int 2007;23(11):1033–44.

3. Backer CL, Holinger LD. A history of pediatric tracheal surgery. World J Pediatr Congenit Heart Surg 2010;1(3):344–63.
4. Sandu K, Monnier P. Congenital tracheal anomalies. Otolaryngol Clin North Am 2007;40(1):193–217.
5. Rutter MJ, Cotton RT, Azizkhan RG, et al. Slide tracheoplasty for the management of complete tracheal rings. J Pediatr Surg 2003;38(6):928–34.
6. Benjamin B, Pitkin J, Cohen D. Congenital tracheal stenosis. Ann Otol Rhinol Laryngol 1981;90(4):364–71.
7. Hoffer ME, Tom LWC, Wetmore RF, et al. Congenital tracheal stenosis: the otolaryngologist's perspective. Arch Otolaryngol - Head Neck Surg 1994;120(4):449–53.
8. Janik JS, Nagaraj HS, Yacoub U, et al. Congenital funnel-shaped tracheal stenosis: an asymptomatic lethal anomaly of early infancy. J Thorac Cardiovasc Surg 1982;83(5):761–6.
9. Wilcox LJ, Schweiger C, Hart CK, et al. Growth and management of repaired complete tracheal rings after slide tracheoplasty. Otolaryngol Head Neck Surg 2019;161(1):164–70.
10. Oshima Y, Yamaguchi M, Yoshimura N, et al. Management of pulmonary artery sling associated with tracheal stenosis. Ann Thorac Surg 2008;86(4):1334–8.
11. Sengupta A, Murthy RA. Congenital tracheal stenosis & associated cardiac anomalies: operative management & techniques. J Thorac Dis 2020;12(3):1184–93.
12. Cantrell JR, Guild HG. Congenital stenosis of the trachea. Am J Surg 1964;108(2):297–305.
13. Kimura K, Mukohara N, Tsugawa C, et al. Tracheoplasty for congenital stenosis of the entire trachea. J Pediatr Surg 1982;17(6):869–71.
14. Idriss FS, DeLeon SY, Ilbawi MN, et al. Tracheoplasty with pericardial patch for extensive tracheal stenosis in infants and children. J Thorac Cardiovasc Surg 1984;88(4):527–36.
15. Tsang V, Murday A, Gillbe C, et al. Slide tracheoplasty for congenital funnel-shaped tracheal stenosis. Ann Thorac Surg 1989;48(5):632–5.
16. Jacobs JP, Elliott MJ, Haw MP, et al. Pediatric tracheal homograft reconstruction: A novel approach to complex tracheal stenoses in children. J Thorac Cardiovasc Surg 1996;112(6):1549–60.
17. Backer CL, Mavroudis C, Dunham ME, et al. Repair of congenital tracheal stenosis with a free tracheal autograft. J Thorac Cardiovasc Surg 1998;115(4):869–74.
18. Kocyildirim E, Kanani M, Roebuck D, et al. Long-segment tracheal stenosis: Slide tracheoplasty and a multidisciplinary approach improve outcomes and reduce costs. J Thorac Cardiovasc Surg 2004;128(6):876–82.
19. Manning PB, Rutter MJ, Lisec A, et al. One slide fits all: The versatility of slide tracheoplasty with cardiopulmonary bypass support for airway reconstruction in children. J Thorac Cardiovasc Surg 2011;141(1):155–61.
20. Grillo HC. Slide tracheoplasty for long-segment congenital tracheal stenosis. Ann Thorac Surg 1994;58(3):613–20.
21. de Alarcon A, Rutter MJ. Cervical slide tracheoplasty. Arch Otolaryngol Head Neck Surg 2012;138(9):812.
22. Richardson C, Friedman SD, Park JS, et al. Comparison of slide tracheoplasty technique on postoperative anatomic outcomes in three-dimensional printed models. Laryngoscope 2022;132(6):1306–12. Published online October 4, 2021.
23. Li C, Rutter MJ. Acquired tracheal stenosis: Cervical slide tracheoplasty. Semin Pediatr Surg 2021;30(3):151058.

24. Abelardo E, Hewitt R, Elliott MJ, et al. Successful surgical repair of complex Christmas-tree pattern tracheo-bronchial anatomy with stenosis. Eur Arch Otorhinolaryngol 2013;270(7):2161–3.

25. Beierlein W, Elliott MJ. Variations in the technique of slide tracheoplasty to repair complex forms of long-segment congenital tracheal stenoses. Ann Thorac Surg 2006;82(4):1540–2.

26. Hagl S, Sebening C, Springer W, et al. Modified sliding tracheal plasty using the bridging bronchus for repair of long-segment tracheal stenosis. Ann Thorac Surg 2008;85(3):1118–20.

27. Ragalie WS, Chun RH, Martin T, et al. Side-to-side tracheobronchoplasty to reconstruct complex congenital tracheobronchial stenosis. Ann Thorac Surg 2017;104(2):666–73.

28. Stock C, Nathan M, Murray R, et al. Modified end-to-end anastomosis for the treatment of congenital tracheal stenosis with a bridging bronchus. Ann Thorac Surg 2015;99(1):346–8.

29. Wang S, Zhang H, Zhu L, et al. Surgical management of congenital tracheal stenosis associated with tracheal bronchus and congenital heart disease. Eur J Cardiothorac Surg 2016;49(4):1201–6.

30. Anton-Pacheco JL, Kalicinski P, Kansy A, et al. Slide tracheoplasty in an infant with congenital tracheal stenosis and oesophageal atresia with tracheoesophageal fistula. Eur J Cardio-Thoracic Surg 2012;42(5):892–3.

31. Kennedy AA, Hart CK, Alarcon A, et al. Slide tracheoplasty for repair of complex tracheoesophageal fistulas. Laryngoscope 2022;132(8):1542–7. Published online August 2, 2021:lary.29785.

32. Provenzano MJ, Rutter MJ, von Allmen D, et al. Slide tracheoplasty for the treatment of tracheoesophogeal fistulas. J Pediatr Surg 2014;49(6):910–4.

33. Wolter NE, Kennedy AA, Rutter MJ, et al. Diagnosis and management of complete tracheal rings with concurrent tracheoesophageal fistula. Int J Pediatr Otorhinolaryngol 2020;133:109971.

34. Kopelovich JC, Wine TM, Rutter MJ, et al. Secondary reverse slide tracheoplasty for airway rescue. Ann Thorac Surg 2016;101(3):1205–7.

35. Sidell DR, Hart CK, Tabangin ME, et al. Revision thoracic slide tracheoplasty: Outcomes following unsuccessful tracheal reconstruction: Revision Slide Tracheoplasty. Laryngoscope 2018;128(9):2181–6.

36. Kutlu C. Modified slide tracheoplasty for the management of tracheobroncopathia osteochondroplastica. Eur J Cardio-Thoracic Surg 2002;21(1):140–2.

37. Tasci E, Ciftci H, Periovi F, et al. Latero-lateral slide tracheoplasty for upper airway stenosis: an 8-year follow-up. J Thorac Cardiovasc Surg 2009;137(1):e44–6.

38. Smith MM, Kou YF, Schweiger C, et al. Congenital absence of tracheal or bronchial rings. Otolaryngol Head Neck Surg 2021;164(2):422–6.

39. Fandiño M, Kozak FK, Verchere C, et al. Modified slide tracheoplasty in a newborn with bronchial and carinal stenosis. Int J Pediatr Otorhinolaryngol 2013;77(12):2075–80.

40. Darr OA, Stone ML, Mitchell MB, et al. Slide tracheoplasty for tracheal cartilaginous sleeve in a patient with apert syndrome. Ann Thorac Surg 2021;112(6): e419–21.

41. Zenner K, Bonilla-Velez J, Johnson K, et al. Slide tracheoplasty to repair stenotic tracheal cartilaginous sleeve with advanced surgical planning. Otolaryngol Head Neck Surg 2020;163(2):391–3.

42. Wertz A, Fuller SM, Mascio C, et al. Slide tracheoplasty: Predictors of outcomes and literature review. Int J Pediatr Otorhinolaryngol 2020;130:109814.

43. Rutter MJ, Willging JP, Cotton RT. Nonoperative management of complete tracheal rings. Arch Otolaryngol Head Neck Surg 2004;130(4):450.

44. Wilcox LJ, Hart CK, de Alarcon A, et al. Unrepaired complete tracheal rings: natural history and management considerations. Otolaryngol Head Neck Surg 2018; 158(4):729–35.

45. Hobbs RD, Moon J, Murala J, et al. Novel suture technique for slide tracheoplasty for the treatment of long-segment tracheal stenosis. Semin Thorac Cardiovasc Surg 2020;32(4):930–4.

46. DeMarcantonio MA, Hart CK, Yang CJ, et al. Slide tracheoplasty outcomes in children with congenital pulmonary malformations: Slide Tracheoplasty and Lung Malformation. Laryngoscope 2017;127(6):1283–7.

47. Chen L, Zhu L, Wang H, et al. Surgical management strategy of slide tracheoplasty for infants with congenital tracheal stenosis. J Thorac Cardiovasc Surg 2022;163(6):2218–28. Published online November 2021:S0022522321015233.

48. Stephens EH, Eltayeb O, Mongé MC, et al. Pediatric tracheal surgery: a 25-year review of slide tracheoplasty and tracheal resection. Ann Thorac Surg 2020; 109(1):148–53.

49. Statham MM, de Alarcon A, Germann JN, et al. Screening and treatment of methicillin-resistant Staphylococcus aureus in children undergoing open airway surgery. Arch Otolaryngol Head Neck Surg 2012;138(2):153–7.

50. Wen W, Du X, Zhu L, et al. Surgical management of long-segment congenital tracheal stenosis with tracheobronchial malacia. Eur J Cardiothorac Surg 2021; 61(5):1001–10 [published online ahead of print, 2021 Dec 23].

51. Yokoi A, Nakao M, Bitoh Y, et al. Treatment of postoperative tracheal granulation tissue with inhaled budesonide in congenital tracheal stenosis. J Pediatr Surg 2014;49(2):293–5.

52. Manning PB, Rutter MJ, Border WL. Slide tracheoplasty in infants and children: risk factors for prolonged postoperative ventilatory support. Ann Thorac Surg 2008;85(4):1187–92.

53. Stramiello JA, Mohammadzadeh A, Ryan J, et al. The role of bioresorbable intraluminal airway stents in pediatric tracheobronchial obstruction: A systematic review. Int J Pediatr Otorhinolaryngol 2020;139:110405.

54. Fujieda Y, Morita K, Otake S, et al. Infectious complications after tracheoplasty for congenital tracheal stenosis: a retrospective comparative study. Pediatr Surg Int 2021;37(12):1737–41.

55. Raake J, Johnson B, Seger B, et al. Extracorporeal membrane oxygenation, extubation, and lung-recruitment maneuvers as rescue therapy in a patient with tracheal dehiscence following slide tracheoplasty. Respir Care 2011;56(8): 1198–202.

56. Butler CR, Speggiorin S, Rijnberg FM, et al. Outcomes of slide tracheoplasty in 101 children: a 17-year single-center experience. J Thorac Cardiovasc Surg 2014;147(6):1783–9.

57. Kaneko N, Hasegawa T. Incidence and risk factor of vocal cord paralysis following slide tracheoplasty for congenital tracheal stenosis: a retrospective observational study. Cardiol Young 2021;12:1–5.

58. Stewart AJ, Butler CR, Muthialu N, et al. Swallowing outcomes in children after slide tracheoplasty. Int J Pediatr Otorhinolaryngol 2018;108:85–90.

59. Alkadhi H, Euler A. The future of computed tomography: personalized, functional, and precise. Invest Radiol 2020;55(9):545–55.

60. Konuthula N, Parikh SR, Bly RA. Robotics in pediatric otolaryngology-head and neck surgery and advanced surgical planning. Otolaryngol Clin North Am 2020;53(6):1005–16.

61. Balakrishnan K, Cofer S, Matsumoto JM, et al. Three-dimensional printed models in multidisciplinary planning of complex tracheal reconstruction: 3D Printed Models in Tracheal Reconstruction. Laryngoscope 2017;127(4):967–70.

62. Arcieri L, Giordano R, Bellanti E, et al. Impact of 3D printing on the surgical management of tracheal stenosis associated to pulmonary sling: a case report. J Thorac Dis 2018;10(2):E130–3.

63. Wootten CT, Belcher R, Francom CR, et al. Aerodigestive programs enhance outcomes in pediatric patients. Otolaryngol Clin North Am 2019;52(5):937–48.

64. Boesch RP, Balakrishnan K, Grothe RM, et al. Interdisciplinary aerodigestive care model improves risk, cost, and efficiency. Int J Pediatr Otorhinolaryngol 2018; 113:119–23.

Enhanced Recovery After Surgery

A Quality Improvement Approach

Shelby Kitchin, BS[a], Vidya T. Raman, MD, MBA[b],
Thomas Javens, BS[c], Kris R. Jatana, MD[c,d],*

KEYWORDS

- ERAS • Enhanced recovery • Surgery • Surgical outcomes • Quality improvement
- Otolaryngology • Pediatric

KEY POINTS

- Enhanced recovery after surgery (ERAS) protocols have been used in many surgical specialties to reduce complications and achieve the best patient outcomes.
- Although numerous studies have investigated these protocols in the adult population, limited studies have been published in pediatric surgical specialties.
- There is a definite opportunity to further develop ERAS protocols in pediatric otolaryngology.

INTRODUCTION

The enhanced recovery after surgery (ERAS) concept was first developed in Denmark in 1990 and is a strategic, multidisciplinary approach to optimizing the care of surgical patients.[1] These protocols aim to optimize the perioperative experience for patients by shortening lengths of stay (LOS), preventing further admissions, reducing complications, and overall creating a more favorable patient experience.[2] ERAS interventions range from the administration of preoperative antibiotic prophylaxis to intraoperative monitoring and checklists, to postoperative pain management, nutrition, ambulation, and more.[3]

Since its incorporation into clinical practice, an abundance of literature supporting the efficacy of ERAS protocols within adult populations has emerged across a vast

[a] University of Cincinnati College of Medicine, 3230 Eden Avenue, Cincinnati, OH 45267, USA;
[b] Department of Anesthesia, Wexner Medical Center at Ohio State University, 410 West 10th Avenue, Columbus, OH 43210, USA; [c] Center for Clinical Excellence, Nationwide Children's Hospital, 700 Children's Drive, Columbus, OH 43205, USA; [d] Department of Otolaryngology-Head and Neck Surgery, Nationwide Children's Hospital and Wexner Medical Center at Ohio State University, 555 South 18th Street, Suite 2A, Columbus, OH 43205, USA
* Corresponding author.
E-mail address: Kris.Jatana@nationwidechildrens.org

Otolaryngol Clin N Am 55 (2022) 1271–1285
https://doi.org/10.1016/j.otc.2022.07.011
0030-6665/22/© 2022 Elsevier Inc. All rights reserved.

number of disciplines, including but not limited to, colorectal surgery, urology, gynecology, and otolaryngology. Still, the application of these protocols to pediatric populations remains somewhat limited, despite these protocols emerging as a mainstay of treatment for pediatric surgical patients.[4] The bulk of this evidence has been explored in pediatric colorectal, gastrointestinal, and urologic procedures. However, the evidence to support the efficacy of ERAS within pediatric otolaryngology exists in limited studies. The purpose of this literature review is to provide a summary of the current data on ERAS and its effectiveness within pediatric otolaryngology.

The PubMed search engine was used to explore publications relating to ERAS. The following search terms were used: enhanced recovery after surgery pediatric, enhanced recovery after surgery pediatric otolaryngology, enhanced recovery after surgery otorhinolaryngology, enhanced recovery after surgery and otolaryngology, enhanced recovery after ear, nose, and throat surgery. Articles were identified and reviewed that assessed ERAS protocols within pediatric surgery and otolaryngology; these are summarized in **Tables 1** and **2**. In addition, in this article, we describe the impact of our Nationwide Children's Hospital (NCH) Pediatric Tonsillectomy Protocol (**Fig. 1**).

DISCUSSION
Enhanced Recovery After Surgery in Pediatric Surgery

In 2020, Brindle and colleagues[3] reviewed the literature to create an evidence-based comprehensive guideline for ERAS within pediatrics. Specifically, they reviewed systematic reviews, randomized controlled trials (RCTs), and observational cohorts to compile data and give recommendations for neonates undergoing intestinal resection. A total of 17 recommendations were included in the guideline, with quality and strengths ranging from very low and weak to high and strong, respectively. Some of the strongest data within this study discussed recommendations for postoperative nutrition, including early enteral feeds and use of breast milk, perioperative communication strategies, such as the use of established checklists, and perioperative analgesia, such as the use of acetaminophen over opioids as well as nasal lingual sucrose/dextrose. This guideline can be applied to neonates ($\geq$37 weeks gestational age) without major comorbidities undergoing intestinal resection surgery within the first 4 weeks of life.

Han and colleagues[5] conducted a prospective case-control study that utilized an ERAS protocol to try to optimize outcomes relating to anesthesia in pediatric patients. Participants included those under 18 years who were undergoing urologic reconstruction and bowel anastomosis, totaling 13 experimental subjects and 26 control subjects. The study focused specifically on optimizing medical management before and immediately on leaving the operating room to reduce the need for opioids postoperatively. This management included regional blocks before incision, and a combination of ketorolac, intravenous (IV) acetaminophen, and ondansetron on leaving the operative room. Outcomes were assessed based on post-anesthetic care unit (PACU) pain score, number of days without opioid use, and the need for opioids on the day of discharge. Their study concluded that the ERAS protocol decreased postoperative pain and the need for opioids in this population with the following results for the control group and experimental group, respectively: those not needing opioids 0% versus 15% ($P = .046$) and maximum PACU pain scores of 3 versus 0 ($P < .001$). The percentage of days without opioids postoperatively was increased in the ERAS group (62% vs 33% in the control). Furthermore, the ERAS protocol

Table 1
Published Pediatric Surgery ERAS Studies

Authors	Surgeries	Patient Populations	Types of Study	# Of Patients	Benefits of Protocol
Han et al,[5] 2021	Urologic reconstruction that included a bowel anastomosis	Pediatric patients	Prospective case-control study	39 total (13 experimental, 26 control)	Decreased postoperative pain and need for opioids, decreased maximum PACU pain scores, decreased requirement for oxygen, no statistical differences in neither anesthesia time nor time to first opioid dose
Brindle et al,[3] 2020	Intestinal resection surgery	Term neonates ($\geq$37 wk gestational age) without major comorbidities within the first 4 wk of life	Literature review	N/A	N/A
Rove et al,[6] 2020	Lower urinary tract reconstruction	Pediatric (ages 4–17 y) and young adult (18–25) patients	Prospective case-control study	192 total (64 experimental, 128 control)	Proposed benefit: significant changes in lengths of stay, readmissions, reoperations, emergency room visits, 90-d complications, pain scores, opioid usage and differences in quality of recovery 9 scores
Yeh et al,[7] 2020	Laparoscopic cholecystectomy	Pediatric and young adult patients ages 0–31 undergoing elective surgery	Prospective study	250 total (145 experimental, 105 control)	Significantly greater rate of SDD, shorter average LOS, reduced use of opioids, earlier average surgery start time. Operative time and rate of 30-d readmissions were not statistically significant.

(continued on next page)

Table 1
(continued)

Authors	Surgeries	Patient Populations	Types of Study	# Of Patients	Benefits of Protocol
Rove et al,[4] 2018	Colon resection, pyeloplasty, pyloromyotomy, fundoplication, hypospadias repair, and nephrectomy	Pediatric patients	Literature review	N/A	N/A
Leeds et al,[8] 2018	Colorectal surgery	Pediatric patients aged >2 y undergoing surgical intervention that incises any gastrointestinal lumen distal to the ligament of Treitz to the anus	Retrospective study	58 total (28 experimental, 30 control)	Increase in formal preoperative education and improved administration of preoperative medication. Readmissions were highest in early implementation group. Children in late implementation group had fewer complications.

Table 2
Published Otolaryngology ERAS Studies

References	Surgeries	Patient Populations	Types of Study	# of Patients	Benefits of Protocol
Zhang et al,[14] 2021	Adenotonsillectomy	Pediatric patients with OSA (2.5 y to 14 y)	Retrospective historical control study	394 total (208 experimental, 186 control)	Significantly lower overall complication rate and incidence of fever for 2 wk of follow-up, less postsurgical pain, better dietary intake at days 1, 3, and 7 after surgery, lower preoperative anxiety scores, no significant change in rates of post-op infection, or pneumonia. Trend toward reduced hemorrhage rates in ERAS group 0.48% vs 2.69%.
Zhang et al,[10] 2021	Laryngeal cancer surgery	Adult patients, 45–75 year old	Randomized controlled trial	80 total (40 experimental, 40 control)	24 h postoperatively, significantly higher pain relief scores, lower perioperative thirst score and hunger score, reduced number of adverse reactions, decreased oral feeding time, and shorted LOS. Statistically insignificant data included length of indwelling catheter time and neck drainage tube time.

(continued on next page)

Table 2
(continued)

References	Surgeries	Patient Populations	Types of Study	# of Patients	Benefits of Protocol
Bertelsen et al,[9] 2020	Free flap reconstruction	Adult patients	Retrospective cohort study (baseline), post-implementation prospective cohort study	122 total (61 experimental, 61 control)	Reduced ventilator days, ICU LOS, vasopressor use, and blood transfusions. Additionally, labor-intensive flap monitoring can be scaled back without adverse effects on near-term perioperative outcomes.
Jandali et al,[11] 2020	Head and neck surgery	Adult patients	Retrospective cohort study	185 total (92 experimental, 93 control)	Decreased narcotic use in the postoperative period and at discharge, improved postoperative analgesia, shortened LOS, decreased time for ambulating postoperatively, shorter time to bolus NG tube feeds, reduced need for PCA narcotics and number of patients requiring refills of narcotic prescription refills within 30 d of operation. No significant difference in ICU LOS, number of ED visits, numbers of readmission within 30 d, and number or hematomas necessitating return to the OR.

Source	Procedure	Population	Study Design	Sample Size	Results
Tan et al,[13] 2021	Tympanoplasty and/or mastoidectomy due to chronic suppurative otitis media	Adult patients with chronic suppurative otitis media between 18 and 65 y of age	Randomized controlled trial	84 total (42 experimental, 42 control)	Optimized surgical scheme, shortened fasting time, reduced post-op pain, and increased the postoperative comfort for the patients, No significant differences in postoperative complications, postoperative hospitalization times, or costs associated with hospitalization.
Won et al,[12] 2019	Head and neck cancer surgery with free-flap reconstruction	Adult patients	Retrospective cohort study (baseline), post-implementation prospective cohort study	89 total (60 experimental, 29 control)	Reduced LOS, reduced start times to ambulation/time to adjuvant chemotherapy/oral. No statistical difference in total surgery duration, free-flap reconstruction duration, and rates of complications (ie, pneumonia, delirium, wound complication, fatality)
Dort et al,[2] 2017	Major head and neck cancer surgery with free-flap reconstruction	Adult patients	Literature review	N/A	N/A

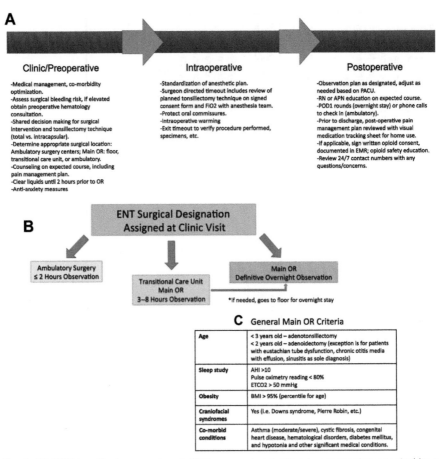

Fig. 1. (A) NCH tonsillectomy protocol; (B) Surgeon designation to appropriate surgical location and observation pathway; and (C) Criteria for surgery in main OR. (*From* Kris Jatana, MD, Columbus, Ohio, USA.)

decreased the need for supplemental oxygen (85% in the control group vs 38% in the ERAS group, $P = .013$). However, the two groups showed no statistical difference in anesthesia time nor the time to first opioid dose in those that required opioids.[5]

A prospective case-control study[6] initiated in 2016 will explore outcomes after implementing ERAS protocols in pediatric urologic populations. Patients aged 4 to 25 years undergoing bladder augmentation, continent ileovesicostomy/appendicovesicostomy, or urinary diversion will be included for an anticipated total of at least 64 experimental and 128 control patients to observe a decrease in mean LOS by 2 days. Primary outcomes will include adherence to ERAS protocols with goals of ≥70%, while secondary outcomes will explore LOS, readmissions, reoperations, emergency room visits, 90-day complications, pain scores, opioid usage, and differences in Quality of Recovery 9 scores. The study commenced enrollment in 2017 with initial aims to have been completed in 2021 and is ongoing. Authors of this study also conducted an educational review[4] in 2018 that described ERAS and compared it with perioperative surgical home (PSH), which is a "concept that encompasses the time from a decision to have surgery to weeks beyond the hospital setting."[4] This review summarizes some widely accepted practices that have been incorporated into ERAS protocols, including the minimization of prolonged fasting preoperatively, favoring minimally invasive surgeries compared to open surgeries, avoidance of opioid anesthesia and nasogastric tubes, avoidance of bowel preparations, and encouraging the maintenance of a euvolemic state in patients perioperatively. This review identified ample evidence to support ERAS among adult populations but a lack of data supporting ERAS protocols in pediatric populations. Lastly, in comparing ERAS to PSH, the study concluded that the two protocols both aim to provide better care at lower costs, but that PSH tends to take a more holistic approach (ie, wider scope) and varies more widely based on institution compared with ERAS protocols which tend to be more guideline-driven and evidence-based.

In another study, Yeh and colleagues[7] implemented an ERAS protocol in elective laparoscopic cholecystectomy within pediatric and young adult populations and did a retrospective review of prospectively collected data from patients before (baseline) and after implementation (AI) of an ERAS protocol. This study included 250 patients ranging from ages 0 to 31. Metrics studied include same-day discharge (SDD), use of opioids, and 30-day emergency department (ED) returns. Interventions included: administration of transdermal scopolamine, scheduled acetaminophen and IV ketorolac and fentanyl as needed, limiting the use of narcotics and IV fluids, scheduled dexamethasone IV at the start of the case, and scheduled ondansetron IV at the conclusion of surgery. Furthermore, early mobilization and early diet advancement were emphasized postoperatively. When patients were ambulating, tolerating diet, and had pain control, they were discharged. The ERAS protocol group had a significantly greater rate of SDD (77.2%) compared with the baseline group (1.9%), a shorter average LOS of 13.6 hours compared with baseline with 27.5 hours ($P<.001$) and significantly reduced use of opioids (morphine equivalents/kg AI 0.36 vs baseline 0.46, $P < .001$) compared with the control group. With regard to surgical start times, patients in the AI group had an earlier average surgery start time of 10:37 AM compared with control with an average surgery start time of 12:22 PM ($P<.001$); this could help to facilitate SDD. Other metrics, including operative time and rate of 30-day readmissions, were not statistically significant.

In 2018 Leeds and colleagues[8] enrolled pediatric colorectal surgery patients into the Pediatric Colorectal pathway, an ERAS protocol, at their institution and assessed 30-day outcomes over 2 years. Patients ranged from 8 to 16 years of age and underwent colorectal surgery with specifications of any patient undergoing surgical intervention that incises any gastrointestinal lumen distal to the ligament of Treitz to the anus. The study included a total of 58 patients, 28 in the experimental group and 30 in the control group. The study resulted in a marked improvement in education (56% vs 0%, $P = .004$) in the preoperative period. In the perioperative period, they also identified improvement in the administration of preoperative gabapentin, acetaminophen, and bisacodyl ($P = .002$, $P = .001$, $P = .025$). Rates of readmission were greatest during the early implementation phase (40%, $P = .029$). In addition, a worsening of complications was observed in this early phase. Both of these findings were significantly insignificant and researchers at this institution hypothesized these changes indicate an adjustment to the new care model.

In pediatric surgery populations, ERAS has shown promising results by displaying success in increasing rates of SDD, reducing the need for opioids postoperatively, and reducing LOS. Readmission rates had not been reduced greatly in the existing data, but they should be explored in further studies.

Enhanced Recovery After Surgery in Otolaryngology

Head and Neck Surgery

Dort and colleagues[2] identified studies and compiled data from 215 papers to identify best practices within head and neck cancer surgery. A total of 17 topic areas, within preoperative, intraoperative, and postoperative care were included. These include preoperative carbohydrate treatment, thromboprophylactic medication, perioperative antibiotics in clean-contaminated procedures, corticosteroid and antiemetic medications, short-acting anxiolytics, goal-directed fluid management, opioid-sparing multimodal analgesia, frequent flap monitoring, early mobilization, and the avoidance of preoperative fasting.

Another center studied the efficacy of an ERAS protocol for free flap reconstruction[9] at their institution. All patients undergoing free flap reconstruction were prospectively enrolled in the ERAS group, and a retrospective control group was created by randomly selecting an equivalent number of patients from a records search of those undergoing free flap surgery between 2009 and 2015. The study compared blood transfusions, complications, 30-day readmission rates, intensive care unit (ICU) and hospital LOS, and costs of hospitalization. The ERAS group underwent less frequent flap monitoring by physicians and had lower rates of intraoperative (70.5% vs 86.8%, $P = .04$) and postoperative (49.2% vs 27.2%, $P = .026$) blood transfusion, were more likely to be off vasopressors (98.3% vs 50.8%, $P < .01$), ventilator support (63.9% vs 9.8%, $P < .01$), and had shorter ICU stays (2.11 vs 3.39 days, $P = .017$). LOS, readmissions, and complication rates did not significantly differ between groups.[9]

In another study,[10] a total of 80 patients were included in the application of an ERAS protocol for the treatment of laryngeal cancer. Participants were randomized into ERAS and control groups (40 cases each). A visual analog scale, general comfort questionnaire, and self-rating Anxiety Scale were used to evaluate the groups before and after surgery. At 24 hour postoperatively, the ERAS group had significantly higher pain relief scores than the control group ($P<.05$). Additionally, the ERAS group had a lower perioperative thirst score (0.15 vs 4.29 in the control group, $P<.001$) and hunger score (0.38 vs 3.44 in the control group, $P<.001$). Other significant metrics included a reduced number of adverse reactions in the ERAS groups (8 vs 16), decreased oral feeding time (4.06 vs 9.06), and shorter postoperative hospital stay (5.91 d vs 11.03 d). Statistically insignificant data included length of indwelling catheter time and neck drainage tube time. Overall, the study concluded that the application of ERAS in laryngeal cancer surgery can improve preoperative hunger and thirst, decrease postoperative pain and improve mental state, shorten LOS, and reduce postoperative adverse reactions.[10]

A different study[11] assessed an ERAS protocol within head and neck surgery populations. A total of 185 patients were included in the study, with 92 ERAS patients and 93 controls. Populations were studied retrospectively to observe differences among groups. The mean morphine equivalent dose given within 72 hours postoperatively was significantly lower in the ERAS group (17.5 ± 46.0 mg vs 82.7 ± 116.1 mg, $P<.001$). Average pain scores in the first 72 hours postoperatively were lower in the ERAS group (2.6 ± 1.8 vs 3.6 ± 1.9; $P<.001$) and the average LOS was shorter for ERAS patients (7.8 ± 4.8 vs 9.7 ± 4.7 days, $P = .008$). Other significant metrics included decreased time for ambulating postoperatively (1.4 vs 2.0 days, $P = .006$), shorter time to bolus NG tube feeds (3.5 vs 5.1 days, $P<.001$), reduced need for PCA narcotics (6.5% vs 18.3%, $P = .028$), and a number of patients requiring refills of narcotic prescription refills within 30 days of operation (6.5% vs 36.6%, $P<.001$). There was no significant difference in ICU LOS between groups, number of ED visits, numbers of readmission within 30 days, and number of hematomas necessitating a return to the operation room (OR).

Won and colleagues[12] investigated two groups undergoing head and neck cancer surgery with free-flap reconstruction before and after the implementation of an ERAS protocol. The ERAS group was observed via a prospective observational cohort study and included 60 patients and the non-ERAS group was retrospectively studied using medical records of patients who had undergone surgery from August 2012 to July 2015 and included 29 patients, for a total of 89 patients. The study compared demographics, comorbidities, LOS, postoperative complications, the starting time of rehabilitation, and postoperative periods before radiotherapy for both groups. The study concluded that hospital LOS was significantly lower for patients in the ERAS protocol group than for patients in the non-ERAS group (30.87 $\pm$ 20.72 days vs 59.66 $\pm$ 40.43 days, $P < .0001$). Furthermore, start times for ambulation, adjuvant chemotherapy, and oral feeds were reduced in the ERAS group. Other differences, including total surgery duration, free-flap reconstruction duration, and rates of complications (ie, pneumonia, delirium, wound complication, fatality) were not statistically significant between ERAS and control groups.

Otology

An RCT[13] evaluated how ERAS protocols optimized surgery in adult patients with chronic suppurative otitis media. A total of 84 patients scheduled for tympanoplasty and/or mastoidectomy due to chronic suppurative otitis media were assigned to the ERAS group or control group. The ERAS group showed a lower Self-Rating Anxiety Scale score (30 [28–31.5] vs 35 [30–43], $P < .05$), a higher General Comfort Questionnaire score (88 [84–100] vs 83 [78.25–92.25], $P < .05$), and a lower Visual Analog Scale score (0 [0–0] vs 1 [0–2], $P < .05$) postoperatively. No significant differences ($P > .05$) were observed between the ERAS group and the control group in postoperative complications, postoperative hospitalization times, or costs associated with hospitalization.

Pediatric Adenotonsillectomy

A 2020 retrospective historical control study[14] of children undergoing adenotonsillectomy explored the effects following ERAS implementation. The study included 394 patients, 208 in the ERAS group, with OSA undergoing adenotonsillectomy. Following implementation, patients in the ERAS group had significantly lower complication rates (10.22% vs 1.92%; $P = .000$) and reduced incidence of fever (4.84% to 0.96%, $P = .029$) for 2 weeks of follow-up compared with the control group. Additionally, patients in the ERAS group had significantly less postsurgical pain scores on days 1, 3, and 7, better dietary intake after surgery, and lower preoperative anxiety scores ($P = .021$). Differences in rates of hemorrhage, wound infection, and pneumonia between ERAS and control groups were not statistically significant in this study.

Nationwide Children's Hospital Pediatric Tonsillectomy Protocol

Our institution has previously developed guidelines for decreasing unanticipated admissions from outpatient surgery centers.[15] With the opening of an off-site ambulatory surgery center 20 miles from our main hospital, it was critical to determine the appropriate scheduling of otolaryngology patients in a main OR (main hospital) location versus ambulatory surgery center.

Our NCH Tonsillectomy Protocol is shown in **Fig. 1A**. We track preoperative bleeding risk screening compliance, unplanned ICU or general admission, opioid prescriptions, opioid doses prescribed, appropriate utilization of a transitional care unit

(TCU), ED, or urgent care returns, nonoperative readmissions, and operative readmissions.

For pediatric patients undergoing tonsillectomy, appropriate preoperative patient assessment for appropriate surgical location and postoperative monitoring is critical. As shown in **Fig. 1**B, our patients follow one of the surgeon-directed care pathways. In 2016, we identified a significant source of poor resource utilization of floor beds and the need for short-term (3–8 hours) of observation of many of our post-op tonsillectomy patients. Historically, we sent all these patients done in the main OR to the inpatient floor and then discharged them later in the day. This required parents to go to admitting, be assigned a floor bed, and more vertical movement of the patient within the institution for short-term observation. In May 2018, we launched a TCU as a hybrid pathway for individualized care for these patients. The TCU is housed within our existing surgery unit in the main OR (same floor), and we utilize existing nursing resources within our perioperative staff. There has been positive feedback from patient satisfaction scores of 4.8/5. This has helped facilitate early discharge home once discharge criteria are met. If a patient in the TCU has a need to stay overnight, then he or she will get admitted to the floor. The TCU anesthetic plan was customized for the concepts of expedited recovery to help facilitate discharge. We have had 2288 patients go through our TCU and 2052 (90%) were discharged home from this unit and none of them were readmitted less than 24 hours. Our overall results of the NCH Tonsillectomy Protocol are best demonstrated from an outcome perspective as shown in **Table 3**. Although we did not track pain scores as Zheng and colleagues,[14] we did demonstrate the decreased need for opioid prescriptions and doses.

Role of Quality Improvement Methodology

Quality improvement (QI) efforts in pediatric otolaryngology at the NCH have identified metrics to track monthly to optimize our care protocols and identify opportunities for improvement. While many ERAS protocols have been geared toward using previously established evidence-based care, Institute for Health Care (IHI) QI methods allow for setting new standards of care and best outcomes by the implementation of unique interventions for improvement. The Plan, Do, Study, and Act methodology can be easily applied to relevant metrics as new interventions are implemented.[16] An example of a control chart as shown in **Fig. 2** demonstrates how specific metrics can be tracked for reducing utilization of inpatient floor beds through the creation of a TCU as a part of an overall protocol. Appropriate surgeon delegation of patients to the TCU can be assessed as shown in **Fig. 3**.

Table 3
Nationwide Children's Hospital Pediatric tonsillectomy protocol outcomes

Outcomes	2021 Results	% Reduction from Baseline[a]
% Patients getting an opioid Rx	11%	↓ 77%
Average # opioid doses per Rx	14.3 doses	↓ 56%
% Patients discharged home from inpatient floor bed	7%	↓ 56%
% ED/UC returns	2%	↓ 51%
% Nonoperative readmission	2%	↓ 59%
% Operative control of hemorrhage readmissions	1.45%	↓ 68%

[a] All metrics with statistically significant reductions ($P < .01$).

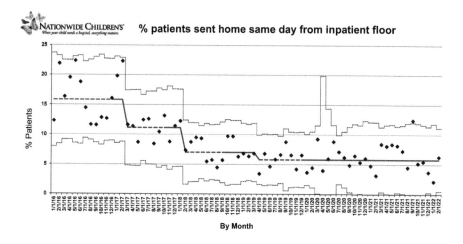

Fig. 2. Control chart demonstrating the reduction in unnecessary utilization of inpatient floor beds for patients needing short-term observation.

As described earlier, ERAS has been used extensively within a number of surgical specialties, including adult and pediatric otolaryngology surgery. This article has summarized some of the current data on the efficacy of ERAS protocols within pediatric surgery, adult head and neck and otology, and pediatric otolaryngology, as well as introduced the protocol at our institution that approaches these protocols from a QI perspective.

In the adult otolaryngology populations studied, ERAS was shown to improve overall patient comfort, reduce LOS, improve postoperative pain. and reduce postoperative complications. Furthermore, dietary intake and postoperative ambulation were

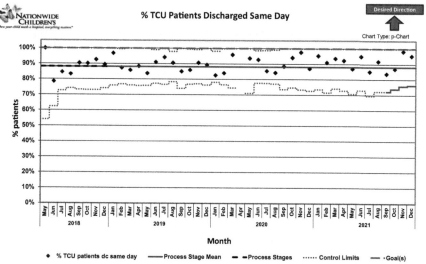

Fig. 3. Control chart of % of patients successfully discharged home same day as surgery from transitional care unit over time.

more optimized in ERAS populations. In both pediatric and adult otolaryngology populations, more data are needed to better assess rates of readmission, postoperative rates of infection, need for reoperation, and more. In pediatric otolaryngology patients specifically, published data continue to be incredibly scarce. Current data in otolaryngology pediatric surgery can reasonably support that ERAS protocols are effective in these populations as well, but further exploration, especially incorporating QI methodology is needed to specifically address LOS, rates of readmission, and postoperative complications. Additionally, as guidelines for pediatric surgery begin to emerge as ERAS protocols have been able to become more standardized within these specialties. The American College of Surgeons Children's Surgery Verification Program supports the utilization of ERAS protocols to optimize pediatric surgical care as they require multidisciplinary coordination and education across the entire perioperative period. Published ERAS protocols are lacking in pediatric otolaryngology, highlighting opportunities within this specific surgical population.

SUMMARY

ERAS is a multidisciplinary approach to improving the experience and outcomes for patients undergoing surgery. Evidence to support the efficacy of ERAS is growing and suggests that consistency of perioperative care can improve the overall perioperative experience for patients, reduce LOS, improve postoperative pain, and so forth. Specifically, in pediatric otolaryngology, published data on ERAS protocols remains incredibly limited. IHI QI methodology can help institutions adjust such protocols to improve perioperative care and patient outcomes.

CLINICS CARE POINTS

- Enhanced recovery after surgery (ERAS) protocols can successfully reduce the length of stay, improve postoperative pain, and reduce postoperative complications after surgery.
- There is little published data on the use of ERAS in pediatric otolaryngology and other pediatric surgical specialties.
- As demonstrated by our Nationwide Children's Hospital Pediatric Tonsillectomy Protocol, quality improvement methodology can be utilized in the development and ongoing modifications of ERAS protocols to maximize their impact on patient care and best outcomes.

DISCLOSURE

The authors have nothing to disclose.

REFERENCES

1. Anesthesiology AAoN. Enhanced recovery after surgery considerations for pathway development and implementation. 2022. Available at: https://www.aana.com/docs/default-source/practice-aana-com-web-documents-(all)/professional-practice-manual/enhanced-recovery-after-surgery.pdf?sfvrsn=6d184ab1_14. Accessed April 1, 2022.
2. Dort JC, Farwell DG, Findlay M, et al. Optimal Perioperative Care in Major Head and Neck Cancer Surgery With Free Flap Reconstruction: A Consensus Review

and Recommendations From the Enhanced Recovery After Surgery Society. JAMA Otolaryngol Head Neck Surg 2017;143(3):292–303.

3. Brindle ME, McDiarmid C, Short K, et al. Consensus Guidelines for Perioperative Care in Neonatal Intestinal Surgery: Enhanced Recovery After Surgery (ERAS. World J Surg 2020;44(8):2482–92.

4. Rove KO, Edney JC, Brockel MA. Enhanced recovery after surgery in children: Promising, evidence-based multidisciplinary care. Paediatr Anaesth 2018; 28(6):482–92.

5. Han DS, Brockel MA, Boxley PJ, et al. Enhanced recovery after surgery and anesthetic outcomes in pediatric reconstructive urologic surgery. Pediatr Surg Int 2021;37(1):151–9.

6. Rove KO, Strine AC, Wilcox DT, et al. Design and development of the Pediatric Urology Recovery After Surgery Endeavor (PURSUE) multicentre pilot and exploratory study. BMJ Open 2020;10(11):e039035.

7. Yeh A, Butler G, Strotmeyer S, et al. ERAS protocol for pediatric laparoscopic cholecystectomy promotes safe and early discharge. J Pediatr Surg 2020; 55(1):96–100.

8. Leeds IL, Ladd MR, Sundel MH, et al. Process measures facilitate maturation of pediatric enhanced recovery protocols. J Pediatr Surg 2018;53(11):2266–72.

9. Bertelsen C, Hur K, Nurimba M, et al. Enhanced Recovery After Surgery-Based Perioperative Protocol for Head and Neck Free Flap Reconstruction. OTO Open 2020;4(2). 2473974X20931037.

10. Zhang H, Mou YK, Liu ZL, et al. [Application of enhanced recovery after surgery in laryngeal cancer surgery with multi-disciplinary team]. Zhonghua Er Bi Yan Hou Tou Jing Wai Ke Za Zhi 2021;56(3):221–8.

11. Jandali DB, Vaughan D, Eggerstedt M, et al. Enhanced recovery after surgery in head and neck surgery: Reduced opioid use and length of stay. Laryngoscope 2020;130(5):1227–32.

12. Won HR, An JY, Lee JJ, et al. The effectiveness of an enhanced recovery after surgery protocol in head and neck cancer surgery with free-flap reconstruction. Ann Surg Treat Res 2019;97(5):239–44.

13. Tan JQ, Chen YB, Wang WH, et al. Application of Enhanced Recovery After Surgery in Perioperative Period of Tympanoplasty and Mastoidectomy. Ear Nose Throat J 2021;100(10_suppl):1045S–9S.

14. Zhang Y, Liu D, Chen X, et al. An enhanced recovery programme improves the comfort and outcomes in children with obstructive sleep apnoea undergoing adenotonsillectomy: A retrospective historical control study. Clin Otolaryngol 2021; 46(1):249–55.

15. Raman VT, Jatana KR, Elmaraghy CA, et al. Guidelines to decrease unanticipated hospital admission following adenotonsillectomy in the pediatric population. Int J Pediatr Otorhinolaryngol 2014;78(1):19–22.

16. Institute for Healthcare Improvement. Available at: http://www.ihi.org. Accessed April 1, 2022.

Healthcare Equity in Pediatric Otolaryngology

Prasanth Pattisapu, MD, MPH[a,b,c,]*, Nikhila P. Raol, MD, MPH[d,e,f]

KEYWORDS

- Health disparities • Health equity • Outcomes • Pediatric otolaryngology

KEY POINTS

- Issues of health equity have been identified in all studied areas of pediatric otolaryngology, but most notably in tonsillectomy, ear tube placement, cochlear implantation, and tracheostomy.
- Within sleep-disordered breathing tonsillectomy, health disparities have been identified for evaluation, management, and outcomes throughout all stages of disease, with racial/ethnic and socioeconomic minorities generally poorer health and outcomes.
- Clinical practice guidelines and other national guidance can reduce health disparities, often through reduction in overuse, as in the FDA warning on codeine following tonsillectomy.
- Future research in pediatric otolaryngology should be specifically purposed to study health disparities, their causes, and potential solutions.

INTRODUCTION

The Institute of Medicine defines disparities in healthcare as a difference in treatment provided to members of different racial (or ethnic) groups that is not justified by the underlying health conditions or treatment preferences of patients,[1] whereas the National Library of Medicine defines health disparities as variation in rates of disease occurrence and disabilities among socioeconomic and/or geographically defined

This article is exempt from IRB determination as no human subjects were involved in the project.

Conflicts of Interest: The authors have nothing to disclose.

[a] Department of Otolaryngology — Head & Neck Surgery, Nationwide Children's Hospital, 700 Children's Drive, Suite T2G, Columbus, OH, USA; [b] Department of Otolaryngology — Head & Neck Surgery, The Ohio State University, Columbus, OH, USA; [c] Center for Surgical Outcomes Research, Nationwide Children's Hospital, Columbus, OH, USA; [d] Department of Otolaryngology—Head and Neck Surgery, Emory University School of Medicine, Atlanta, GA, USA; [e] Department of Pediatrics, Emory University School of Medicine, Atlanta, GA, USA; [f] Division of Pediatric Otolaryngology, Children's Healthcare of Atlanta, Atlanta, GA, USA

* Corresponding author. Department of Otolaryngology – Head & Neck Surgery, Nationwide Children's Hospital, 700 Children's Drive, Suite T2G, Columbus, OH.

E-mail address: prasanth.pattisapu@nationwidechildrens.org

Otolaryngol Clin N Am 55 (2022) 1287–1299
https://doi.org/10.1016/j.otc.2022.07.006
0030-6665/22/© 2022 Elsevier Inc. All rights reserved.

population groups.[2] Regardless of the precise definition, universal agreement exists that healthcare disparities result in inequitable health outcomes. In the pediatric population, these disparities may be attributed to numerous patient factors, including race, ethnicity, sex, gender, socioeconomic status, insurance status, and caregiver health literacy, and provider factors, such as implicit bias.[3] Because more knowledge is accrued regarding pediatric health inequity, changes in health policy are essential to help close the gap.

In 2003, a survey study was published in *Pediatrics* demonstrating the disparity in access to care for tonsillectomy, with 97% of surveyed otolaryngologists reporting they would see privately insured children who needed tonsillectomy in consultation, compared with 27% of publicly insured children.[4] Thus was born health disparities research in pediatric otolaryngology. During the past 2 decades, as health services research and studies using claims data have grown, health disparities research has grown significantly. Areas in which disparities have been noted include diagnosis, management, and outcomes of obstructive sleep apnea (OSA)/sleep-disordered breathing (SDB), recurrent acute and chronic otitis media, sensorineural hearing loss (SNHL), and respiratory failure/tracheotomy. In this article, we discuss what is known about health disparities in the pediatric otolaryngology patient population and potential targets for improving equitable outcomes.

SLEEP-DISORDERED BREATHING AND ADENOTONSILLECTOMY

With approximately 500,000 procedures performed every year, tonsillectomy is one of the most studied topics in pediatric otolaryngology.[5,6] As such, disparities research on pediatric tonsillectomy and related conditions is robust and nuanced. Across this research, disparities have been found by race, ethnicity, socioeconomic status, insurance coverage, and distance from the hospital. Disparities have been identified in all stages of illness, from baseline severity to posttreatment outcomes. Additionally, new guidelines related to pediatric tonsillectomy care have narrowed some health disparities, providing hope that similar evidence-based standards can be set in other areas of otolaryngology to improve care and reduce disparities.

Sleep-disordered Breathing

A variety of racial and ethnic disparities have been identified in pediatric sleep, including in use of bedtime, length of sleep on weeknights, and relative distribution of sleep stages.[7] However, especially important to the pediatric otolaryngologist are the numerous differences seen in the prevalence and management of SDB. A systematic review in 2011 demonstrated that across a variety of racial, ethnic, and socioeconomic measures, minority groups tended to have more severe SDB in several studies.[8] Non-Hispanic black patients are 3 to 4 times as likely to have SDB as white patients.[9,10] Black patients also have more severe OSA, even when controlling for comorbidities.[9,11]

In addition to race, neighborhood characteristics are a major factor in sleep apnea disparities. Among children aged 2 to 8 years, patients were more likely to have OSA and had a higher severity of OSA if they originated from census tracts with greater poverty, higher population density, and a higher percentage of single-parent families, even when clinical comorbidities are considered.[12–14] In the analysis by Wang and associates,[13] when these measures of neighborhood disadvantage are accounted for, racial disparities are no longer significant. This suggests that racial disparities in SDB/OSA may be mediated by social determinants of health at the neighborhood level.

Polysomnography

After evaluation for SDB, racial and socioeconomic disparities can exist in completing a preoperative polysomnogram (PSG). Pecha and colleagues found that white children with SDB underwent tonsillectomy without preoperative PSG more often than black, Hispanic, or other race patients. In all, racial/ethnic minority status was associated with increased us of PSG or no intervention as initial management.[15] This may be because PSGs are often obtained for patients with more severe disease. As noted, SDB severity is associated with racial/ethnic and socioeconomic minority status.[7–11] However, once evaluated by an otolaryngologist, recent research has not demonstrated disparities in whether surgery or polysomnography was recommended.[16–18] Importantly, although, socioeconomic status and overall social vulnerability was associated with a 60% to 65% decrease in likelihood of attending an otolaryngology referral.[16] Considered together, this research suggests that some of the greatest disparities in pediatric SDB occur before the initial evaluation, through either polysomnography or an otolaryngologist.

Additionally, the same analysis showed statistically significant delays in time to obtaining said PSG, an average of 44.8 days for non-Hispanic white patients compared with 49.9, 51.7, and 51.0 days for black, Hispanic, and other races, respectively.[15] Although this difference may not be clinically significant, a study by Boss and colleagues demonstrated very long delays for publicly insured patients obtaining a PSG for SDB compared with privately insured patients, 141 versus 49.9 days, respectively.[18] Furthermore, PSG completion has been shown to be negatively associated with distance from the sleep center.[19] However, Knaus and colleagues found no differences in time to PSG according to race/ethnicity, insurance status, rural/urban status, or language.[17] Even more surprising, Yan and colleagues lower social vulnerability was associated with a *higher* rate of polysomnography completion among patients recommended the study.[16] This variability suggests that local demographics, policies, clinical processes, or other factors may play a role in the ease of obtaining polysomnography for different groups. It thus highlights the importance of monitoring one's individual clinical environment to evaluate and intervene in disparities that may exist.

Tonsillectomy Utilization

Whatever the upstream causes, disparities in tonsillectomy utilization have long been established, with fewer tonsillectomies being performed in racial/ethnic and socioeconomic minorities. Although these disparities were demonstrated more than a decade ago,[8] more recent research has examined these trends through larger studies and national databases with finer detail.

As before, Pecha and colleagues demonstrated more white patients undergoing tonsillectomy without PSG compared with black and Hispanic patients. On multivariable analysis, they also showed that black and Hispanic patients were 28% less likely than white counterparts to receive any intervention (PSG or surgery).[15] Cooper and colleagues examined state ambulatory and state inpatient databases and found that white patients were more likely to undergo tonsillectomy for recurrent tonsillitis compared with black and Hispanic patients, who were more likely to undergo tonsillectomy for SDB. However, for either indication (or overall), white patients had a higher utilization than black or Hispanic patients, and nonmetropolitan patients had a higher utilization than metropolitan patients.[20] A single-institution study by the same group showed increased utilization among nonmetropolitan patients compared with metropolitan patients could be explained by a higher population of black patients in metropolitan areas and more white patients in nonmetropolitan areas.[17] By contrast, the multistate analysis was able to stratify race and metropolitan status and found both to have a distinct influence on utilization.[20]

Echoing a trend that disparities are local phenomena, Yan and colleagues found contrasting results.[21] Although Cooper's team found that rural (nonmetropolitan) status was associated with higher tonsillectomy utilization,[20] Yan's team found rural status led to a 30% decrease in the rate of undergoing tonsillectomy.[21] However, unlike other analyses, their study included a greater population of black patients in the rural areas compared with urban (35% vs 24%).[21] One might expect social determinants of health to elucidate the relationship between race/ethnicity, rural/urban status, and tonsillectomy utilization, although at least one large single-institution study failed to find an association between a patient's neighborhood deprivation and tonsillectomy indication.[22]

In a rare study of how disparities might be reduced, Heller and colleagues examined state ambulatory and inpatient databases for all pediatric tonsillectomies in Florida and South Carolina. They examined whether there was a change in tonsillectomy utilization by race/ethnicity in association with the 2011 American Academy of Otolaryngology-Head and Neck Surgery Clinical Practice Guidelines on tonsillectomy and polysomnography before tonsillectomy.[23–25] Strikingly, they found that the guidelines were associated with a decrease in tonsillectomy utilization among white patients without a decrease for black or Hispanic patients, effectively narrowing known disparities among these groups.[23] This result provides some hope that standardization of care through clinical practice guidelines may be an effective tool for reducing health disparities.

Tonsillectomy Outcomes

After patients undergo surgery, there are differences in outcomes. However, whether these differences represent disparities themselves or downstream effects of other disparities is not always clear. For example, the Childhood Adenotonsillectomy Trial (CHAT)—the landmark randomized controlled trial of early adenotonsillectomy versus watchful waiting for 6 months for OSA—found that for either arm of the study, black patients had lower resolution of OSA than other patients. They also found that black patients were less likely to complete the study.[26] Additional study of the CHAT data showed that black patients had more severe OSA when measured on PSG.[11] Although there may be biologic differences in SDB for black patients, there are also associations with asthma and obesity.[10,27,28] These factors may play a direct role in poorer SDB/OSA outcomes after adenotonsillectomy even separate from factors like access to care, health literacy and other structural inequities.[29–31]

Whatever risk factors contribute to poor resolution of SDB/OSA in black patients may play a similar role in higher perioperative respiratory complications in those same patients. Indeed, black patients had a higher rate of respiratory complications than other patients (35% vs 24%), out of more than 300 consecutive patients undergoing tonsillectomy for SDB in one study. This difference was also noted specifically for major respiratory complications (22% vs 14%) but not for nonrespiratory complications.[32] This difference may be an effect of increased asthma, obesity, or other medical conditions in black patients. However, in a study of pediatric inpatient admissions, black children were 50% more likely to have respiratory complications of tonsillectomy than other patients. Interestingly, this difference was relatively unchanged after adjustment by age, gender, OSA, obesity, sickle cell anemia, or asthma, suggesting that these factors cannot explain the difference.[33] Therefore, the respiratory complications following adenotonsillectomy likely represent a true health disparity warranting further investigation.

In addition to respiratory complications, there are disparities in resource utilization following adenotonsillectomy. For example, black and Hispanic children are more likely to meet criteria for inpatient admission (ie, stay for more than "2 midnights") after adenotonsillectomy compared with white children. Public insurance was similarly associated with inpatient stay compared with private patients, who were more likely to undergo ambulatory surgery.[34] Lloyd and colleagues found that black children were readmitted more often than white children following pediatric tonsil surgery for reasons other than bleeding. Their single-institution study also found that readmissions were higher if a child came from a zip code where more than 10% of the population lived below the poverty level or where less than 25% of parents achieved a college education.[35] Bhattacharya and Shapiro connected the state ambulatory surgery, inpatient and emergency department to study readmissions after tonsillectomy. They found that both black patients and Hispanic patients had 11% and 17% higher odds of readmission, respectively, following tonsillectomy than non-Hispanic white patients. Patients from the lowest income quartile had an approximately 50% higher risk of readmission than those from the highest quartile.[36]

Racial/ethnic or socioeconomic differences are less commonly identified for post-tonsillectomy hemorrhage. Studies on racial disparities have found no difference in bleeding after adenotonsillectomy for any race or ethnicity.[32,33,36] Language barriers were similarly not associated with increases in posttonsillectomy hemorrhage.[37] One study identified a statistically significant effect of poverty on emergency room (ER) visits for posttonsillectomy hemorrhage, with patients from the lowest income quartile having about 30% higher risk for hemorrhage than those from the highest income quartile. However, this could in part reflect an increased propensity to use the ER for bleeding concerns rather than an actual difference in bleeding, given that the same study showed a higher revisit rate for poorer patients for all causes.[36] Another study found no effect of socioeconomic factors on bleeding rates.[35]

Tonsillectomy Pain and Opioid Use

Disparities in posttonsillectomy pain management are a concern but they take a different form than disparities in other aspects of pediatric SDB or tonsillectomy. However, there is a concerted effort to reduce opioid use following pediatric adenotonsillectomy.[38] This is partly not only due to concerns for opioid-related respiratory depression in SDB patients following surgery[39,40] but also due to a general concern to reduce often-excessive opioid prescribing amid a national opioid epidemic.[41,42] However, implicit bias has been shown to affect pediatric pain management, and these biases are often associated with inadequate pain management in racial and ethnic minority patients.[43–45] Perhaps, it is due to this balance that Chavez and colleagues did not find differences by race in opioid prescribing after pediatric tonsillectomy. This contrasts with their overall finding for pediatric surgical procedures that black patients received fewer opioid prescriptions and an associated longer length of stay than white patients.[46]

Additionally, there may be biologic differences in opioid response by race/ethnicity that must be considered to avoid disparities. For example, Sadhasivam and colleagues observed black and white children following adenotonsillectomy with a standardized pain management protocol. They found higher ratings of pain among black patients with a higher risk of opioid-related side effects in white patients.[47] Donaldson and colleagues evaluated perioperative pain management for children undergoing adenotonsillectomy alongside a separate clinical trial. They found that parent-reported pain was higher for Hispanic patients than non-Hispanic white patients. However, they also found a stronger relationship between reported pain and opioid use among white patients suggesting that they were more likely to use opioids to manage pain.[48] In another study by

Jimenez and colleagues of 47 white and 47 Latino children undergoing tonsillectomy and adenoidectomy, Latino patients received 30% less opioid analgesics than white patients and received more short-acting medications. Their analysis had incomplete results for pain reporting but this study suggests disparities in management.[49]

However, with the previously mentioned respiratory concerns of opioids, increased prescribing among white patients may represent overprescribing in that population (ie, a disparity against white patients). For example, before 2013, white children received more prescriptions for codeine following tonsillectomy than black children.[50] However, in February 2013, the Food and Drug Administration (FDA) issued a black box warning regarding children undergoing tonsillectomy and/or adenoidectomy.[51] Following the FDA warning, disparities in codeine prescribing were severely reduced, with white patients receiving fewer codeine prescriptions than before the warning. Similarly, more patients from large or medium metropolitan areas received codeine prescriptions following adenotonsillectomy before 2013, with a narrower difference following the FDA warning.[50] As before with clinical practice guidelines on tonsillectomy,[23–25] this finding is further hope that evidence-based national guidance can help reduce health disparities in pediatric tonsillectomy.

OTITIS MEDIA AND TYMPANOSTOMY TUBE PLACEMENT

With acute otitis media (AOM) being the second most common illness diagnosed in children and tympanostomy tube placement being the most common pediatric procedure, such as tonsillectomy, this is another area that is frequently studied in pediatric otolaryngology. Indications for tubes, utilization of procedures and antibiotics, risk factors for surgery, and guideline adherence are among the topics that have been explored, with some studies evaluating disparities within each of these topics.

Diagnosis and Medical Management

Racial and ethnic disparities have been demonstrated in both diagnosis and management of otitis media. Smith and Boss's 2010 systematic review demonstrated racial disparities in diagnosis of AOM and chronic otitis media with effusion (COME), although there was no clear race that was the outlier in diagnosis.[52] However, disparities have been noted in antibiotic prescriptions for recurrent AOM (RAOM) once a child does present to the office for evaluation,[53] as well as choice of broad-spectrum antibiotics,[54] with black children less likely to receive any antibiotics, as well as broad-spectrum antibiotics, for AOM.

Tympanostomy Tube Placement

Disparities have also been noted in the receipt of tympanostomy tubes, with children in high-poverty neighborhoods more likely to receive tubes for COME and those in low-poverty neighborhoods for RAOM.[55] In addition, publicly insured children tend to receive evaluation for tubes at an older age[56] and have a higher rate of loss or change in insurance, resulting in increased time between consultation and surgery.[57] Interestingly, race as a sole risk factor has not been shown to lead to significant disparities in tympanostomy tube placement.[55,56,58] Together, these data suggest that changes in policy affecting insurance, as well as improved education of clinicians and caregivers may improve disparities in the management of AOM and COME.

SENSORINEURAL HEARING LOSS AND COCHLEAR IMPLANTATION

With 2 to 3 out of 1000 children diagnosed with hearing loss at birth in the United States,[59] hearing loss is a condition frequently seen and managed by the pediatric otolaryngologist. Management may consist of monitoring, amplification, classroom accommodations, or surgery. Disparities in hearing loss identification and management have been noted across several patient characteristics, including race/ethnicity, socioeconomic status, insurance, and area of residence.

Diagnosis

Given the diversity of the US population, genetic testing for hearing loss in its current form may not detect variants that are thought to cause hearing loss. Florentine, Rouse, and colleagues demonstrated that variants of unknown significance that were not included identified as pathogenic/likely pathogenic are more likely to be found in black and Hispanic children when compared with Asian and white, and the expansion of diagnostic criteria may allow for more children of black/Hispanic races to receive a definitive diagnosis.[60] Furthermore, they highlighted that inclusion of minorities in studies on SNHL would help close the gap in identifying genetic causes of hearing loss.[61] Population-level studies have confirmed the racial/ethnic and economic disparities seen in workup and the need for more education and standardization around management.[62] Fowler and colleagues showed that even cytomegalovirus (CMV) prevalence is significantly higher in black and multiracial children when compared with white, Hispanic, and Asian children by 3-fold to 9-fold. Although they did not find a difference in rates of SNHL diagnosed at birth, given that CMV can lead to progressive hearing loss,[63] surveillance is critical to prevent disparities in identification of hearing loss.

Although disparities will likely take time and multidisciplinary interventions in order to see an improvement, Cedars and colleagues were able to demonstrate how the use of a school-based screening using otoacoustic emissions after failed conditioned play audiometry reduced referrals and disparities while improving identification of hearing loss and follow-up. This demonstrates the need for buy in from multiple stakeholders to adequately deliver equitable care.[64]

Cochlear Implantation

Significant disparities have been demonstrated in rates of cochlear implantation, as well as in time to evaluation and surgery. In a 2005 study, Stern and colleagues initially demonstrated that rates of cochlear implantation were significantly lower for black and Hispanic children (odds ratio [OR] 0.1 and 0.28, respectively) compared with white and Asian children (OR 1.0 and 0.93, respectively),[65] which was shown again on a 2022 study from Fujiwara and colleagues.[66] Furthermore, this study also showed that those with public insurance were more likely to be implanted after 2 years of age, and for each 1-year increase in maternal high school education in a given hospital referral region, there is a significant increase in the percentage of cochlear implants performed before 2 years of age in that region.[66] In DeVries's study, public insurance was associated with significant delays in all aspects of assessment (vestibular, speech, developmental, and implant profile) and in time to implant after evaluation.[67] Wiley and colleagues demonstrated that children with married parents were more likely to make it to the cochlear implant team evaluation after being identified as candidates for implantation,[68] with these 2 studies highlighting the disparity created by lower education level and less social support. Finally, even after implantation, Tolan and colleagues demonstrated that publicly insured patients required more time to achieve the same degree of sound recognition and imitation using Ling-6 scores as privately insured patients, illustrating that disparities must be addressed at each step of the process in order to achieve equity.[69]

Some studies have offered potential interventions to help reduce the disparities associated with cochlear implantation. These interventions include comprehensive Medicaid coverage; increased provider-counseling about cochlear implant benefits with a focus on rural, single-parent, and non-English speaking caregivers; and improved early detection through newborn screening.[70] As with other efforts to affect disparities, policy change is key to seeing a measurable improvement in these inequities.

Tracheotomy

More than 4000 pediatric tracheotomies are performed annually in the United States, with a high associated immediate and delayed mortality. Although efforts to improve related outcomes for these patients have been longstanding, including development of multidisciplinary programs for management and expert consensus statements, the study of disparities in this population is more nascent.

Similar to other conditions in pediatric otolaryngology, multiple factors may contribute to disparities in tracheotomy outcomes. For instance, Johnson and colleagues evaluated rates of tracheotomy placement and associated outcomes, finding that black infants were disproportionately more likely to undergo tracheotomy due to more prematurity and bronchopulmonary dysplasia, whereas overall outcomes of decannulation, neurocognitive delay, and mortality did not differ among races.[71] However, Liao and colleagues' study using Area Deprivation Index as a marker for communities with low and high disadvantage did demonstrate that patients from high disadvantage communities have longer hospital length of stay, total median cost, and relative risk of prolonged hospitalizations.[72] Additional studies have demonstrated increased time to decannulation in lower socioeconomic status groups[73] and higher risk of intensive care unit readmissions in black children.[74] Although it is difficult to draw conclusions based on these data due to the paucity, early research does suggest that disparities may exist and may be most influenced by socioeconomic status. Improving caregiver education and resources available to these families, both through hospital systems and the government, may help address many of the inequities seen.

Conducting Disparities Research in Pediatric Otolaryngology

As seen in many of the referenced studies, disparities are numerous in pediatric otolaryngology and are attributable to various factors. When studying disparities, one should conduct these studies with the primary intention of evaluating healthcare inequity. Use of a classification system, such as PROGRESS, which incorporates the place of residence, race/ethnicity/culture/language, occupation, gender/sex, religion, education, socioeconomic status, and social capital, can remind one to focus on the various characteristics that may play a role in disparate outcomes.[75] PROGRESS-Plus, an extension of PROGRESS, includes personal, relational, and time-dependent characteristics in that these fluid individual qualities can contribute to health inequity.[75] In today's landscape, specific tools for studies evaluating disparities exist, including updated PRISMA and CONSORT guidelines with equity extensions for systematic reviews/meta-analyses and randomized-controlled trials, respectively.[3] Approaching these studies through a lens of equity will assure that equity itself remains the primary outcome measure for that study.

SUMMARY

Health inequities and healthcare disparities are prevalent in pediatric otolaryngology and can be attributed to race, socioeconomic status, insurance status, caregiver education, primary language spoken, and social support, among others. Various interventions have been suggested to mitigate disparities, with the most successful efforts engaging multiple stakeholders. Continued research in this area is needed, and established tools to conduct high-quality disparities research should be used to maintain the focus on healthcare inequities.

CLINICS CARE POINTS

- Inequities in delivery of healthcare in pediatric otolaryngology have been identified across multiple health conditions, including obstructive sleep apnea, sensorineural hearing loss, and otitis media.

- Specific research focused on identifying and reducing disparities is needed to address health inequity.

- Multi-level systemic interventions will be needed to reduce health disparities. However, modest improvements in disparities in otolaryngology have been seen from standardization of care through clinical practice guidelines or other national regulations.

- Future research in disparities in otolaryngology should use an existing framework for studying equity, such as PROGRESS, or revised guidelines specific to the study of health equity, such as PRISMA and CONSORT. These guidelines help ensure that equity remains the primary outcome and focus of the research.

REFERENCES

1. Nelson A. Unequal treatment: confronting racial and ethnic disparities in health care. J Natl Med Assoc 2002;94(8):666–8.
2. US National Library of Medicine. MeSH Browser. 2021. Available at: https://meshb.nlm.nih.gov/record/ui?ui=D054624. Accessed August 5, 2022.
3. Megwalu UC, Raol NP, Bergmark R, et al. Evidence-based medicine in otolaryngology, part XIII: health disparities research and advancing health equity. Otolaryngol Head Neck Surg 2022;166(6):1249–61.
4. Wang EC, Choe MC, Meara JG, et al. Inequality of access to surgical specialty health care: why children with government-funded insurance have less access than those with private insurance in Southern California. Pediatrics 2004; 114(5):e584–90.
5. Hall MJ. Ambulatory Surgery Data From Hospitals and Ambulatory Surgery Centers: United States, 2010, Natl Health Stat Report, (102), 2017, 15, Available at: https://www.cdc.gov/nchs/data/nhsr/nhsr102.pdf. Accessed August 5, 2022.
6. Karaca Z, McDermott K. High-volume invasive, therapeutic ambulatory surgeries performed in hospital-owned facilities, 2016 #252 [internet]. Rockville (MD): Agency for Healthcare Research and Quality; 2019. Available at: https://www.hcup-us.ahrq.gov/reports/statbriefs/sb252-Invasive-Ambulatory-Surgeries-2016.jsp.
7. Smith JP, Hardy ST, Hale LE, et al. Racial disparities and sleep among preschool aged children: a systematic review. Sleep Health 2019;5(1):49–57.
8. Boss EF, Smith DF, Ishman SL. Racial/ethnic and socioeconomic disparities in the diagnosis and treatment of sleep-disordered breathing in children. Int J Pediatr Otorhinolaryngol 2011;75(3):299–307.
9. Redline S, Tishler PV, Schluchter M, et al. Risk factors for sleep-disordered breathing in children. Associations with obesity, race, and respiratory problems. Am J Respir Crit Care Med 1999;159(5 Pt 1):1527–32.

10. Rosen CL, Larkin EK, Kirchner HL, et al. Prevalence and risk factors for sleep-disordered breathing in 8- to 11-year-old children: association with race and prematurity. J Pediatr 2003;142(4):383–9.

11. Weinstock TG, Rosen CL, Marcus CL, et al. Predictors of obstructive sleep apnea severity in adenotonsillectomy candidates. Sleep 2014;37(2):261–9.

12. Brouillette RT, Horwood L, Constantin E, et al. Childhood sleep apnea and neighborhood disadvantage. J Pediatr 2011;158(5):789–95.e1.

13. Wang R, Dong Y, Weng J, et al. Associations among neighborhood, race, and sleep apnea severity in children. a six-city analysis. Ann Am Thorac Soc 2017; 14(1):76–84.

14. Spilsbury JC, Storfer-Isser A, Kirchner HL, et al. Neighborhood disadvantage as a risk factor for pediatric obstructive sleep apnea. J Pediatr 2006;149(3):342–7.

15. Pecha PP, Chew M, Andrews AL. Racial and ethnic disparities in utilization of tonsillectomy among medicaid-insured children. J Pediatr 2021;233:191–7.e2.

16. Yan F, Pearce JL, Ford ME, et al. Examining associations between neighborhood-level social vulnerability and care for children with sleep-disordered breathing. Otolaryngol Head Neck Surg 2022;166(6):1118–26.

17. Knaus ME, Koppera S, Lind MN, et al. Sociodemographic differences in care plans and time to treatment among children being considered for adenotonsillectomy. Otolaryngol Head Neck Surg 2022;166(6):1106–17.

18. Boss EF, Benke JR, Tunkel DE, et al. Public insurance and timing of polysomnography and surgical care for children with sleep-disordered breathing. JAMA Otolaryngol Head Neck Surg 2015;141(2):106–11.

19. Radhakrishnan D, Knight B, Gozdyra P, et al. Geographic disparities in performance of pediatric polysomnography to diagnose obstructive sleep apnea in a universal access health care system. Int J Pediatr Otorhinolaryngol 2021;147: 110803.

20. Cooper JN, Koppera S, Boss EF, et al. Differences in Tonsillectomy Utilization by Race/Ethnicity, Type of Health Insurance, and Rurality. Acad Pediatr 2021;21(6): 1031–6.

21. Yan F, Levy DA, Wen CC, et al. Rural Barriers to Surgical Care for Children With Sleep-Disordered Breathing. Otolaryngol Head Neck Surg 2022;166(6):1127–33.

22. Cheung AY, Kan KY, Jang S, et al. Socioeconomic variables as a predictor of indication for pediatric adenotonsillectomy. Int J Pediatr Otorhinolaryngol 2020;136: 110181.

23. Heller MA, Lind MN, Boss EF, et al. Differences in tonsillectomy use by race/ethnicity and type of health insurance before and after the 2011 tonsillectomy clinical practice guidelines. J Pediatr 2020;220:116–24.e3.

24. Baugh RF, Archer SM, Mitchell RB, et al, American Academy of Otolaryngology-Head and Neck Surgery Foundation. Clinical practice guideline: tonsillectomy in children. Otolaryngol Head Neck Surg 2011;144(1 Suppl):S1–30.

25. Roland PS, Rosenfeld RM, Brooks LJ, et al, American Academy of Otolaryngology—Head and Neck Surgery Foundation. Clinical practice guideline: Polysomnography for sleep-disordered breathing prior to tonsillectomy in children. Otolaryngol Head Neck Surg 2011;145(1 Suppl):S1–15.

26. Marcus CL, Moore RH, Rosen CL, et al. Childhood adenotonsillectomy trial (CHAT). A randomized trial of adenotonsillectomy for childhood sleep apnea. N Engl J Med 2013;368(25):2366–76.

27. Redline S, Tishler PV, Hans MG, et al. Racial differences in sleep-disordered breathing in African-Americans and Caucasians. Am J Respir Crit Care Med 1997;155(1):186–92.

28. Rudnick EF, Walsh JS, Hampton MC, et al. Prevalence and ethnicity of sleep-disordered breathing and obesity in children. Otolaryngol Head Neck Surg 2007;137(6):878–82.

29. Cooper LA, Hill MN, Powe NR. Designing and evaluating interventions to eliminate racial and ethnic disparities in health care. J Gen Intern Med 2002;17(6):477–86.

30. Bisgaier J, Rhodes KV. Auditing access to specialty care for children with public insurance. N Engl J Med 2011;364(24):2324–33.

31. Flores G, Olson L, Tomany-Korman SC. Racial and ethnic disparities in early childhood health and health care. Pediatrics 2005;115(2):e183–93.

32. Thongyam A, Marcus CL, Lockman JL, et al. Predictors of perioperative complications in higher risk children after adenotonsillectomy for obstructive sleep apnea: a prospective study. Otolaryngol Head Neck Surg 2014;151(6):1046–54.

33. Kou YF, Sakai M, Shah GB, et al. Postoperative respiratory complications and racial disparities following inpatient pediatric tonsillectomy: A cross-sectional study. Laryngoscope 2019;129(4):995–1000.

34. Kou YF, Mitchell RB, Johnson RF. A Cross-sectional Analysis of Pediatric Ambulatory Tonsillectomy Surgery in the United States. Otolaryngol Head Neck Surg 2019;161(4):699–704.

35. Lloyd AM, Behzadpour HK, Schonman I, et al. Socioeconomic factors associated with readmission following pediatric tonsillectomy. Int J Pediatr Otorhinolaryngol 2021;151:110917.

36. Bhattacharyya N, Shapiro NL. Associations between socioeconomic status and race with complications after tonsillectomy in children. Otolaryngol Head Neck Surg 2014;151(6):1055–60.

37. Plocienniczak M, Rubin BR, Kolli A, et al. Outcome disparities and resource utilization among limited english proficient patients after tonsillectomy. Ann Otol Rhinol Laryngol 2021. 34894211061996.

38. Barrette LX, Harris J, De Ravin E, et al. Clinical practice guidelines for pain management after tonsillectomy: systematic quality appraisal using the AGREE II instrument. Int J Pediatr Otorhinolaryngol 2022;156:111091.

39. Subramanyam R, Varughese A, Willging JP, et al. Future of pediatric tonsillectomy and perioperative outcomes. Int J Pediatr Otorhinolaryngol 2013;77(2):194–9.

40. Mahant S, Hall M, Ishman SL, et al. Association of National Guidelines with tonsillectomy perioperative care and outcomes. Pediatrics 2015;136(1):53–60.

41. Gaither JR, Shabanova V, Leventhal JM. US National Trends in Pediatric Deaths From Prescription and Illicit Opioids, 1999-2016. JAMA Netw Open 2018 Dec 7; 1(8):e186558.

42. Horton JD, Munawar S, Corrigan C, et al. Inconsistent and excessive opioid prescribing after common pediatric surgical operations. J Pediatr Surg 2019;54(7):1427–31.

43. Sabin JA, Greenwald AG. The influence of implicit bias on treatment recommendations for 4 common pediatric conditions: pain, urinary tract infection, attention deficit hyperactivity disorder, and asthma. Am J Public Health 2012;102(5):988–95.

44. Hoffman KM, Trawalter S, Axt JR, et al. Racial bias in pain assessment and treatment recommendations, and false beliefs about biological differences between blacks and whites. Proc Natl Acad Sci U S A 2016;113(16):4296–301.

45. Green CR, Anderson KO, Baker TA, et al. The unequal burden of pain: confronting racial and ethnic disparities in pain. Pain Med 2003;4(3):277–94.

46. Chavez LJ, Cooper JN, Deans KJ, et al. Evaluation of racial disparities in postoperative opioid prescription filling after common pediatric surgical procedures. J Pediatr Surg 2020;55(12):2575–83.

47. Sadhasivam S, Chidambaran V, Ngamprasertwong P, et al. Race and unequal burden of perioperative pain and opioid related adverse effects in children. Pediatrics 2012;129(5):832–8.

48. Donaldson CD, Jenkins BN, Fortier MA, et al. Parent responses to pediatric pain: the differential effects of ethnicity on opioid consumption. J Psychosom Res 2020;138:110251.

49. Jimenez N, Seidel K, Martin LD, et al. Perioperative analgesic treatment in Latino and non-Latino pediatric patients. J Health Care Poor Underserved 2010;21(1):229–36.

50. Lawrence A, Cooper JN, Deans KJ, et al. Effects of the FDA Codeine Safety Investigation on Racial and Geographic Disparities in Opioid Prescribing after Pediatric Tonsillectomy and/or Adenoidectomy. Glob Pediatr Health 2021;8:1–11.

51. U.S. Food and Drug Administration. FDA Drug Safety Communications: Safety review update of codeine use in children; new Boxed Warning and Contraindication on use after tonsillectomy and/or adenoidectomy. [Internet]. [cited 2022 May 30]. Available at: https://www.fda.gov/media/85072/download. Accessed August 5, 2022.

52. Smith DF, Boss EF. Racial/ethnic and socioeconomic disparities in the prevalence and treatment of otitis media in children in the United States. Laryngoscope 2010;120(11):2306–12.

53. Gerber JS, Prasad PA, Localio AR, et al. Racial differences in antibiotic prescribing by primary care pediatricians. Pediatrics 2013;131(4):677–84.

54. Fleming-Dutra KE, Shapiro DJ, Hicks LA, et al. Race, otitis media, and antibiotic selection. Pediatrics 2014;134(6):1059–66.

55. Nieman CL, Tunkel DE, Boss EF. Do race/ethnicity or socioeconomic status affect why we place ear tubes in children? Int J Pediatr Otorhinolaryngol 2016;88:98–103.

56. McCoy JL, Dixit R, Lin RJ, et al. Impact of patient socioeconomic disparities on time to tympanostomy tube placement. Ann Otol Rhinol Laryngol 2022;131(2):182–90.

57. Schwartz M, Shah R, Wetzel M, et al. Relationship between insurance type and delays in tympanostomy tube placement. Ann Otol Rhinol Laryngol 2021;130(2):142–7.

58. Chang JE, Shapiro NL, Bhattacharyya N. Do demographic disparities exist in the diagnosis and surgical management of otitis media? Laryngoscope 2018;128(12):2898–901.

59. National Institute on Deafness and Other Communication Disorders. Quick Statistics About Hearing [Internet]. 2021 [cited 2022 Jun 1]. Available at: https://www.nidcd.nih.gov/health/statistics/quick-statistics-hearing. Accessed August 5, 2022.

60. Florentine MM, Rouse SL, Stephans J, et al. Racial and ethnic disparities in diagnostic efficacy of comprehensive genetic testing for sensorineural hearing loss. Hum Genet 2022;141(3–4):495–504.

61. Rouse SL, Florentine MM, Taketa E, et al. Racial and ethnic disparities in genetic testing for hearing loss: a systematic review and synthesis. Hum Genet 2022;141(3–4):485–94.

62. Qian ZJ, Chang KW, Ahmad IN, et al. Use of Diagnostic Testing and Intervention for Sensorineural Hearing Loss in US Children From 2008 to 2018. JAMA Otolaryngol Head Neck Surg 2021;147(3):253–60.

63. Fowler KB, Ross SA, Shimamura M, et al. Racial and ethnic differences in the prevalence of congenital cytomegalovirus infection. J Pediatr 2018;200: 196–201.e1.

64. Cedars E, Kriss H, Lazar AA, et al. Use of otoacoustic emissions to improve outcomes and reduce disparities in a community preschool hearing screening program. PLoS One 2018;13(12):e0208050.

65. Stern RE, Yueh B, Lewis C, et al. Recent epidemiology of pediatric cochlear implantation in the United States: disparity among children of different ethnicity and socioeconomic status. Laryngoscope 2005;115(1):125–31.

66. Fujiwara RJT, Ishiyama G, Ishiyama A. Association of socioeconomic characteristics with receipt of pediatric cochlear implantations in California. JAMA Netw Open 2022;5(1):e2143132.

67. DeVries J, Ren Y, Purdy J, et al. Exploring factors responsible for delay in pediatric cochlear implantation. Otol Neurotol 2021;42(10):e1478–85.

68. Wiley S, Meinzen-Derr J. Access to cochlear implant candidacy evaluations: who is not making it to the team evaluations? Int J Audiol 2009;48(2):74–9.

69. Tolan M, Serpas A, McElroy K, et al. Delays in sound recognition and imitation in underinsured children receiving cochlear implantation. JAMA Otolaryngol Head Neck Surg 2017;143(1):60–4.

70. Omar M, Qatanani A, Kaleem SZ, et al. Sociodemographic disparities in pediatric cochlear implantation access and use: a systematic review. Laryngoscope 2022; 132(3):670–86.

71. Johnson RF, Brown CM, Beams DR, et al. Racial influences on pediatric tracheostomy outcomes. Laryngoscope 2022;132(5):1118–24.

72. Liao K, Chorney SR, Brown AB, et al. The impact of socioeconomic disadvantage on pediatric tracheostomy outcomes. Laryngoscope 2021;131(11):2603–9.

73. Smith MM, Hart CK, Benscoter DT, et al. The impact of socioeconomic status on time to decannulation among children with tracheostomies. Otolaryngol Head Neck Surg 2021;165(6):876–80.

74. Slain KN, Barda A, Pronovost PJ, et al. Social factors predictive of intensive care utilization in technology-dependent children, a retrospective multicenter cohort study. Front Pediatr 2021;9:721353.

75. O'Neill J, Tabish H, Welch V, et al. Applying an equity lens to interventions: using PROGRESS ensures consideration of socially stratifying factors to illuminate inequities in health. J Clin Epidemiol 2014;67(1):56–64.

Quality Improvement Methodology

Jennifer M. Lavin, MD, MS[a,b,]*, Jonathan B. Ida, MD, MBA[a,b]

KEYWORDS

- Quality improvement • Improvement science • Change management • SQUIRE

KEY POINTS

- Proper execution of quality and safety initiatives require study of the problem, use of improvement methodology, measuring success, and sustaining change.
- Measurement plans in quality improvement often involve use of statistical process control methods over traditional statistics, allowing for the study of data over time.
- Change management principles are highly utilized in quality improvement as successful initiatives require stakeholder buy-in for adaptation and sustainment.
- Publication of quality improvement findings in the literature should follow SQUIRE format as it highlights foundational assumptions made and contextual elements impacting success or failure of an improvement initiative.

INTRODUCTION

Around the turn of the twenty-first century, a series of publications from the Institute of Medicine (IOM) highlighted the urgent need to improve patient safety and quality improvement (PSQI) in the United States.[1–3] In their calls to action, the IOM defined 6 principles of health care quality (**Table 1**) and emphasized systems level approaches to PSQI, marking the beginning of the modern discipline of quality and safety in health care. With growth of the discipline, methodologies were adapted from manufacturing giving structure to the process of quality improvement.[4]

Today, PSQI is a central focus of hospitals and health systems who often have teams dedicated to the discipline. Physician champions are essential to the success of such teams, given their clinical expertise and degree of influence with both patients and institutional administrative processes. Because of the fact that pediatric otolaryngologists interface with multiple different specialties in inpatient, outpatient, and operating room settings, they are well positioned to be influential in improvement initiatives.

[a] Division of Pediatric Otolaryngology-Head and Neck Surgery, Ann & Robert H. Lurie Children's Hospital of Chicago, 225 East Chicago Avenue, Box #25, Chicago, IL 60611, USA;
[b] Department of Otolaryngology - Head and Neck Surgery, Northwestern University Feinberg School of Medicine, 676 North St. Claire Street Suite 1325, Chicago, IL 60611, USA
* Corresponding author.
E-mail address: jlavin@luriechildrens.org

Otolaryngol Clin N Am 55 (2022) 1301–1310
https://doi.org/10.1016/j.otc.2022.07.008
0030-6665/22/© 2022 Elsevier Inc. All rights reserved.

oto.theclinics.com

Table 1	
The institute of medicine domains of quality	
Safe	Free from Harm
Effective	Providing evidence-based treatment. Avoiding treatment when not indicated
Patient-centered	Care that respects patient needs, preferences, and values
Timely	Reducing unnecessary delay
Efficient	Avoiding waste. Includes supplies, energy, and so on. Ensures right patient, right treatment/test/procedure
Equitable	Care that is not varied based on patient demographic profile

Within the past decade, otolaryngologists demonstrated such leadership potential through high-profile initiatives that have streamlined outpatient clinic flow, improved safety of tracheostomy care, expedited diagnosis of critical emergency diagnoses, and improved efficiency in high-volume procedures.[5–11]

In order to have success in PSQI, however, the physician leader must be deliberate about improvement processes. The problem must be clearly defined with a structured aim, interventions must be based on rigorous study of the problem, and measures must assess the full spectrum of interventions, including assessment of unintended consequences. Once complete, the initiative must have a plan for sustained change. In addition to following fundamentals of quality improvement, physician leaders must also have a basic understanding of change management in order to ensure that their interventions are supported by frontline staff and executives. Finally, dissemination of knowledge in the form of scholarly publication should be strongly considered, so care can be improved across institutions.

INTERVENTION PLANNING
Defining the Problem

As one embarks on a quality improvement initiative, one of the initial steps is selection and definition of the problem that is to be solved. Often, ideal problems are those that everyone knows exist but many have come to accept. Other times, they can be identified through local-level quality dashboards or through reports generated by registries such as the American College of Surgeons National Surgery Quality Improvement Program (ACS-NSQIP). Having a working knowledge of institutional and local-level priorities as delineated in fiscal year or short-term plans may aid in leveraging resources for one's project.

Problems should be defined using a concise problem statement that describes the gap between current state and ideal future state, who is affected, and the consequences of inaction. Clearly worded problem statements can be used to create a "burning platform" for change and to provide a foundation for assembly of stakeholders.

Establishing Aims

Once the problem is defined, an aim statement helps narrow the focus of what is to be improved. Using the acronym SMART helps to create an aim statement that is structured with an established timeline and that provides a framework for future measurement plan (**Fig. 1**). It is here that one can also define what is considered "in scope" and "out of scope" for the project.

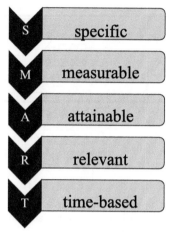

Fig. 1. SMART can be used as an acronym for drafting aim statements that fully delineate what the improvement team expects to achieve.

Stakeholder Analysis

In order to be successful in intervention design and implementation, a comprehensive, multidisciplinary team of stakeholders must be assembled. Stakeholders may include executive leadership, physicians, nurses, technicians, pharmacists, patients/families, facilities engineers, information technology specialists, data analysts, and so forth. Creation of a comprehensive group of stakeholders aids in the design of interventions that are useable and effective across all disciplines and helps drive genuine engagement and acceptance of changes due to ownership of intervention design. Such acceptance increases the chance of sustainability over time.

Study of the Problem

One of the most common pitfalls that is encountered in quality improvement is the tendency to prematurely design interventions without adequately understanding the problem. Failure to understand root causes risks creation of interventions that are "work-arounds," which may further complicate patient care systems. Study of the problem may be quantitative through review of internal or registry data or may be qualitative such as via "pain-point" interviews of front-line stakeholders. Problems can then be mapped onto tools such as Fishbone Diagrams that help identify and categorize gaps and their underlying causes (**Fig. 2**).

Quality Improvement Methodologies

Quality improvement is most successful when one implements established methodologies for improvement. An exhaustive discussion of methodologies is beyond the scope of this article, but among the most commonly used include Model for Improvement and Six Sigma.[12–16] Model for Improvement uses iterative Plan, Do, Study, Act (PDSA) cycles to achieve improvement. A commonly used method in Six Sigma is to implement Define, Measure, Analyze, Improve, Control (DMAIC) cycles. On occasion, Kaizen can be used as a methodology for rapid improvement cycles.[17] Often, selection of improvement methodology is made through what is typically utilized in one's institutional setting; however, if methods are not established in a work unit, it is recommended that one methodology be adopted and then followed. Proper utilization will

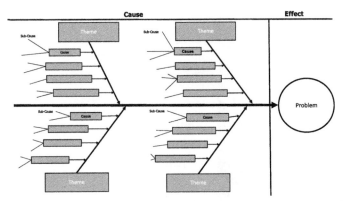

Fig. 2. A fishbone diagram is an improvement tool used to map out contributing factors to a problem. Major categories of underlying causes are placed in the boxes labeled "themes" with causes and subcauses being mapped below.

help ensure that improvements will follow an organized process with plans for measurement and sustainability.

INTERVENTIONS

Once a problem has been fully defined, aims are clearly stated, and stakeholders are assembled, interventions can then be designed and implemented. To aid in selection of interventions, tools such as Key Driver Diagrams—which are developed using fishbone diagrams—can help ensure that interventions map to gaps identified during study of the problem (**Fig. 3**). When selecting interventions, one must consider and balance strength of intervention, ease of implementation, potential for impact, and sustainability. Often these aspects may be at odds with one another necessitating compromise. Tools such as impact versus effort matrices may be helpful in determining selected interventions.

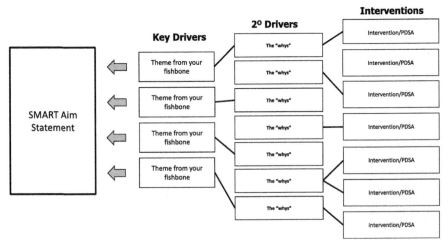

Fig. 3. Fishbone diagrams can be used to populate key driver diagrams. Interventions can then be designed and mapped to the secondary drivers as depicted on the diagram, ensuring that interventions address root causes.

Strength of interventions has been thoroughly studied in quality improvement.[18] Systems with more automated change are more likely to be effective, as they do not rely on human factors. In an initiative to standardize postoperative adenotonsillectomy care, Studer and colleagues[5] utilized order sets with automatically selected non-opioid pain regimens to reduce utilization of opioids. Forcing functions is another effective means of change. For example, lines for blood pressure cuffs have different connectivity than Leur locks so they cannot be accidently attached to intravenous lines. Other strategies such as creation of checklists and standardized protocols are also strong interventions.[19] Conversely, communication (such as e-mails, posted signs, and so forth) and educational interventions are considered weak, as they may go unnoticed and are susceptible to knowledge atrophy and turnover of personnel. Strength of intervention is often correlated with sustainability, provided that the intervention itself does not require excessive use of resources.

When considering ease of implementation, one must factor in resources required as well as the potential for buy-in by frontline staff. For example, for an intervention to improve bedside care involving a 100-question checklist that took 15 minutes to complete, the intervention may be strong, but it will likely be too onerous to be useable. Proper involvement of stakeholders in intervention design will aid in determining ease of implementation.

Depending on the resources required, implementation of simultaneous interventions may be advantageous as they can be utilized to address multiple key drivers. In addition, redundancy in interventions may increase the likelihood of improvement. If resource limitations hinder the ability to implement simultaneous interventions, iterative cycles of change can alternatively be utilized to improve quality. Should the success of these interventions prove interdependent, then these can be planned as conditional based on success of prior iterations.

MEASUREMENT PLAN
Measure Selection

To assess the impact of interventions, one must develop a measurement plan. Measures help determine if an intervention was associated with an improvement effort and consist of a numerator and a denominator. Some measures are standard and require no definition, such as length of stay or 30-day readmissions. Nonstandard measures require formal definition of a numerator and denominator. Measures most commonly used in quality improvement are categorized into outcome, process, and balancing types. Outcome measures assess the "end point." In some circumstances such as those regarding rare events or events that occur in the distant future, outcome measures may have limited value. In these instances, intermediate outcome measures may be favorable. For example, in the care of a patient with diabetes mellitus type II, development of blindness is an outcome measure with limited value given average time to develop. Instead, hemoglobin A1C can be tracked as an intermediate outcome and marker of good control.

In addition to outcome measures, process measures are utilized to assess success of a quality intervention. A process measure examines whether an activity is performed. An example of process measure is rate of utilization of an order set or completion of a care bundle. When used in conjunction with outcome measures, process measures help lend credence to an argument that an intervention actually led to change. Say, for example, a quality project was designed to reduce tracheostomy-associated pressure ulcers, and the intervention was implementation of an electronic medical record–based checklist for tracheostomy care. If tracheostomy wound incidence decreased and checklist utilization was high, it is conceivable that the checklist helped improve tracheostomy care. If, on the other hand, examination of the process measure of checklist completion rate revealed low frequency of completion, it is likely that some external drivers were associated with the observed decrease in pressure injuries.

The last measure that is frequently used in quality improvement endeavors is the balancing measure. Balancing measures assess for unintended consequences that may occur during intervention implementation. They may reveal an opportunity cost that, despite success of the intervention, may make it unsustainable. For example, if an otolaryngology team wanted to adopt an extended, procedure-specific, surgical safety checklist for airway surgery, a balancing measure may be poor adherence, checklist completion time, or operative time.

In addition to assessing impact of the intervention, a quality improvement measurement plan should take into account study of interventions. In doing this, one is assessing whether the interventions were impactful, practical, and sustainable. Generally, study of interventions can occur through process and balancing measures. In addition, qualitative study through conducting interviews of frontline staff allows for additional assessment of intervention impact.

Methods of Measurement

Once measures have been selected, one must next determine the method and frequency of measurement. Methods for measurement vary and can include manual observation, manual or automatic data extraction from the electronic medical record, extraction from administrative databases, review of registry reports, and so forth. Frequency of measurement depends on frequency of events being studied, resources available, and difficulty of extraction. When feasible, regular tracking via automatically updated dashboards provides the best opportunity to assess intervention sustainability.

Statistical Analysis

Analysis of measured data can occur using traditional statistics or through statistical process control (SPC) methods. SPC methods employ the use of run charts and control charts to study data over time. Using these methods helps provide insight into whether an intervention led to improvement and whether the improvement is sustained over time, making them the preferred statistical analysis plan in quality improvement.[20] Although control charts require more advanced statistical analysis and specialized software, run charts can be accomplished with minimal training and standard graphing methods (**Fig. 4**).

SUSTAINING CHANGE

After completion of a quality improvement project, one must have a plan to assess for sustainability. Efforts made to design an intervention and measurement plan that has the potential for long-term viability at improvement initiative outset will facilitate sustainability. Advance planning for resource need, identification of program leaders, and specific determination of how "success" is defined is imperative. Selection of strong interventions avoids change that is susceptible to staff turnover or the Hawthorne effect (change in behavior based on the perception that one is being observed).[21] Reconvening the improvement team at preset intervals after intervention implementation will also aid in assessment of progress, identification of barriers to continued success, and selection of potential future iterative cycles of change. Long-term, one should consider meeting annually to assess the impact of large-

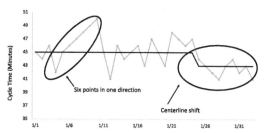

Fig. 4. Hypothetical run chart depicting clinic cycle time. The centerline is calculated as the median of the baseline datapoints. Variation around the mean is deemed common cause variation. A run of 6 points in a single direction suggests special cause variation. Centerline shifts occur if 8 points lie on the same side of the centerline, designating a significant change in the system.

scale interventions, as well as the potential effects of external influences on the intended improvement.

CHANGE MANAGEMENT

Change is difficult, and change that imparts meaningful improvement in quality generally requires an organizational split from long-sustained practices and the perceived benefits of established culture. Furthermore, organizations are by no means singular-minded, but rather an agglomeration of individuals, representing a milieu of multiple perspectives and experiences. Thus, every change initiative is presented with a series of challenges in development, implementation, execution, and sustainment, which go beyond the quality of the project and its potential outcome.

It has been estimated that as many as 70% of organizational change initiatives fail, and although this figure has been challenged, it is clear that many such initiatives do fail.[22,23] The reasons for this have been extensively studied, and the field of implementation science has codified many steps by which change efforts can be optimized, as alluded to aforementioned, and these steps are readily available for further review.[24] But there are important considerations surrounding even these steps, a kind of "reading between the lines" of the steps for change management.

Institutional Support

The choice of projects and outcome goals are critically important to the ultimate ability to implement change. Ensuring that projects align well with institutional goals is certainly important, but just as important is the messaging that surrounds the proposed project and its organizational deliverables. In general, health care organizations have a series of key pillar goals that tend to be common across organizations: quality care and outcomes, profitability, efficiency, access, and so forth. Creating a narrative regarding the meaningful impacts of the project outcome on one of these must be a priority in project planning. Going beyond the burning platform to recruit support among executives, managers, leaders, and frontline personnel can do far more for the ultimate success of a project than meticulous planning.

Executive Sponsorship

Identifying a key executive leader who recognizes the value of and believes strongly in the proposed effort provides the team with support with a broader institutional view than many team members. A good executive sponsor helps the team avoid potential institutional pitfalls, highlight potential collaborators or synergisms, provide alignment among distinct workgroups, mobilize resources, and maintain support and dialogue among the executive team. Regular updates to executive sponsors engage these individuals in the process, while updating them and providing a forum in which to inform them of team needs.

Change Adaptation

It is well known that individuals on a team adapt to change at different rates,[25] which means that implementation is a type of primary sustain phase during which individuals of varying support or resistance for the change gradually adapt to the new process. A clear pitfall in this area is to expect quick adaptation from all or to misinterpret the activities of early adapters as successful implementation. Open and honest conversations at the outset of project planning and throughout implementation can provide team leaders with information on whom resistance to change will be strongest and can provide important insight into how well the affected groups have adapted.

PUBLISHING QUALITY IMPROVEMENT INITIATIVES

Similar to traditional research, the dissemination of knowledge in scholarly publication facilitates large-scale improvements that can cross institutions and should be seen as the duty of the academic otolaryngologist. Contrary to traditional research, quality improvement publication should follow SQUIRE format.[26] The primary differentiating elements of SQUIRE publications are highlighted as follows.

Rationale

Rationale is defined by SQUIRE as the "Informal or formal frameworks, models, concepts and/or theories used to explain the problem, any reasons or assumptions that were used to develop the interventions, and why the interventions were expected to work."[26] It can be seen as analogous to the hypothesis in traditional research articles. The investigators should use the rationale to justify the proposed interventions selected and frequently will guide the reader into understanding proposed measures. One helpful way to depict rationale is using the if…then…so that… framework. In other words, if the root cause of a problem is _____, then doing _____ will improve the problem so that _____.

Context

As quality improvement must be understood within the confines of the work unit in which an intervention is being performed, context is an essential element to quality improvement writing. In this section, one highlights elements of the work environment where the intervention is being carried out. Common contextual elements include the care setting (inpatient, outpatient, tertiary care, number of beds, and so forth) as well as factors such as staffing/personnel models, relevant structural elements of the workspace, workplace cultural trends, and so forth. Defining context helps the reader understand the setting in which the interventions occurred, and it permits interpretation of whether such interventions may be feasible in his/her own work unit. Although context is first introduced in the methods section, contextual elements are frequently referenced throughout the entire article, as they provide insight into why the intervention worked/did not work, the sustainability of the intervention, and adaptability to alternate settings.

Study of Interventions

Study of interventions is an element of the methods section of SQUIRE writing that is a means of assessing whether an intervention itself led to change. In addition, study of interventions also investigates whether there are opportunity costs that may make an intervention unsustainable, whether there are unintended benefits warranting continuation of an intervention despite limited outcome improvement, and whether there are generalizable features that may make the intervention applicable in other settings. It is often conducted by careful selection of process and balancing measures but may also be performed using qualitative study, for example, via field notes or interviews of frontline staff or patients.

SUMMARY

Quality improvement has become a well-developed scholarly field in medicine. The otolaryngologist has the potential to be a leader in the PSQI realm due to his/her interfacing with multiple different services and settings. A strong foundation in basic principles and methodologies of improvement is essential to success, and the otolaryngologist must be deliberate in the study of the problem, selection of interventions, and measurement plan. A foundation in change management principles will aid the otolaryngologist in recruiting executive and front-line support, especially if interventions represent large departures from standard practice. Once complete, dissemination of knowledge in scholarly writing allows for the work to be adapted to multiple settings, improving patient care beyond the confines of the otolaryngologist's work unit.

CLINICS CARE POINTS

- Proper methodology, using models such as model for improvement or six sigma, should be employed when undertaking improvement initiatives.

- Measure success or failure of an initiative using a combination of outcome, process and balancing measures to fully understand the success and impact if an intervention.

- Interventions selected should favor forcing functions or automation over educational or communication-based intervention to enhance sustainability.

REFERENCES

1. Chassin MR, Galvin RW. The urgent need to improve health care quality. Institute of Medicine National Roundtable on Health Care Quality. JAMA 1998;280:1000–5.
2. Institute of Medicine Committee on Quality of Health Care. in A. In: Kohn LT, Corrigan JM, Donaldson MS, editors. To err is human: building a safer health system. Washington (DC): National Academies Press (US)Copyright 2000 by the National Academy of Sciences. All rights reserved.; 2000.
3. Institute of Medicine Committee on Quality of Health Care in A. Crossing the quality chasm: a new health system for the 21st century. Washington (DC): National Academies Press (US) Copyright 2001 by the National Academy of Sciences. All rights reserved.; 2001.
4. Nicolay CR, Purkayastha S, Greenhalgh A, et al. Systematic review of the application of quality improvement methodologies from the manufacturing industry to surgical healthcare. Br J Surg 2011;99:324–35.

5. Studer A, Billings K, Thompson D, et al. standardized order set exhibits surgeon adherence to pain protocol in pediatric adenotonsillectomy. Laryngoscope 2021; 131:E2337–43.

6. Lavin JM, Wiedermann J, Sals A, et al. Electronic medical record-based tools aid in timely triage of disc-shaped foreign body ingestions. Laryngoscope 2018;128: 2697–701.

7. Lavin JM, Sawardekar A, Sohn L, et al. Efficient postoperative disposition selection in pediatric otolaryngology patients: a novel approach. Laryngoscope 2021; 131(Suppl 1):S1–10.

8. Yang CJ, Bottalico D, Philips K, et al. Improving the pediatric floor discharge process following tonsillectomy. Laryngoscope 2022;132:225–33.

9. Huddle MG, Tirabassi A, Turner L, et al. application of lean sigma to the audiology clinic at a large academic center. Otolaryngol Head Neck Surg 2016;154:715–9.

10. Swegal WC, Iwata AJ, Chang SS. Developing a patient driven head and neck cancer care pathway. Head Neck 2019;41:1094–5.

11. Ong T, Liu CC, Elder L, et al. the trach safe initiative: a quality improvement initiative to reduce mortality among pediatric tracheostomy patients. Otolaryngol Head Neck Surg 2020;163:221–31.

12. Courtlandt CD, Noonan L, Feld LG. Model for improvement - Part 1: a framework for health care quality. Pediatr Clin North Am 2009;56:757–78.

13. Crowl A, Sharma A, Sorge L, et al. Accelerating quality improvement within your organization: applying the Model for Improvement. J Am Pharm Assoc (2003) 2015;55:e364–74 [quiz: e375-366].

14. Randolph G, Esporas M, Provost L, et al. Model for improvement - part two: measurement and feedback for quality improvement efforts. Pediatr Clin North Am 2009;56:779–98.

15. de Koning H, Verver JPS, van den Heuvel J, et al. Lean six sigma in healthcare. J Healthc Qual 2006;28:4–11.

16. Niñerola A, Sánchez-Rebull MV, Hernández-Lara AB. Quality improvement in healthcare: six sigma systematic review. Health Policy 2020;124:438–45.

17. Goyal S, Law E. An introduction to Kaizen in health care. Br J Hosp Med (Lond) 2019;80:168–9.

18. Scott I. What are the most effective strategies for improving quality and safety of health care? Intern Med J 2009;39:389–400.

19. Haynes AB, Weiser TG, Berry WR, et al. A surgical safety checklist to reduce morbidity and mortality in a global population. N Engl J Med 2009;360:491–9.

20. Perla RJ, Provost LP, Murray SK. The run chart: a simple analytical tool for learning from variation in healthcare processes. BMJ Qual Saf 2011;20:46–51.

21. Srigley JA, Furness CD, Baker GR, et al. Quantification of the Hawthorne effect in hand hygiene compliance monitoring using an electronic monitoring system: a retrospective cohort study. BMJ Qual Saf 2014;23:974–80.

22. Hammer M, Champy J. Reengineering the corporation: a manifesto for business revolution. New York: Harper Business; 1994.

23. Tasler N. Stop using the excuse "organizational change is hard". Periodical [serial online]. Boston, MA: Harvard Business Review; 2017.

24. Kotter JP. Leading change. Boston: Harvard Business School Press; 1996.

25. Rogers EM. Diffusion of innovations. New York: Free Press; 2003.

26. Ogrinc G, Davies L, Goodman D, et al. SQUIRE 2.0 (Standards for QUality Improvement Reporting Excellence): revised publication guidelines from a detailed consensus process. BMJ Qual Saf 2016;25:986–92.

Principles of Adult Learning
Tips for the Pediatric Otolaryngologist

Eric A. Gantwerker, MD, MMSc[a,b], Gi Soo Lee, MD, EdM[c,d,*]

KEYWORDS

- Faculty development • Learning strategies • Adult learning theory
- Cognitive load theory • Experiential learning • Self-efficacy • Deliberate practice
- Surgical training

KEY POINTS

- Adult learners have important differences from children in how they approach and participate in learning experiences.
- By engaging with adult learning principles, such as respecting autonomy, prior knowledge, a need for problem-focused learning, and embracing the proximal application of the content, faculty can improve the learning experience for their trainees.
- By keeping trainees at the upper end of their abilities and constantly challenging them with deliberately difficult tasks, faculty can maximize the efficiency and efficacy of their teaching.
- Chunking complex tasks into smaller component parts can improve the trainees' ability to focus and remember and prevent them from getting easily overwhelmed.
- Increasing trainee confidence (self-efficacy) in a particular domain can have a direct effect on improving performance even without improved skill development.

INTRODUCTION

Humans are innately programmed to learn. Throughout development, children are constantly interacting with their world, incessantly placing everything in their mouths and throwing objects off their highchairs to try to uncover the secrets of the world around them. As children grow to school age, they enter a world of education defined and prescribed by higher authorities. This formal education continues through high school and college; at some point, a transit ion occurs, and learning becomes focused

[a] Department of Otolaryngology, Cohen Children's Medical Center/Long Island Jewish Medical Center at Northwell Health, 430 Lakeville Road, New Hyde Park, NY 11042, USA; [b] Department of Otolaryngology, Zucker School of Medicine at Northwell/Hofstra, Hempstead, NY, USA; [c] Department of Otolaryngology and Communication Enhancement, Boston Children's Hospital, 300 Longwood Avenue, Boston, MA 02115, USA; [d] Department of Otolaryngology - Head and Neck Surgery, Harvard Medical School, 25 Shattuck Street, Boston, MA 02115, USA
* Corresponding author.
E-mail address: Gi.Lee@childrens.harvard.edu

Otolaryngol Clin N Am 55 (2022) 1311–1320
https://doi.org/10.1016/j.otc.2022.07.009
0030-6665/22/© 2022 Elsevier Inc. All rights reserved.

on their own specific interests. The enjoyment of learning stems from the pursuits and satisfactions of these curiosities. Teaching in this adult phase of learning has important differences from the pedagogical principles followed in K-12 education. One particular researcher is noted for advancing and studying these differences, namely, Malcolm Knowles.

DISCUSSION

Knowles forwarded the concept of *andragogy* and the principles of adult learning theory (ALT). He noted that children and adults differ in several important ways when it comes to education:[1–3]

1. Motivations—Adults learn because they are intrinsically motivated to do so.
2. Need to know—Adults need to understand why they need to learn something.
3. Autonomy—Adults prefer to be responsible and take charge of their own learning.
4. Prior knowledge and skills—Adults learn with a repository of fundamental knowledge, skills, and experience that should be leveraged in educational experiences.
5. Readiness to learn—Adults need to have a perceived deficit and/or recognize an immediate application of the learning.
6. Orientation to learning—Adults engage with learning situationally and learn better with problem-focused content.

Learning theories are important to understand, as they can not only describe phenomena, but guide pediatric otolaryngologists in their training practices for trainees, patients, and colleagues alike. The authors will couch these theories in common educational experiences (surgeries and didactics) and discuss practical applications for everyday use.

Adult Learning Theory in Practice

Putting ALT to practice requires an understanding of and respect for all the principles discussed earlier. Trainees need context as to why they are learning something and how this will apply to future practice. For example, learning about the concept of partial pressures of gases early in medical school is irrelevant until students understand how it applies to arterial blood gases when caring for patients in the intensive care unit. Trainees should be offered autonomy and agency when it comes to their learning. This includes allowing them to choose when and where they want to learn, what they desire to learn, and what resources they want to utilize, such as videos, articles, simulations, and so forth. Because not everyone learns best through a single style or resource, individuals should be provided a curated list of the best resources from which to choose.

Faculty should never assume that trainees do not possess any advanced knowledge or skill. For instance, the failure is assuming that a second-year junior resident cannot place an endoscopic suture. Teaching knowledge or skills that have already been mastered is ineffective; this can be mitigated by allowing the trainees to demonstrate their knowledge or skill before the educational experience. Readiness to learn is identified by directly asking the trainees what their strengths and weaknesses are regarding a certain topic and then providing external feedback as they navigate that task. Consider asking trainees, before starting a case, what their comfort level is performing specific aspects of the case and what they want to work on. This will be highlighted further later when discussing self-efficacy (SE) and deliberate practice. The principle of orientation to learning dictates that a didactic lecture void of context or practical application will not be received as well as a clinically oriented case or a discussion of a problem while actively involving the audience. Adult learners tend to learn better if actively engaged in problem-solving than when listening passively to a lecture.

Four other relevant core theories are the concepts of SE, the zone of proximal development (ZPD), the reducibility hypothesis, and chunking.

Self-efficacy

SE was described by Albert Bandura in the 1980s as part of social cognitive theory and portrays how people develop social, emotional, and cognitive abilities and behaviors. SE is the self-perceived confidence in one's ability to perform a certain task that is informed by prior performance, external feedback, emotional states, and vicarious learning opportunities.

Importantly, SE mediates goal setting, motivation, and performance. SE increases the likelihood of persistence on task, improved task performance, and willingness to take on difficult tasks as opposed to avoiding them (**Fig. 1**).[4,5]

Consider basketball as an example. Players' confidence in making a single free throw shot may be high, but their confidence in making 10 consecutive free throws might be low. The likelihood of successfully making the first free throw is higher simply because the SE is higher; similarly, the likelihood of making 10 consecutively is low. If players increased their SE in making 10 shots (eg, through mental rehearsal), they would have a higher likelihood of actually making them despite no change in skill level.

This requires insight into their own abilities and can be affected by events, outcomes, and external influences (feedback). SE also influences trainees' desires to learn. All attendings have seen residents with respectable skills but low confidence that ultimately results in poor performance (the reverse has been universally seen as

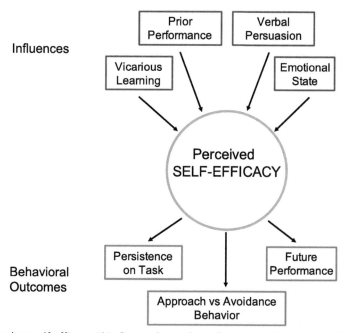

Fig. 1. Bandura self-efficacy. This figure shows the influences and outcomes of perceived self-efficacy as originally described by Bandura and colleagues

well). As confidence increases, performance should follow. This phenomenon also occurs by developing skills through practice (deliberate practice) but is importantly distinct.

Zone of proximal development

Lev Vygotsky described the zone of promxial development (ZPD) in 1978 as the *zone of assisted ability* of students as they progress from novices to experts in a certain domain. Above this zone are tasks that individuals cannot accomplish even with scaffolding (ie, assistance), and below this zone are tasks that they can complete independently (**Fig. 2**A). The ideal is to maintain trainees at the upper edge of this zone and provide occasional assistance (scaffolding) as the task difficulty increases. This sustains the optimum level of activation or stress that results in maximally efficient learning (**Fig. 2**B). Importantly, tasks beyond their abilities (upper zone) will lead to frustration, stagnation, and often negative emotional responses. Tasks below this zone introduce learning inefficiency and can lead to boredom and disengagement.[6]

In the context of surgery, it is important to remain relatively agnostic to residents' training years because skill levels may vary above or below the expectation. In practice, this means inquiring, before a case, where trainees are along their continuum of learning for that case and where they want to be after. During the case, the attending can recalibrate the plan based on their actual skills to keep them at the leading edge of their ZPD. Intuitively, this provides graduated responsibilities within a case that continuously stretches a trainee's abilities. Engaging trainees in tasks on the upper edge of the ZPD maximizes their learning and is termed "desirably difficult tasks."

Maintaining trainees within their ZPD and constantly challenging them will increase engagement and keep them focused on mastery along the *line, speed, and beauty* continuum. This is an expression borrowed from the sport of boxing. On the *line,* fighters learn the basic steps and skills to box.

Once the fundamental elements are individually mastered, they are then combined sequentially. *Speed* refers to integrating the skills and improving efficiency in execution. *Beauty* refers to making it look easy and elegant. In surgical training, this concept also rings true. Trainees must first learn the individual steps of the procedures and be

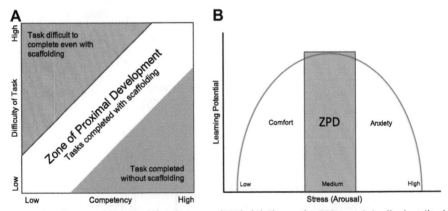

Fig. 2. (*A, B*) Zone of proximal development (ZPD). (*A*) Shows the ZPD as originally described by Vygotsky and colleagues and shows the tasks that learners can complete with assistance in the middle with those that are too challenging above the zone, and those that they can complete independently below the ZPD. (*B*) Shows the stress/arousal that exists within the ZPD that can maximize learning potential avoiding disengagement below and anxiety above the optimal zone.

able to perform them sequentially. Then they then must learn to operate efficiently. Once the execution becomes autonomous, they can then focus on making it look easy and elegant. Utilizing this framework allows for consistent and stepwise growth for trainees.

Notably, early in training, assessing trainees' current abilities and allowing them to struggle safely is paramount. Learning happens best during this struggle as they try to problem solve independently—a construct known as desirable difficulty. For the attending, this means not just "taking the surgery away from them" but, instead, being patient as they navigate through their own struggles. During a struggle, the attending can step in to nudge them just past the point of current stagnation (scaffolding) but then must relinquish control back to them to allow them to continue operating. Confiscating the surgery from them does not allow for problem-solving development and can negatively impact their confidence.

In the current era of time constraints and emphasis on surgical safety, trainees should be directed to select certain aspects of the surgery that *they* want to focus on. Steer away from easy tasks once they have mastered them. In tonsillectomy, for example, the attending can prep the educational session by first inserting the mouth gag and suspending the patient; this allows the trainee to then focus on the actual task of removing the tonsils. Once all the individual steps are mastered on the *line,* the trainee can concentrate on the *speed:* efficiency of movement, the anticipation of subsequent steps, and so on, all in the effort to be maximally efficient with surgical time. Finally, once efficiency is achieved, the experience can focus on making it look easy and effortless. By utilizing this format, the attending never stops pushing the residents' abilities as they move toward complete mastery of the entire surgery.

It is critical to note that where a trainee is on the line, the speed and beauty continuum will vary for each procedure at any given time. Therefore, a senior resident could be working on making a tonsillectomy beautiful, making a tympanoplasty more efficient, and learning the basic steps of a tracheal resection simultaneously. By keeping that resident in his or her ZPD for each unique surgery, learning will always continue and be most effective.

Reducibility hypothesis

The reducibility hypothesis is a subtheory of cognitive load theory (CLT). Further, CLT, described by John Sweller, states that the amount of mental capacity available to learn a new intellectual task is a finite resource and an individual's capacity to learn the task is dependent on the (1) difficulty of the material itself (intrinsic load), (2) how the material is presented (extrinsic load), and (3) the amount of effort required to learn that information (germane load) (**Fig. 3**).[7] Practically speaking, a trainee's ability to learn a very complex task, such as a new surgical procedure, is not just dependent on the task itself but also on *how* it is presented to them. Managing cognitive load is important to make the learning process most efficient and efficacious.

The reducibility hypothesis dictates that complex tasks are simply a conglomeration of smaller tasks that add up to the whole.[8] Therefore, one easy method of managing the intrinsic load is to divide a task into smaller components that are easier to assimilate. For tonsillectomy these "chunks" could include inserting the mouth gag, placing a catheter as a palate retractor, removing the tonsils sequentially (which can be broken down even further), achieving hemostasis, and then removing all equipment. Each of these larger chunks can be further divided into smaller, more manageable tasks. Removing a tonsil entails grasping the tonsil, retracting, incising mucosa, exposing the plane, retracting, developing the plane, cauterizing vessels, and so forth. The steps can be as granular as desired.

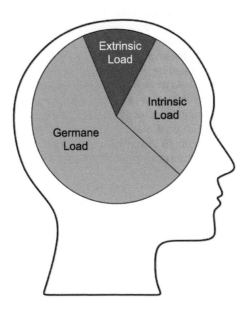

Fig. 3. Cognitive load theory (CLT). This figure shows an overview of CLT as described originally by Sweller and colleagues. Depicted are the components of total cognitive load, including intrinsic (complexity of the learning content), extrinsic (how the content is presented), and germane (effort involved in integrating that content into their knowledge base) loads. One must manage the intrinsic, minimize the extrinsic, and maximize the germane load for effective and efficient learning.

Chunking theory

The concept of breaking apart tasks into smaller elements stems from the chunking theory developed by Chase and Simon in 1973. Their original studies investigated differences between novices and experts in memory tasks and utilized the game chess as the medium to learn, recognize, and implement maneuvers and strategies.[9] The theory helped explain various phenomena in chess expertise using simple mechanisms; the use of this concept applies to other domains of expertise in the arts (playing the violin), sports (swinging a golf club), and professions (performing surgery).

Chunking in surgery is best demonstrated when the trainee performs tasks in *reverse* order. For example, the attending begins and removes the entire tonsil except for the attachment to the inferior pole. The trainee then completes the tonsillectomy. For the next case, the trainee takes over earlier and releases the capsule from midpole down to completion. During the third case, the attending identifies only the plane and allows the trainee to remove the entire tonsil. Finally, the trainee identifies and develops the plane, and removes the entire tonsil. This reverse sequence accomplishes several things. First, the trainee experiences early success and develops a sense of achievement by completing the surgery (increasing SE). Confidence improves with each iteration because the trainee completes the operation multiple times *even before he or she ever started it.*

Furthermore, as identifying the plane is typically the most difficult task in tonsillectomy, it is reserved for the final iteration once the trainee has already gained higher confidence and skill.

This is in stark contrast to how many faculty teach surgery from beginning to end. In this format, when difficulties are encountered, the surgery is often "taken away" from the trainee. The lack of completion or sense of accomplishment is often detrimental to the trainee decreasing SE and affecting future performance.

For subsequent encounters, the attending should meet with the trainee before the next clinical case to identify areas of decreased competence or SE within a procedure. Once identified, the attending can begin and perform the procedure right up to the identified task and then permit the trainee to step in. This allows the trainee to maximize the germane load (the effort required to perform the difficult chunked task) while minimizing the extrinsic load (the remaining easier portions of the case). Constantly altering the tasks keeps the trainee at the edge of their abilities. This deliberate practice of areas of weakness is much more efficient than repeating the entirety of procedures without focus.

Once all the essential steps of the procedure are mastered, the trainee then focuses on efficiency and, lastly, on making the surgery look easy. Finally, the surgeon can task the trainee to teach a more junior trainee. This is the ultimate step to achieving mastery. This last step also respects the adult learning principles of autonomy (they are choosing the task to focus on when teaching), activation of prior knowledge (they are drawing from skills already learned), and problem-focused learning. The overriding concept is to continuously challenge the trainee instead of mindlessly having them complete surgeries they have already mastered. Peer teaching then allows the trainee to consolidate their own knowledge/skills and identify any remaining gaps to help guide future training sessions.

Experiential learning, retrieval practice, and adult learning theory

Much has been discussed about procedural training. However, cognitive tasks are also in the purview of the surgeon as a teacher. For example, consider polysomnograms (PSGs). Although many trainees reduce PSG knowledge to simply recognizing the apnea-hypopnea index, PSGs are much more than that. As adult learners have abundant prior knowledge and tend to learn better when educational experiences are problem-focused, learning through doing is a much more efficient and efficacious way to teach. This introduces the concept of experiential learning or active learning as described by David Kolb.

Kolb described adult learning as a cycle of having a concrete experience, reflecting on the experience (reflective observation), learning from the experience (abstract conceptualization), and reapplying that learning into practice (active experimentation).[10] To assimilate information, adults use these experiences, reflect on what may have happened, create a working theory, and then actively experiment with their current conceptual understanding to further refine their understanding of the information by revolving around the cycle again and again (**Fig. 4**). This methodology is most effective in an active and engaging learning environment.

By cycling through this process, trainees are participating in retrieval practice, also called the testing effect. Humans have a habit of forgetting. They will forget 50% of newly presented information within 20 minutes of learning it. After 1 day, they forget two-thirds of what was learned just the day prior.[11,12] Retrieval practice is the attempt to blunt the forgetfulness curve (**Fig. 5**) by accessing information and reintroducing it into working memory. By activating prior knowledge and assimilating new information, a new memory is created, and information is strengthened or consolidated. Constantly challenging trainees to apply newly learned information improves their ability to consolidate this information and lessen the decay.[13]

To understand PSGs, instruct trainees to read actual sleep studies instead of lecturing about them, even if they have never seen a PSG before. Ideally, they should

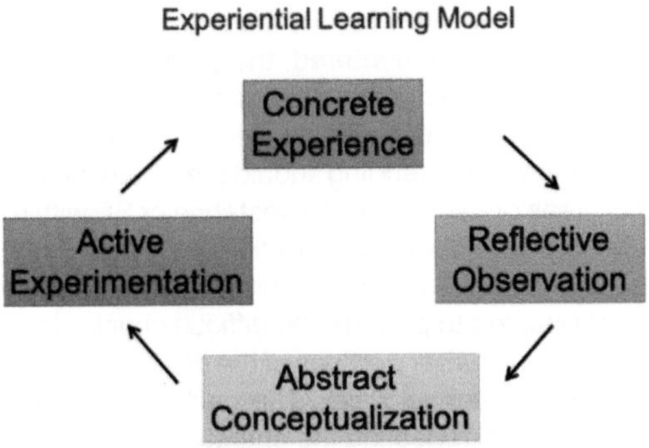

Experiential Learning Model

Concrete
Experience

Reflective
Observation

Abstract
Conceptualization

Active
Experimentation

Fig. 4. Kolb's learning cycle. This figure shows the experiential learning model also known as Kolb's cycle as originally described by Kolb and colleagues. The learner progresses from concrete experience to reflective observation to abstract conceptualization to active experimentation as they cycle through this model.

have prestudied or familiarized themselves with the PSG components—a concept known as a *flipped classroom*. By attempting to interpret PSGs, they will calibrate their current abilities and self-identify knowledge gaps. The attending can activate prior knowledge about sleep [eg, rapid eye movement (REM) sleep induces relative hypotonia; as a result, REM sleep may exhibit more obstructive events than non-REM sleep]. Some trainees may know sleep laboratory equipment and can discuss what information is derived from those biosensors. Others may know fluid dynamics and understand how an upstream obstructive site in the nose can affect downstream sites dynamically. Once each section of the PSG is discussed, the group can review it by interpreting a new PSG in its entirety.

Utilizing social learning theory, separate trainees into small groups to facilitate sharing of information and collaborative discussion. Once they have a deeper understanding of the information, they can then present it to the greater group. This serves to maintain active engagement through problem-focused exercises, increases SE in their ability to analyze studies, and utilizes retrieval practice to consolidate and assimilate new information.

These various learning theories and techniques can be applied to *any* surgical procedure or clinical construct. In review, consider myringotomy and tube placement.

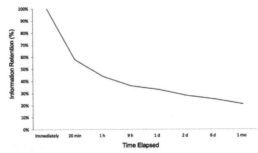

Fig. 5. Ebbinghaus forgetfulness curve. This figure shows the Ebbinghaus forgetfulness curve that shows knowledge retention drastically decreases over the immediate minutes to hours to days after initial exposure to learning material.

The surgical steps are clear: insert a speculum, introduce operating microscope, perform cerumenectomy, inspect tympanic membrane, make myringotomy, suction fluid, place tube at the edge of incision, insert and seal the tube, and place ear drops. For a novice trainee, using the principles described, the attending would perform everything until the ear tube was positioned with one edge in the myringotomy. The trainee would then insert the tube and complete the procedure. The next time the trainee with position and seat the tube in the myringotomy made by the attending. And so forth until the trainee can perform the entire procedure independently. Next, the attending concentrates on teaching efficiency of movement and, ultimately, making it look easy. To maintain the edge of the ZPD, the attending can then require the trainee to perform the procedure with a two-hand technique similar to that used for tympanoplasty or middle ear surgery. They can be tasked to teach younger trainees.

SUMMARY

ALT, as described by Malcolm Knowles, contrasts children (pedagogy) and adults (andragogy) in their learning environments and preferences. Knowles describes the primarily intrinsic motivations, the need to know why they are learning something, the need for autonomy, the desire to build on prior knowledge and skills, and a need to identify a perceived deficit and/or see an immediate application of the learning. SE describes the confidence in one's ability to perform a certain task. Increasing a resident's confidence can have a direct positive influence on performance. This can be achieved by reverse-order training of "chunks," or smaller component steps of the procedure. Faculty can maximize the growth of the trainee but sustaining them at the edge of their abilities, allowing them to struggle safely, and providing them deliberately difficult tasks to complete.

Understanding the principles and theories that are well recognized in adult learning can have a major impact on learning and teaching today. In an era with time constraints and ever-dwindling experiential learning opportunities, the focus should be on maximizing the efficiency and efficacy of everyday teaching. The concepts discussed will provide faculty with more tools to transform trainees' learning experiences. This, ultimately, allows them to teach the next generation how to invoke these strategies, forever propagating better teaching practices.

CLINICS CARE POINTS

- Adult learners have important differences from children in how they approach and participate in learning experiences.

- By engaging adult learning principles ,such as respect for autonomy, prior knowledge, a need for problem-focused learning, and embracing the proximal application of the content, faculty can improve the learning experience for their trainees.

- By maintaining trainees at the upper end of their abilities and constantly challenging them with deliberately difficult tasks, faculty can maximize the efficiency and efficacy of their teaching.

- Chunking complex tasks into smaller component parts can improve the trainees' ability to focus and remember and prevent them from getting easily overwhelmed.

- Increasing trainee confidence in a particular domain can have a direct effect on improving performance even without improved skill development.

DISCLOSURE

Dr E.A. Gantwerker works part-time for a medical video game company that engages in continuing medical education (Level Ex, Inc) and is the CEO and founder of an educational technology consulting company (MedEd Innovations, LLC). He is also the vice president of a medical education for a video surgical journal (CSurgeries. com). None of these entities provided any financial support or had any influence, review, or control of any of the content of this article. No financial support or conflicts of interest to declare for Dr G.S. Lee.

REFERENCES

1. Knowles MS, Holton EF, Swanson RA. The adult learner. Vol 24.; 2011.
2. Taylor DCM, Hamdy H. Adult learning theories: implications for learning and teaching in medical education: AMEE Guide No. 83. Med Teach 2013;35(11): e1561–72.
3. Moore K. The three-part harmony of adult learning, critical thinking, and decision-making Kyle Moore. J Adult Educ 2010;39(1):1–10. Availabl at: http://www.eric.ed.gov/ERICWebPortal/detail?accno=EJ917394.
4. Bandura A. Self-efficacy mechanism in human agency. Am Psychol 1982;37(2): 122–47. https://doi.org/10.1037/0003-066X.37.2.122.
5. Maddux JE. Albert bandura self-efficacy: the exercise of control. Vol 43.; 1998.
6. Vygotsky LS. Mind and Society: The Development of Higher Psychological Processes.; 1978. doi:(Original manuscripts [ca. 1930-1934]).
7. Sweller J. Cognitive load theory , learning difficulty , and instructional design. Learn Instr 1994;4:295–312. https://doi.org/10.1016/0959-4752(94)90003-5.
8. Lee FJ, Anderson JR. Does learning a complex task have to be complex?: a study in learning decomposition. Cogn Psychol 2001. https://doi.org/10.1006/cogp.2000.0747.
9. Chase WG, Simon HA. Perception in chess. Cogn Psychol 1973;4(1):55–81.
10. Kolb DDavid A. Kolb on Experiential Learning. 1983. Availabl at: Www.Infed.Org/Biblio/b- Explrn.Htm.
11. Ebbinghaus H. Memory: a contribution to experimental psychology. New York: New York Teach Coll Columbia Univ; 1885 (translated by HA ruger & CE bussenues, 1913).
12. Subirana B, Bagiati A, Sarma S. On the forgetting of college academics: at "Ebbinghaus Speed". Edulearn17 Proc 2017;1(068):8908–18.
13. Roediger HL, Butler AC. The critical role of retrieval practice in long-term retention. Trends Cogn Sci 2011;15(1):20–7.

Pediatric Otolaryngology in COVID-19

Scott Rickert, MD[a],*, Reza Rahbar, DMD, MD[b,c]

KEYWORDS

- COVID-19 • Pediatric otolaryngology • Pediatric ear • Nose and throat

KEY POINTS

- Managing children has several unique features, which potentially increase COVID-19 exposure risk to the provider, including a high frequency of upper respiratory tract infections, asymptomatic carries, and poor patient compliance with a routine examination.
- By its very nature, otolaryngologists have a unique set of conditions that make providers particularly vulnerable to upper respiratory pathogens, including close physical proximity of the examination to the pharynx and the practice of aerosol-generating procedures.
- There are many features of COVID-19 infection that manifest in the pediatric population postinfection including anosmia/hyposmia, dysgeusia, MIS-C, and long COVID-19.
- Many system-based initiatives instituted in hospitals across the country have helped to mitigate risks and improve the patient experience.
- With the advent of new technologies for remote examination and integrated electronic medical records, this hybrid model will provide a high level of satisfaction for patients and families who can get access to their health care provider more easily from multiple avenues in a convenient set.

INTRODUCTION

While the majority of attention to the health care impact of COVID-19 has focused on adult first responders and critical care providers, the pandemic has had a profound effect on the entire health care industry, including the pediatric otolaryngology community. As a result of resource limitations and social distancing measures, the day to day practice of pediatric otolaryngology was been abruptly altered, requiring rapid adaption to provide safety to the patients and the practitioners, as well as provide quality care to patients in need. The result of these adaptations has included the

[a] Division of Pediatric Otolaryngology, Department of Otolaryngology, Pediatrics, and Plastic Surgery, Hassenfeld Children's Hospital at NYU Langone, NYU Langone Health, 240 East 38th Street, New York, NY 10016, USA; [b] Center for Airway Disorders, Neck and Skull Base Surgery Program, Harvard Medical School; [c] Department of Otolaryngology & Communication Enhancement, 333 Longwood Avenue, Boston, MA 02115, USA
* Corresponding author.
E-mail address: scott.rickert@nyulangone.org

Otolaryngol Clin N Am 55 (2022) 1321–1335
https://doi.org/10.1016/j.otc.2022.07.020
0030-6665/22/© 2022 Elsevier Inc. All rights reserved.

oto.theclinics.com

further development of telemedicine, elaborate protective protocols to allow for limited exposure to potential aerosol-generating procedures (AGP) for both patients and practitioners, and engaging in a national discussion regarding how to resume "normal" practice following the peak of the pandemic while continuing to provide safe and efficient care. Several consequences of COVID-19 infection manifested in the pediatric otolaryngology community are discussed and highlighted including anosmia, dysgeusia, hearing loss, MIS-C symptoms, and long COVID-19 symptoms.

The objective of this article is to highlight the unique ramifications of COVID-19 on pediatric otolaryngology, with a focus on the immediate and potential long-term shifts in practice.

Initial Diagnosis and Safety Protocols in Care for the Pediatric Patient and the Practitioners

In early March 2020, COVID-19 began its historic pandemic spread across the world. Unusual viral illnesses eventually identified as COVID-19 were discovered as early as November 2019 in China and January 2020 in the US. The widespread discovery of COVID-19 was identified in March 2020 and predominant spread at that time was communal based. Initial symptoms included include fever (43%–98%), cough (68%–82%), fatigue (38%–44%), sore throat (13.9%–17.4%), dry cough (59.4%), and sputum production (28%–33%).[1] Common inflammatory markers were noted to be elevated including increased values of C-reactive protein (75%–93%), lactate dehydrogenase (27%–92%), and erythrocyte sedimentation rate (up to 85%).[2]

As this respiratory-based virus began to cause a significant increase in hospitalizations particularly in the adult population, there was a concerted effort to curb the spread of the virus. As those sick with COVID-19 initially presented to the hospital for care, much of the initial concerted effort to contain COVID-19 was focused on hospital-based care and protection. While the vast majority of the patients initially presenting to the hospital with COVID-19 were adults, there was a minority of children, particularly children with complex preexisting diseases, who also needed care for COVID-19-related respiratory issues in a hospital-based setting. In 2020, a review of 72314 cases from China identified less than 2% of the cases under 19 years of age and 1% of cases in patients under 10 years of age.[3] It was determined that the vast majority of pediatric patients had much milder symptoms than adults and 15% of pediatric patient in Wuhan were asymptomatic[4] which presented its own risk in asymptomatic spread through the pediatric population. The true prevalence of asymptomatic children is most likely underreported.[5] There was an initial 14.8% rate of mortality in those over 80 years there was a 0% reported mortality in children under 9.[6]

As COVID-19 has evolved, the prevalence in children has evolved. Currently in the United States, children <18 years of age account for approximately 13.3% of laboratory-confirmed COVID-19 cases. Even with this increase in prevalence, the number of hospitalizations remains preponderantly small compared with adults with COVID-19.[7,8]

Initial efforts were made in a two-pronged approach: implementation of safety strategies to keep patients and practitioners safe and remote care through telemedicine to provide safe distance and curb the spread of COVID-19.

Initially, COVID-19 did not spread in a uniform manner internationally and pockets around the world were more dramatically impacted than others. Initially impacted communities included China, Italy, Iran, Seattle, New York, Spain, and France. In March 2020, the worldwide community of pediatric otolaryngologists began to share information via WhatsApp and through national and international societies. Local experiences with COVID-19 as well as protocols for safety and continued care of patients with COVID-19 were shared. This worldwide distribution of information allowed the pediatric otolaryngology community to implement national and local strategies to enhance safety and care for patients throughout the pandemic. IPOG (International Pediatric Otolaryngology Group) acted as the main working group to share guidelines and protocols across society. IPOG consists of several member pediatric otolaryngology groups including ANZSPO (Australian and New Zealand Society of Pediatric Otolaryngology), APOG (Asia Pacific Pediatric Otolaryngology Group), ASPO (American Society of Pediatric Otolaryngology), ESPO (European Society of Pediatric Otolaryngology), IAPO (Interamerican Association of Pediatric Otolaryngology), PENTAFRICA (Pediatric Ear, Nose, and Throat in Africa). An IPOG compiled and shared document in April 2020 included discussions of many urgent aspects of otolaryngology care including otolaryngology case classification, management and operative protocols of urgent cases, preprocedural testing for COVID-19, ethical decision making during COVID-19, and PPE use during COVID-19 with particular emphasis on aerosol-generating procedures.[9] (https://cdn.ymaws.com/aspo.us/resource/resmgr/covid_19/ipog_covid_report_april_14.pdf) (**Fig. 1**)

In May 2020, ASPO issued a societal statement in regards to aerosol-generating procedures (AGPs), suggesting that safety should be of utmost importance for COVID-19 unknown or positive patients, and providers should wear a gown, gloves, N95 mask, or powered air-purifying respirators (PAPR) and face shield (or equivalents) during an AGP either in the ambulatory or surgical setting. In communities with high prevalence of COVID-19 infections, unknown patients with COVID-19 undergoing AGPs with higher risk of aerosol transmission should be managed with proper isolation precautions, including maximal PPE and limiting the procedure to essential personnel.[10]

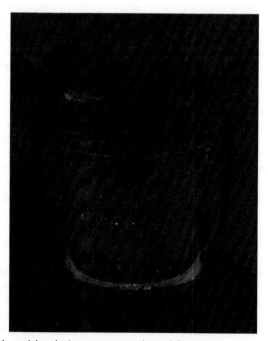

Fig. 1. Aerosolized particles during surgery and need for PPE.

https://cdn.ymaws.com/aspo.site-ym.com/resource/resmgr/covid_19/aspo_c-19_ppe_statement_fina.pdf.

Many strategies that were shared included strategies for personal protection equipment in the operating room as well as the outpatient facilities. As COVID-19 is a respiratory-based virus, pediatric otolaryngologists are a particularly vulnerable specialty to viral exposure from pharyngeal/laryngeal exams. To prevent further spread, a great deal of strategic effort was employed in the personal protection of the patient and the practitioners. As hospital-based protocols were established, they were shared as best practices with communities that had not been impacted by the initial wave of COVID-19. While some communities were able to implement best practices, resources were not uniform from institution to institution and were limited in many cases. In New York City (and many other communities) in March/April 2020, there was an extreme shortage of surgical N95 masks for the health care community's needs. These single-use masks were reused and reprocessed as was necessary[11] with limited data to support the use.[12] This practice placed health care workers in danger of contaminating themselves or others when doffing or donning the reused or reprocessed personal protection equipment (PPE) and nationally was advocated to only reuse and reprocess in times of critical shortage of equipment.[11] Advocacy from the national and international community (such as IPOG and ASPO) for quality personal protection equipment was paramount to engage in providing adequate PPE to ensure that the safety of the patient and practitioners was at the forefront. In pediatric otolaryngology particular concern was for airway evaluation in the COVID-19 + patient or the COVID-19 unknown patient in the operating room or outpatient setting. Similarly, any airway intervention such as open airway surgery or tracheotomy in the COVID-19 + patient was carefully planned to provide as much safety as possible given the risk of contamination to the health care team. Data from the adult literature were used as a proxy for the care of the pediatric patients. For tracheotomy, the key recommendations to provide adequate safety in airway surgery included minimizing aerosolizing during the procedure include cauterization, providing paralysis to avoid coughing, ventilation only with cuff inflation, and stopping ventilation before entering the airway.[13] Posttracheotomy care had recommendations of keeping the cuff inflated, use in-line suction, and delay tracheostomy tube change until COVID-19 has passed. Additionally, every effort should be made to avoid disconnecting the circuit before manipulating the airway.[14]

A four-institution North American pediatric hospital collaboration on safety in aerosol-generating procedures (AGPs) was published to provide guidance for all COVID-19 airway interventions. This combined approach of enhanced draping and use of SIM to optimize care and safety prior to operating room intervention provided a framework for all pediatric otolaryngologists to safely take care of their most critical airways.[15,16]

Similar efforts and insights were provided by the experts at Great Ormond Street giving practical insights into safety in laryngoscopy/bronchoscopy.[17] **(Fig. 2)**

Impact of COVID-19 on the Care for the Pediatric Patient

As the prevalence of COVID-19 continued to increase throughout the United States and the rest of the world, many patients were understandably concerned with exposure to COVID-19 and began to isolate. This isolation may have helped to prevent COVID-19 from further community spread but frequently delayed needed medical and surgical care. Routine otolaryngologic care was postponed and complex issues lingered for those in need, frequently becoming more complex with delays in care. This delay in medical and surgical care often manifested in delays in developmental

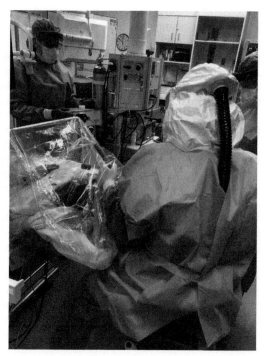

Fig. 2. Airway evaluation with protective PPE and protective covering over the airway.

milestones and learning goals. As schools turned to remote learning, this isolation and less robust learning environment adversely affected children's ability to progress at a typical rate and adversely affected children's mental and physical health.[18–20] It is estimated due to remote schooling during the 2020-2021 year, students are on average 5 months behind on mathematics and 4 months behind on reading[21] for the school year and 35% of parents very or extremely concerned about their children's mental health.[21]

In terms of otolaryngologic issues, children with unresolved chronic otitis media continued to have speech delay and language deficits. Children with unresolved sleep-disordered breathing and/or obstructive sleep apnea continued to have poor sleep and unrestful sleep resulting in poor performance and decreased learning at remote schooling. While the initial reaction of isolation was wise in its ability to limit the community spread of COVID-19, it adversely impacted children's mental and physical health dramatically.

With this data in hand, many system-based initiatives began in hospitals throughout the world to help mitigate risks and improve the patient experience to encourage patients to take care of their medical needs. As each system is unique, the approaches have been unique to the individual system. Most quickly adapted the safety protocols for aerosol-generating procedures with judicious use of PPE including N95 or equivalent masks or powered air-purifying respirators (PAPR) in their ambulatory and inpatient settings. In addition to personal protective equipment for both practitioners and patients, the general concept of a better and safer patient experience is to screen patients prior to visit to identify their medical needs as well as to screen patients for their and other patients' safety. 95% of surveyed institutions used nasopharyngeal PCR and/or symptoms for screening prior to operative intervention.

This enhanced screening of patients in combination with judicious social distancing helped to mitigate the spread of COVID-19 during routine office visits as well as operative experiences.

Telemedicine has acted as a powerful adjunct to in-person visits and helps to initiate medical care and carefully plan a further treatment plan. This has added a necessary bridge to the care of the patient allowing patients who may not feel comfortable with the current pandemic to elicit medical advice and decide on the next steps. Once telemedicine has been initiated, the decision to continue remotely or follow with in-person visitation can be timed appropriately as the examination is limited in the remote setting.

If in-person visitation is needed, screening procedures aim to reduce risks to patients and practitioners for those coming to the office or operating room. Nearly all pediatric otolaryngology practices screen symptomatology and temperature routinely. A survey of COVID-19 and reopening strategies was conducted in May 2020 and at the time, screening tools used included temperature (87%), fever (81%) dry cough (84%), respiratory symptoms (86%) were used often, while muscle aches (42%), fatigue (36%), headache (35%), and loss of taste/smell (49%) were less used.[22]

95% of institutions screen and/or objectively test (via PCR) within 48 hours prior to office-based AGP procedure or any operative surgical procedure to ensure a COVID-19 negative patient (within the error of the test). Any screening or objective test that is found to be positive typically warrants rescheduling unless it is considered an emergency and unavoidable. This process allows for the office and the operating room to mitigate risks and protect both patients and practitioners.

Other endeavors to mitigate risk include allowing only 1 parent and no siblings to accompany patients to visits/operations, decreasing overall clinic volumes, adequate social distancing in the waiting rooms, and allowing time for air circulation to adequately clear the exam rooms of potential contamination help to keep the office setting safer to cross-contamination.

As the pandemic has continued and evolved, small adjustments to individual institutional screenings have occurred as informed by the evolving data: PCR tests have adjusted from a deep nasal swab to a more anterior nasal swab; family may not be limited in their ability to visit with a patient but masks may still be required at all hospital-based settings. Most institutions still require masked interactions and preoperative testing as the rates of community-based COVID-19 remain high.

The development of COVID-19-based vaccinations has been a large step forward in the overall safety and protection of the community during this pandemic. Several vaccinations have been created and many proved to be very effective in preventing transmission of the initial strains of COVID-19. As the virus has evolved, some vaccines have proved less effective in newer strains of COVID-19 virus. Initially, the vaccines were approved for emergency use and subsequently have gotten full FDA approval. These vaccines include Comirnaty and Pfizer-BioNTech COVID-19 Vaccine, Spikevax and Moderna COVID-19 Vaccine, and Janssen COVID-19 Vaccine. In 2021, Moderna and Pfizer were approved for vaccination for children 12 and over. Subsequently, Pfizer and Moderna have just recently been approved for the vaccination of children 6 months and older.

National leadership at the American Academy of Pediatrics and ASPO[23] have encouraged all children eligible to obtain vaccination to help prevent further community transmission, aid in herd immunity and prevent severe disease from COVID-19 infection (https://aspo.us/resource/resmgr/aspo_covid19_statement_sept_.pdf).

COVID-19-Specific Symptoms Within Pediatric Otolaryngology

Generalized pediatric symptomatology of COVID-19 and treatment

Pediatric patients with COVID-19 typically have much milder symptoms than their adult counterparts. As a primarily respiratory virus, COVID-19 presented most typically with a fever, followed by cough, rhinorrhea, and sore throat. Other symptoms include headache, diarrhea, vomiting, and myalgias.[23–25] In an international study of COVID-19-affected children, 242158 children were identified with COVID-19 between January and June 2020 with 9769 (4%) hospitalized with COVID-19.[26] Dyspnea, anosmia, and GI symptoms were the more common than those with an influenza diagnosis during the same timeframe. There are potentially multiple explanations as to why children are infected less frequently and severely than adults. Children have a lower prevalence of comorbidities that are associated with severe disease.[27] Also, children more often get colds (coronaviruses) and have higher coronavirus antibody levels than adults. Antibodies directed against seasonal coronaviruses may confer some protection. Pneumonia and hypoxemic were the most common diagnoses of hospitalized patients at up to 23% and 15%, respectively. Anosmia was uncommon at 0.8-1.5% in all patients and MIS-C was uncommon at 0.5–3% in all patients and 0.6-7% in hospitalized patients.[26] Compared to influenza diagnosed at the same time, the incidence of pneumonia, hypoxemia, and MIS-C was higher in the COVID-19 population than the influenza population. Treatment plan for nonhospitalized pediatric patients continues to be conservative supportive care as most will recover very quickly and many are asymptomatic, to begin with. In hospitalized patients, corticosteroids and H2 blockers were the most common treatment plans. Antithrombotic therapy was more common in the US than internationally. Antibiotics and vitamin supplements were used infrequently.

Anosmia/hyposmia, dysgeusia. Anosmia can occur from postviral syndromes and has frequently been noted to have occurred with coronaviruses and rhinoviruses. Edema and congestion of the olfactory cleft cause conductive temporary loss which is common in rhinosinusitis. COVID-19 appears to cause anosmia despite mild rhinorrhea and mild congestion, suggesting that there is a sensorineural component to its origin. A recent meta-analysis of articles notes that the pooled prevalence of smell loss (anosmia or hyposmia) is 77% by objective measures and 44% by subjective measures.[28]

Dysgeusia can also be affected by postviral inflammation. As smell and taste are closely interlinked that it is not surprising that the incidence of anosmia and dysgeusia is similar at 5% in adults.[29] Anosmia and/or dysgeusia are not common symptoms found in the pediatric COVID-19 + population at 0.8–1.5%[26] and can be present without respiratory symptoms in children.[30] Because of this presentation, it is important to consider the loss of smell or taste without respiratory symptoms as a strong predictor of COVID-19 if present.[30] Most do improve with time but olfactory training is the primary method for restoring anosmia/hyposmia. Limited centers advocate for pharmacotherapy including the intranasal application of sodium citrate and vitamin A, as well as systemic use of omega-3 and zinc.[31] Recovery of taste and smell has been variable in the amount of recovery and timeframe for recovery. Further research is underway in the treatment of smell and taste disordered in regard to COVID-19.

Multisystem inflammatory disorder in children. Multisystem inflammatory disorder in children (MIS-C) is a sequela of COVID-19 and most commonly affects young, school-aged children and is characterized by persistent fever, systemic hyperinflammation, and multisystem organ dysfunction. Initially identified in the UK in April 2020, by the end of June 2020 more than 1000 children had been diagnosed with MIS-C.[32] Overall, MIS-C is relatively uncommon, affecting 0.5% to 3.1% of all patients diagnosed with

COVID-19 but up to 0.9% to 7.6% of those hospitalized with COVID-19. In a separate cohort study, researchers found recently that 11% of children with COVID-19 admitted to hospitals in the United Kingdom developed MIS-C.

Per the US CDC and WHO MIS-C is defined as having a previous COVID-19 infection in conjunction with persistent fever, multi-organ dysfunction, and elevated inflammatory markers. MIS-C notes to have similar symptoms of Kawasaki disease or cytokine storm and was initially misdiagnosed as such. Patients with MIS-C most likely present with fever (100%), gastrointestinal symptoms (60–100%), rash (45–76%), conjunctivitis (30–81%), mucous membrane involvement (27–76%), Neuro symptoms (headache, confusion) (29–58%), respiratory symptoms (21–65%), sore throat (10–16%), and lymphadenopathy (6–16%).[33,34]

In otolaryngology, there have been reports of posterior pharyngeal edema masquerading as retropharyngeal abscess with lymphadenopathy. Retropharyngeal edema may be due to altered lymphatics in the setting of MIS-C inflammation.[35] In terms of treatment, 2 large separate studies used IVIG with or without glucocorticosteroids and had conflicting results. One showed benefit with IVIG[36] and lower risk of cardiovascular dysfunction while the other showed no difference.[37] Time to treatment appears to be of the essence as the significant inflammatory response may make delayed treatments less effective.[38] (**Fig. 3**)

Long COVID-19 and consequences

Long COVID-19 is a general term for persistent symptoms from COVID-19 beyond 2 months of initial symptoms, and includes brain fog, trouble remembering, fatigue, and mood swings. In one recent study, approximately 40% of previously COVID-19 + children experienced long COVID-19 symptoms, while 27% of controls exhibited similar symptoms.[39] It is believed that as COVID-19 appears to affect different children differently, post–COVID-19 symptoms affect children differently. Careful coordination of care between health care, school care, and home care is essential to best take care of these complex recovery periods.

The long-term consequences of the COVID-19 pandemic remains largely unknown. The role of future generations may be affected by widespread COVID-19 infection similar to the widespread immune response of those who went through the 1918 flu pandemic.[40]

It is fully possible that early exposure to COVID-19 may prime one's immune system to a proinflammatory state for future severity of COVID-19 strains.[41] Further research is needed to best understand the longer-term consequences of early COVID-19 infections.

Impact on the Practitioner and the Health Care Team

By its very nature, the otolaryngology specialty has a unique set of conditions that make providers particularly vulnerable to upper respiratory pathogens. After all, we are "ear, nose, and throat" specialists and we spend our entire work day literally "in the face" of our patients. There is an abundance of information, suggesting that AGPs are a risk factor for exposure to a high viral burden, thus putting otolaryngologists at high risk of contracting the infection. The unique risk of close patient contact and AGPs has resulted in the necessity to take immediate steps to mitigate risk to providers. In the pediatric otolaryngology community, this has meant the rapid adoption of telemedicine for evaluating patients and the development of elaborate protocols to mitigate the risk of exposure to AGPs.

There are several unique features of pediatric otolaryngology practice that have made these changes particularly challenging. Firstly, children are inherently more

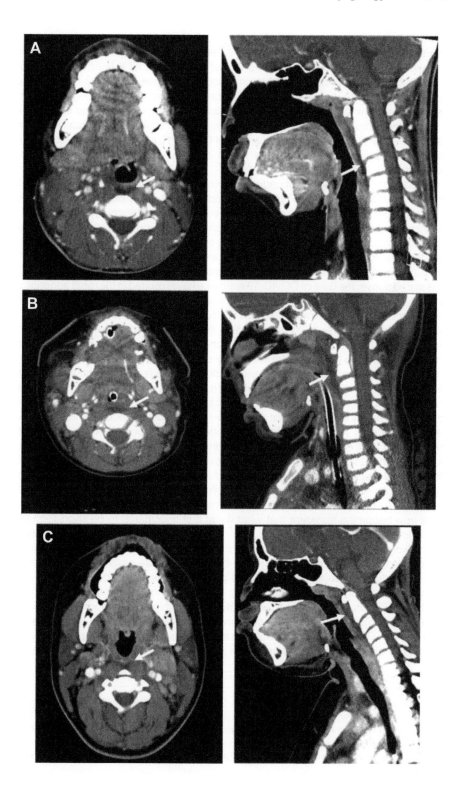

susceptible to viral upper respiratory tract infections (URI) and their sequelae. Whereas it is easy to set criteria to avoid seeing adult patients with URI symptoms and wait until they recover, this is impractical for children as it is often the reason why they need to be seen. It would be impractical to obtain COVID-19 testing for all patients with a "runny nose" who need to be examined in the office. If that were possible, we know that COVID-19 testing has a false negative rate of at least 3–5% in best-case circumstances.[42,43] In addition, current scientific evidence suggests that children may be asymptomatic carriers of COVID-19 of up to 15%,[4] which would indicate that prescreening for illness would not help to mitigate potential risk to providers.

An additional unique feature of pediatric otolaryngology practice is that in a pediatric practice the children are often not "willing participants" in the examination process. This creates additional risk to providers as even a basic oral cavity or nasal exam can turn into an aersol generating event as children who do not want to participate end up crying, screaming, gagging, coughing, or spitting. To make matters more complex, the examination process most often requires close contact with not only the child but also their caregiver, creating additional exposure risk to the provider.

As stated above, the risks of COVID-19 exposure have resulted in the rapid adoption of telemedicine and enhanced safety protocols when physical contact with the patient becomes necessary. While telemedicine has for the most part become a great immediate solution for patient access,[44,45] it is significantly limited by the same challenges that practitioners face with an in-person office visit; the child is often not a "willing participant" and if they refuse to open their mouth, there is only so much that can be evaluated virtually. Even with a fully compliant child on telemedicine, there is limited information that can be obtained in the remote setting particularly if it is the first visit. In addition, much of pediatric otolaryngology practice is focused on otologic complaints and at this point, there is no uniformly available replacement for the in-person otologic exam. While this is an evolving process, most institutions have developed protocols that incorporate screening ± COVID-19 testing, social distancing measures, and cleaning protocols to minimize the risk of exposure to health care providers when an in-person visit is needed. With the advent of vaccination for children and its widespread adoption, the combination of judicious use of telemedicine and safe controlled in-person encounters allow for quality medical care and decreased anxiety from the patient and family.

It is now becoming apparent that what we at first anticipated to be short-term adaptations to practice, are likely to be with us for the foreseeable future. Therefore, it is very likely that the practice of pediatric otolaryngology will permanently become a hybrid of virtual and in-person visits, even beyond the acute crisis. The hybrid model does offer several advantages to both the patient and the practitioner in this time of unease. Its widespread use helps families obtain initial medical care and treatment despite trepidation. It allows a patient–doctor relationship to develop despite the distance. It helps the practitioner to triage those with more serious issues and to streamline their care. Currently, its disadvantages are that it is time-consuming and limited in its ability to elicit a quality examination of the patient. Remote adapted technology

Fig. 3. Retropharyngeal phlegmon present in COVID-19 + children. (**A-C**) Axial and sagittal imaging of retropharyngeal edema of 3 cases of MIS-C. (*From* Daube A, Rickert S, Madan RP, Kahn P, Rispoli J, Dapul H. Multisystem inflammatory syndrome in children (MIS-C) and retropharyngeal edema: A case series. Int J Pediatr Otorhinolaryngol. 2021 May;144:110667. https://doi.org/10.1016/j.ijporl.2021.110667. Epub 2021 Mar 4. PMID: 33752089; PMCID: PMC7931672.)

such as otologic cameras for the visualization of the tympanic membrane and recorded video of sleep and breathing have helped to enhance the remote exam but still are limited. On a positive note, as we develop technologies to overcome the examination limitations of telemedicine, this may become an attractive alternative for many patients (and providers) as it will significantly reduce the time commitment, travel, school time lost, and cost related to an in-person visit.

Impact on Pediatric Otolaryngology Practices

The entire world has seen an economic contraction and the otolaryngology community has not been immune to this fact. Much of what we do is "quality of life" management rather than immediately necessary life preservation.[46] This is even more apparent in general pediatric otolaryngology practice, where complex, life-threatening and/or cancer diagnoses represent only a minority of cases and where the "bread and butter" management is largely geared to improve patient comfort (ear infections), hearing (ear fluid) or sleep (adenotonsillar hypertrophy). During the acute phase of the COVID-19 pandemic, both office-based visits and elective surgical practice abruptly ceased, essentially arresting the financial pipeline of otolaryngology practices primarily treating children. Even 2 years into the pandemic as we reintegrate into the clinics and the operating room, volumes are lower than they were pre–COVID-19 and may be for the foreseeable future for a variety of reasons including enhanced safety protocols, parental fear of taking their child to the doctor and lost family income and/or insurance.

In addition to significantly reduced revenue, pediatric surgical practices in the United States have largely been left behind their adult counterparts in receiving government financial relief made available to Medicare but not Medicaid providers. To make matters worse, the majority of pediatric otolaryngologists practice in hospital-based settings and have, thus been unable to obtain the small business loans available to others specialists who practice in a private practice setting. The net result of these financial constraints has led to significantly reduced practice incomes leading to decreased personal incomes for physicians and the necessitation of reducing the cost by arresting new hires and/or furloughing employees as well as the reduction of expenses related to nonessential activities (meetings, dues, and so forth). While the volumes are slowly returning, adaptations to a new working environment of more remote workforce will yield more permanent shifts in the health care landscape. A hybrid model of telemedicine and in-person care is the most likely solution. With the advent of new technologies for remote examination and integrated electronic medical records, this hybrid model will provide a high level of satisfaction for patients and families who can get access to their health care provider more easily from multiple avenues in a convenient setting.

In summary, while the post–COVID-19 framework of pediatric otolaryngology practice is unknown, it is highly likely that the new normal of pediatric otolaryngology will incorporate telemedicine, enhanced safety protocols, new indications for direct patient contact, and reduced patient volumes. This hybrid model of practice should continue to deliver high-quality care and multiple avenues of access. It remained to be seen how the post–COVID-19 landscape will affect pediatric otolaryngology practices nationwide as the recovery has been slow but continues to improve with time.

CLINICS CARE POINTS

- National leadership at the American Academy of Pediatrics and ASPO[23] have encouraged all children eligible to obtain vaccination to help prevent further community transmission, aid in herd immunity and prevent severe disease from COVID-19 infection.

- Treatment plan for nonhospitalized pediatric patients continues to be conservative supportive care as most will recover very quickly and many are asymptomatic, to begin with.
- In hospitalized patients, corticosteroids and H2 blockers were the most common treatment plans. Antithrombotic therapy was more common in the US than internationally. Antibiotics and vitamin supplements were used infrequently.
- Recovery of taste and smell has been variable in the amount of recovery and timeframe for recovery. Further research is underway in the treatment of smell and taste disordered in regard to COVID-19.
- Multisystem inflammatory disorder in children (MIS-C) is a sequela of COVID-19 and most commonly affects young, school-aged children and is characterized by persistent fever, systemic hyperinflammation, and multisystem organ dysfunction.
- Time to treatment appears to be of the essence as the significant inflammatory response may make delayed treatments less effective. It is believed that as COVID-19 appears to affect different children differently, post–COVID-19 symptoms affect children differently.
- Careful coordination of care between health care, school care, and home care is essential to best take care of these complex recovery periods.
- The post–COVID-19 framework of pediatric otolaryngology practice is unknown, it is highly likely that the new normal of pediatric otolaryngology will incorporate telemedicine, enhanced safety protocols, new indications for direct patient contact, and reduced patient volumes.
- This hybrid model of practice should continue to deliver high-quality care and multiple avenues of access.

DISCLOSURE

The authors have nothing to disclose.

REFERENCES

1. Wang D, Hu B, Hu C, et al. Clinical characteristics of 138 hospitalized patients with 2019 novel coronavirus-infected pneumonia in Wuhan, China. JAMA 2020; 323:1061–9.
2. Lippi G, Plebani M. Laboratory abnormalities in patients with COVID-2019 infection [published online March 3, 2020]. Clin Chem Lab Med. https://doi.org/10.1515/cclm-2020-0198.
3. Wu Z, McGoogan JM. Characteristics of and important lessons from the coronavirus disease 2019 (COVID-19) outbreak in China: summary of a report of 72 314 cases from the Chinese Center for Disease Control and Prevention. JAMA 2020; 323:1239–42. https://doi.org/10.1001/jama.2020.2648.
4. Lu X, Zhang L, Du H, et al. SARS-CoV-2 infection in children. N Engl J Med 2020. https://doi.org/10.1056/NEJMc2005073.
5. Nikolopoulou GB, Maltezou HC. COVID-19 in Children: Where do we Stand? Arch Med Res 2022;53(1):1–8. https://doi.org/10.1016/j.arcmed.2021.07.002 [Epub 2021 Jul 6. PMID: 34311990; PMCID: PMC8257427].
6. Dong Y, Mo X, Hu Y, et al. Epidemiological characteristics of 2143 pediatric patients with 2019 coronavirus disease in China. Pediatrics 2020. https://doi.org/10.1542/peds.2020-0702.
7. American Academy of Pediatrics. Children and COVID-19: State-Level Data Report. Available at: services.aap.org/en/pages/2019-novel-coronavirus-covid-19-infections/children-and-covid-19-state-level-data-report/2021. Accessed August 15, 2022.

8. ASPO statement on vaccination. 2021. Available at: https://aspo.us/resource/resmgr/aspo_covid19_statement_sept_.pdf. Accessed August 15, 2022.

9. IPOG COVID report April 14. 2020. Available at: https://cdn.ymaws.com/aspo.us/resource/resmgr/covid_19/ipog_covid_report_april_14.pdf. Accessed August 15, 2022.

10. ASPO PPE statement May. 2020. Available at: https://cdn.ymaws.com/aspo.site-ym.com/resource/resmgr/covid_19/aspo_c-19_ppe_statement_fina.pdf. Accessed August 15, 2022.

11. Toomey EC, Conway Y, Burton C, et al. Extended use or reuse of single-use surgical masks and filtering face-piece respirators during the coronavirus disease 2019 (COVID-19) pandemic: a rapid systematic review. Infect Control Hosp Epidemiol 2021;42(1):75–83. https://doi.org/10.1017/ice.2020.1243 [Epub 2020 Oct 8. PMID: 33028441; PMCID: PMC7588721].

12. Chirico F, Nucera G, Magnavita N. COVID-19: protecting healthcare workers is a priority. Infect Control Hosp Epidemiol 2020. https://doi.org/10.1017/ice.2020.148.

13. Wei WI, Tuen HH, Ng RWM, et al. Safe tracheostomy for patients with severe acute respiratory syndrome. Laryngoscope 2003;113:1777–9.

14. Harrison L, Ramsden J, Winter S, et al. Tracheostomy guidance during the COVID-19 Pandemic. ENT UK. 2020. Available at: https://www.entuk.org/tracheostomy-guidance-during-covid-19-pandemic. Accessed August 15, 2022.

15. Francom CR, Javia LR, Wolter NE, et al. Pediatric laryngoscopy and bronchoscopy during the COVID-19 pandemic: a four-center collaborative protocol to improve safety with perioperative management strategies and creation of a surgical tent with disposable drapes. Int J Pediatr Otorhinolaryngol 2020;134:110059. https://doi.org/10.1016/j.ijporl.2020.110059.

16. IPOG COVID Report April 14. 2020. Available at: https://cdn.ymaws.com/aspo.us/resource/resmgr/covid_19/ipog_covid_report_april_14.pdf. Accessed August 15, 2022.

17. Frauenfelder C, Butler C, Hartley B, et al. Practical insights for paediatric otolaryngology surgical cases and performing microlaryngobronchoscopy during the COVID-19 pandemic. Int J Pediatr Otorhinolaryngol 2020;134:110030 [Epub 2020 Mar 30. PMID: 32278168; PMCID: PMC7142686].

18. Dunton GF, B Do SD. Wang Early effects of the COVID-19 pandemic on physical activity and sedentary behavior in children living in the US. BMC Public Health 2020;20:1–13.

19. Xie X, Xue Q, Zhou Y, et al. Mental health status among children in home confinement during the coronavirus disease 2019 outbreak in Hubei Province, China. JAMA Pediatr 2020;174:898–900.

20. Zhang J, Shuai L, Yu H, et al. Acute stress, behavioural symptoms and mood states among school-age children with attention-deficit/hyperactive disorder during the COVID-19 outbreak. Asian J Psychiatr 2020;51. Article 102077.

21. COVID-19 and education: The lingering effects of unfinished learning. Available at: https://www.mckinsey.com/industries/education/our-insights/covid-19-and-education-the-lingering-effects-of-unfinished-learning. Accessed August 15, 2022.

22. Rickert SM. COVID and reopening strategies in pediatric otolaryngology, May. 2020. Available at: https://www.surveymonkey.com/results/SM-7239F57N7. Accessed August 15, 2022.

23. Götzinger F, Santiago-García B, Noguera-Julián A, et al. COVID-19 in children and adolescents in Europe: a multinational, multicentre cohort study. Lancet Child Adolesc Health 2020;4:653–61.

24. Parri N, Magistà AM, Marchetti F, et al. Characteristic of COVID-19 infection in pediatric patients: early findings from two Italian Pediatric Research Networks. Eur J Pediatr 2020;179:1315–23.

25. King JA, Whitten TA, Bakal JA, et al. McAlister Symptoms associated with a positive result for a swab for SARS-CoV-2 infection among children in Alberta. CMAJ 2021;193:E1–9.

26. Duarte-Salles T, Vizcaya D, Pistillo A, et al. Thirty-day outcomes of children and adolescents with COVID-19: an international experience. Pediatrics 2021; 148(3). e2020042929. [Epub 2021 May 28. PMID: 34049958].

27. Dorjee K, Kim H, E Bonomo R. Dolma Prevalence and predictors of death and severe disease in patients hospitalized due to COVID-19: A comprehensive systematic review and meta-analysis of 77 studies and 38,000 patients. PLoS One 2020;15. Article e0243191.

28. Hannum ME, Ramirez VA, Lipson SJ, et al. Objective sensory testing methods reveal a higher prevalence of olfactory loss in COVID-19-positive patients compared to subjective methods: a systematic review and meta-analysis. Chem Senses 2020;45(9):865–74.

29. Mao L, Wang M, Chen S, et al. Neurological Manifestations of Hospitalized Patients with COVID-19 in Wuhan, China: a retrospective case series study. Available at SSRN:. 2020. Available at: https://doi.org/10.2139/ssrn.3544840.

30. Mak PQ, Chung K-S, Wong JS-C, et al. Anosmia and ageusia: not an uncommon presentation of COVID-19 infection in children and adolescents. Pediatr Infect Dis J 2020;39:e199–200.

31. Neta FI, Fernandes ACL, Vale AJM, et al. Pathophysiology and possible treatments for olfactory-gustatory disorders in patients affected by COVID-19. Curr Res Pharmacol Drug Discov 2021;2:100035 [Epub 2021 Jun 5. PMID: 34870148; PMCID: PMC8178068].

32. Levin M. Childhood multisystem inflammatory syndrome—a new challenge in the pandemic. N Engl J Med 2020;383. https://doi.org/10.1056/NEJMe2023158NEJMe2023158–NEJMe2023158.

33. Whittaker E, Bamford A, Kenny J, et al. Clinical characteristics of 58 children with a pediatric inflammatory multisystem syndrome temporally associated with SARS-CoV-2. JAMA 2020;324:259.

34. Feldstein LR, Rose EB, Horwitz SM, et al. Multisystem inflammatory syndrome in U.S. children and adolescents. N Engl J Med 2020;383:334.

35. Daube A, Rickert S, Madan RP, et al. Multisystem inflammatory syndrome in children (MIS-C) and retropharyngeal edema: a case series. Int J Pediatr Otorhinolaryngol 2021;144:110667 [Epub 2021 Mar 4. PMID: 33752089; PMCID: PMC7931672].

36. McArdle AJ, Vito O, Patel H, et al. Treatment of multisystem inflammatory syndrome in children. N Engl J Med 2021;385(1):11–22 [Epub 2021 Jun 16. PMID: 34133854; PMCID: PMC8220965].

37. Son MBF, Murray N, Friedman K, et al.Multisystem inflammatory syndrome in children — initial therapy and outcomes. N Engl J Med. 10.1056/NEJMoa2102605

38. DeBiasi RL. Immunotherapy for MIS-C - IVIG, Glucocorticoids, and Biologics. N Engl J Med 2021;385(1):74–5 [Epub 2021 Jun 16. PMID: 34133878; PMCID: PMC8362545].

39. Rutter MJH. Difficult questions about long COVID in children. :S2352-4642(22) 00167-5. Lancet Child Adolesc Health 2022. https://doi.org/10.1016/S2352-4642(22)00167-5 [Epub ahead of print. PMID: 35752193; PMCID: PMC9221929].

40. Chuah CXP, Lim RL. MIC. Chen Investigating the legacy of the 1918 influenza pandemic in age-related seroepidemiology and immune responses to subsequent influenza A(H1N1) viruses through a structural equation model. Am J Epidemiol 2018;187:2530–40.
41. Holuka C, Merz MP, Fernandes SB, et al. The COVID-19 pandemic: does our early life environment, life trajectory and socioeconomic status determine disease susceptibility and severity? Int J Mol Sci 2020;21:5094.
42. Parikh SR, Bly RA, Bonilla-Velez J, et al. Pediatric otolaryngology divisional and institutional preparatory response at seattle children's hospital after COVID-19 regional exposure. Otolaryngol Head Neck Surg 2020;162(6):800–3.
43. Vinh DB, Zhao X, Kiong KL, et al. An overview of COVID-19 testing and implications for otolaryngologists. Head Neck 2020;42(7):1629–33.
44. Ning AY, Cabrera CI, D'Anza B. Telemedicine in otolaryngology: a systematic review of image quality, diagnostic concordance, and patient and provider satisfaction. Ann Otol Rhinol Laryngol 2020. https://doi.org/10.1177/0003489420939590. 3489420939590.
45. Mukerji SS, Liu YC, Musso MF. Pediatric otolaryngology workflow changes in a community hospital setting to decrease exposure to novel coronavirus. Int J Pediatr Otorhinolaryngol 2020;136:110169.
46. Sobol SE, Preciado D, Rickert SM. Pediatric Otolaryngology in the COVID-19 Era. Otolaryngol Clin North Am 2020;53(6):1171–4 [Epub 2020 Aug 19. PMID: 32951900; PMCID: PMC7437513].

Printed and bound by CPI Group (UK) Ltd, Croydon, CR0 4YY

03/10/2024

01040473-0020